Drug Treatment in Psychiatry

Drug Treatment in Psychiatry
A guide for the community mental health worker

Peter Tyrer
MD FRCP FRCPsych MFPHM
Professor of Community Psychiatry
Imperial College School of Medicine at St Mary's, London

Phil Harrison-Read
MB BSc PhD MRCPsych
Consultant Psychiatrist
Park Royal Centre for Mental Health, Central Middlesex Hospital, London

Elizabeth Van Horn
BM MRCPsych
Clinical Research Fellow
Imperial College of Medicine at St Mary's, St Charles Hospital, London

with a chapter on substance abuse by Dr Nicholas Seivewright

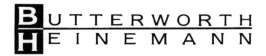

Butterworth-Heinemann
Linacre House, Jordan Hill, Oxford OX2 8DP
A division of Reed Educational and Professional Publishing Ltd

ᴿ A member of the Reed Elsevier plc group

OXFORD   BOSTON   JOHANNESBURG
MELBOURNE   NEW DELHI   SINGAPORE

First published 1997

© Reed Educational and Professional Publishing Ltd 1997

British Library Cataloguing in Publication Data
A catalogue record for this book is
available from the British Library

ISBN 0 7506 2251 2

Library of Congress Cataloguing in Publication Data
A catalogue record for this book is
available from the Library of Congress

Data manipulation and artwork creation by David Gregson Associates, Beccles, Suffolk
Printed in Great Britain by Biddles Ltd, Guildford and King's Lynn

Contents

Preface

There is a need for a guide to the major drugs used in mental health practice, not primarily for the psychiatrist and general practitioner, but for other professionals and carers involved in treating mental illness in the community. There are many books that address the medical readership, and the original edition of this book, *Drugs in Psychiatric Practice*, published in 1982, was one of these (Tyrer, 1982). In writing for a wider readership, the authors have tried to avoid lapsing into jargon or Latin or Greek medical terms that need a glossary before they can be understood. We have concentrated on the practical aspects of drug treatment whilst attempting to avoid writing a mere catalogue of the drugs available, or at the opposite extreme, a comprehensive textbook of drug treatment.

We suspect that we have not fully succeeded in covering all the subjects for which a guide would be helpful, but we hope we have illuminated some of the important issues. We also hope that our medical colleagues will understand why we have done this, and not feel upset that we have disclosed too many secrets of our trade. In our task we have been helped greatly by members of the two community mental health teams with which we have worked (the Early Intervention Service in Paddington and North Kensington, and the Community Intervention Project in Brent), who have commented on different versions of the manuscript. Rebekah Brummell and Geraldine O'Neill have worked hard to fashion our contributions into a readable and unified form. Errors we hope are few but we would be very willing to hear from any readers about them and any other suggested improvements or omissions. We would also like to hear about any points of dissent or disagreement with our views, which we suspect may be more numerous. If so, this would seem to us to be entirely in keeping with the fact that community psychiatry continues to represent both the 'cutting edge' and the 'melting pot' of mental health care.

Peter Tyrer
Phil Harrison-Read
Elizabeth Van Horn
June 1997

Introduction

The practice of medicine used to be very specialized. Doctors who wished to make a name for themselves decided early on in their careers that they must concentrate on one part of the body, one organ system or one discipline within the subject. Similarly, those who entered the nursing, physiotherapy, occupational therapy and psychological professions were also trained to perform a specific set of tasks. It was assumed that only through specialization could professionals attend adequately to the range of problems presented by patients. As a corollary, as there was such a wide range of problems suffered by patients it would be unlikely that one individual could have the expertise to solve them all.

Exactly similar thinking affected industries in which a wide range of skills and tasks were involved. For example, in the automotive industry, people were trained to perform specific tasks – tightening the chassis nuts, fitting a transmission system, assembling doors – and this work was rarely, if ever, shared by others. The disadvantage of this arrangement was exemplified by its inflexibility in practice. If one person in the car assembly team was ill for any length of time all members had to stop work. There were also major difficulties over work status and pay and the term 'demarcation disputes' became synonymous with poor industrial practice in the 1970s. As a consequence the notion of team working developed in which people covered for each other and had a range of skills, some trained to a greater extent than others, but together making for much greater flexibility and co-operation.

The caring professions have now followed suit. One of the reasons why this trend has accelerated recently is that all aspects of community health care have to be much more flexible and resourceful than hospital care. It is easy to have a strict and limited schedule of activities for staff in a hospital in which all grades work on the same clinical problems. In the community, there is often only one person who has to make important decisions about a wide range of problems, under pressure of time and with no-one else to consult. We therefore need every community worker, and a wide variety of voluntary workers, to have key skills that can be drawn on when needed, together with the ability to recognize when further help is required and from where it should be obtained.

Community psychiatry exemplifies this new approach. Whereas in the past anyone deemed to show any form of odd behaviour was admitted to hospital 'for observation' where the hierarchy of professions could gaze on them and assess them at leisure, in community care we now have much less time, but have the advantage of assessing people in the situations where they live and interact with their relatives, friends and neighbours (Kingdon, 1994). We have also learnt to integrate our treatment to a much better extent than in the past. Instead of (ultimately sterile) arguments over whether drugs or psychological treatments are most effective in a particular condition, we now try to identify the circumstances in which each form of treatment may be of value, and also assess when they are most effective in combination.

With this in mind, it is easy to see why a book on drug treatment for the community psychiatric professional (and indeed others without professional qualifications) is of potential value. It is also likely that such a book would not have been thought possible even ten years ago. The notion that doctors are or should be the only personnel in the psychiatric team who know about drug treatment has been a long time dying, and even now, some of our medical colleagues may think that we are doing the equivalent of selling the family silver in betraying some of our secrets to our fellow professionals who do not prescribe drugs. They argue that before long nurses and occupational therapists will be demanding that they too should prescribe the drugs that doctors now guard as their sole prerogative. This seems to us unlikely. However, if patients who are the recipients of our different treatment approaches have at some level to assimilate them in order to be helped, surely it behoves us to be aware of, and knowledgeable about, each other's methods and practices.

Whether this change takes place depends on whether those of us involved in mental health use our knowledge wisely and well. The evidence to date suggests we do. Mental health professionals are quite capable of judging the limits of their particular skills and the need for drug therapy, and in integrated community teams there is little difficulty in combining these approaches (Falloon and Fadden, 1993).

In order to move towards an integrated approach to mental health care, including drug treatments, we need information that is free of jargon and easy to follow, remember and implement in practice; these requirements are the aim of this book. As much as possible we have tried to put ourselves in the position of the community health worker, and have been helped in this by having close involvement with community professionals. We should like to pay particular acknowledgement to the staff of the Early Intervention Service in Paddington and North Kensington and the Community Intervention Project in Brent who have stimulated much of our thinking on this subject during joint work over the past eight years. The many examples of clinical management given throughout this book make this clearer. We hope that these examples and the illustrations of team working will give other community workers the confidence to work similarly and to encourage their medical colleagues to collaborate in the same way. This will not always be an easy task. For a nurse to question the prescription of a certain drug by a doctor may be perceived as excessively challenging, and certainly a few years ago, this might have automatically led to a reprimand. We are certainly not recommending uninformed interference in the way in which drug treatments are used by psychiatrists. It is only when the community mental health worker has accumulated a body of knowledge, e.g. on the detection of adverse effects, the understanding of dosage and response, and the indications for drug therapy, that their suggestions are likely to be useful and taken seriously.

The community worker is in an excellent position to ensure the success of drug treatment. Repeatedly we refer in this book to *compliance*, the extent to which patients take their drug as prescribed. Although the doctor will inevitably play an important part in this, the nurse, psychologist, occupational therapist, relative or friend who enjoys the confidence of the patient can have a major effect on whether or not drug treatment is taken according to the doctor's prescription. The community worker who knows the rationale of drug treatment is in a much better position to ensure the patient's compliance in most cases. Admittedly, psychiatrists who prescribe drugs still have an unfortunate image, somewhat unfairly promoted by the media, of lacking interest in their patients as people, and of taking every opportunity to test out medicines on their unsuspecting patients. The impression is sometimes given that the doctors know too little about these medicines and only prescribe them to satisfy their own intellectual curiosity or to suppress behaviour that is considered offensive. Psychiatrists can do their best to extinguish some of these prejudices, but the task will remain much easier if it is supported by other members of the community mental health team who fully agree with the decision to use drug treatment, and indeed, have been party to its introduction.

Sometimes those people who work in the community and support the idea of drug treatment are accused of slavishly following the medical model of care. We hope that in the pages that follow we can demonstrate this to be false. A 'medical model' is often used as a term of abuse to imply narrow-minded attitudes that are excessively biological in orientation. In contrast, we support an extension of the medical model to a comprehensive collaborative one in which knowledge of disease and its mental manifestations, understanding of dynamic processes, the interplay of social and cultural factors and understanding of cognitive and behavioural influences all interact at different times in the course of illness (Tyrer and Steinberg, 1993).

We are very conscious that a little learning can be a dangerous thing, and so we have tried to cover as comprehensively as possible the range of conditions and drug treatments in community practice that a community health worker is liable to experience. This involves some theoretical knowledge about drug action which may be more difficult to assimilate than some of the more practical aspects of drug treatment. However, both are useful and we hope that the reader will appreciate this. We have also followed what may be considered an unduly medical approach to describing one particular problem in community psychiatric practice, that of diagnosis. We emphasize that diagnosis, despite its great limitations in psychiatry, is important in selecting treatment, and that all community mental health workers should have some knowledge of its principles and main categories. We have linked the chapters describing these diagnoses in a way that reflects clinical practice. For many conditions we know that drug treatment is of limited value and has a very poor base of knowledge. Nevertheless, we have included the whole range of psychiatric disorders, including those of personality, because it is as valuable to know of conditions for which there is no useful drug treatment as to know where specific drug treatments are effective and readily available.

We have enjoyed writing this book and hope that you enjoy reading it. We have tried to keep the references to a minimum and to give suggestions for further reading that are easy to obtain. We hope that this book will have value as both a reference text and also as a stimulus for future investigation of a subject that is likely to become an essential part of the knowledge base of every practitioner in mental health.

The justification for drug treatment

Drug treatment can be very helpful to people suffering mental health problems, and sometimes drugs are the only form of treatment that is likely to make a significant impact in practice. Drug treatments are particularly useful for helping specific mental health complaints or 'symptoms', and in serious states of mental ill-health, drugs may be invaluable for reducing severe distress and emotional turmoil, together with the major disturbances of thinking, feeling and behaviour that mental health problems can produce. Once established on effective drug treatment, the person with mental health problems may be much more accessible to other kinds of help, ranging from practical support to sophisticated forms of psychotherapy.

Although it is usual for doctors to have sole responsibility for prescribing drug treatments used in mental health care, it is a great asset if other professionals in a community mental health team (and everyone else in the role of a carer) are as well informed as possible about the issues involved. This will encourage and empower them to become involved in discussions about medication for their clients, and to make best use of their own specialist skills by optimizing the integration of different treatment approaches. Knowing about drug treatment will help promote a freer discussion amongst the multiprofessional team, demystifying the role of the doctor in this context, and also helping to work against the artificial boundaries that often exist between professionals working within teams. In the well-informed multiprofessional team, it should not be possible to get away with the 'doctor knows best' attitude, but neither will the medical members of the team be so easily marginalized into the limited role of diagnostic experts and prescribers at the expense of their other roles in the assessment and treatment of patients.

Another reason for all team members to know as much as possible about drug treatment in mental health work is to counteract tendencies either to overvalue or to underestimate the usefulness of drug treatments. The media often seem to publicize new 'wonder drugs' or other apparently amazing advances in psychiatric treatment, and from the attitudes of some doctors, one might sometimes believe that these claims were justified. However, experienced mental health workers have only to consider their own experience, and that of their clients, to realize that there are no miracle drug cures in psychiatry. Nonetheless, without the availability of effective drug treatments, most of the modern advances in social psychiatry and community mental health care would not have been possible.

Even more strikingly, most people with mental health problems are less than enthusiastic about taking drug treatments prescribed by their general practitioner or psychiatrist. The exceptions are addictive drugs such as minor tranquillizers (benzodiazepines) and stimulant anti-depressants or appetite suppressant drugs such as the amphetamines which doctors often wish they had never started prescribing in the first place. In contrast, self-medication for emotional problems or 'bad nerves' with drugs such as alcohol, nicotine or cannabis is widespread. Not surprisingly, the reasons for this curious state of affairs are complex, and are concerned with the whole experience of being a 'psychiatric patient', and not just with the perceived direct effects of taking prescribed psychoactive (mind-altering) drugs. This chapter examines the rationale for using psychiatric drug treatments and some of the ethical issues involved. First, however, a brief historical review of drug treatment in mental health care will help to put into perspective the principles and practices that are relevant today.

The drug revolution in psychiatry

Psychiatry in the first half of the twentieth century was dominated by therapeutic nihilism when it came to dealing with those severe forms of mental disorder known as the psychoses. Schizophrenic and other psychotic patients were usually found to be beyond the reach of the new psychotherapeutic methods of Freud and others, which principally relied on helping people's mental distress by removing hidden doubts and conflicts in their thinking and feeling. Although people with psychoses certainly appeared to have many 'psychic knots', it seemed difficult or impossible to untangle these by trying to gain insight through psycho-analysis. Indeed in many people with psychosis, psychoanalysis appeared to make their condition worse.

By default, therefore, predominantly physical methods of treatment such as drugs and restraint were increasingly advocated for dealing with psychotic patients. Although it had been shown a hundred years earlier that humane and personal attention could do much to help the distress of psychotic patients, most psychiatrists in the early years of the twentieth century continued to tackle the problems of the severely mentally ill by using regimens of harsh physical restraint and containment. The widespread use of drugs like bromides, opiates, paraldehyde and barbiturates, which all have relatively non-specific depressant effects on the brain, was justified by psychiatrists not because these drugs were particularly helpful for reducing mental disorder and distress, but largely because patients were more easily managed by overworked and ill-trained attendants. The likely detrimental effects of these depressant drugs only added to the physical and social impoverishment of the patients' environment, and not surprisingly a poor prognosis was generally accepted as inevitable.

One of the reasons why remedies such as homoeopathy became so popular was that they virtually avoided the use of drugs, as only very small dosages with no possible side-effects were administered. As most of the traditional drugs that were available did more harm than good (nowadays we would say they had a low benefit/risk ratio), famous psychiatrists of the past, such as John Conolly and Samuel Tuke, achieved distinction through their humanity of care and by avoiding the use of drugs wherever possible. It was only in those hospitals in which excessive control and constraint were used that the old drugs were deemed necessary in large measure.

The failure of psychiatrists to find any effective physical remedies for helping serious mental illness had produced by the 1930s two somewhat paradoxical effects. Firstly, there was a general belief that all mental illnesses, including the psychoses, could only ultimately be understood in psychodynamic terms, even though psychodynamic therapies had been decidedly ineffective in practice. Secondly, it encouraged psychiatrists to try even more drastic and ill-conceived means of physical treatment for the seriously mentally ill. Treatments such as psychosurgery and insulin coma therapy, if they had any benefit at all, probably did so as a result of the extra care and personal attention that was necessary in order to administer them to patients. However, electroconvulsive therapy (ECT) was developed at about this time, and this certainly represented the first major advance in the physical treatment of the psychoses, especially those disorders where there was a marked disturbance of mood as well as a loss of contact with reality. Although today ECT remains a controversial treatment, careful evaluation of modern ECT has confirmed that it is an effective although short-term treatment which is relatively safe in severe forms of mental illness (Gregory et al., 1985), even though the mechanism of its therapeutic effect is poorly understood.

This dispiriting state of affairs in psychiatry continued into the 1950s when the start of a remarkable new era coincided with the chance discovery of drugs that had specific beneficial effects in severe mental illness. Nearly all of the original drug prototypes introduced in the late 1940s and 1950s are still regarded as important treatments today. The first specific psychotherapeutic agent to be used was lithium, which is still as popular as ever with psychiatrists, mainly as a preventative treatment in severe recurrent affective disorders (manic-depressive illness, see Chapter 7). Perhaps the most important prototypical psychotherapeutic drug is chlorpromazine, which despite its broad spectrum of actions in the brain and body (pharmacological non-selectivity) emerged in 1952 as the first specific antipsychotic drug treatment. For many, the introduction of chlorpromazine heralded a drug revolution in mental health care. About the same time as chlorpromazine was introduced, the trend towards greatly increasing numbers of people in mental hospitals began to reverse. This was probably as much due to a general feeling of therapeutic optimism and concern over the harmful effects of institutional care as to the direct and specific benefits of the drug on people with psychotic illnesses. Although not a cure, drugs like chlorpromazine enabled symptoms of severe mental illness to be specifically brought under control with relatively little impairment in alertness, unlike the 'blunderbuss' actions of the old drugs. The result was that people who had previously been severely incapacitated by chronic mental symptoms were able to return to a more normal way of life, within the limitations imposed by the irreducible impairments and disabilities of their mental illness. However, it was realized from the start that social reforms in promoting community care were equally if not more important than the direct benefits resulting from the new drugs, and this is still the case (Hafner, 1987).

Even at this early stage, there was unfortunately a tendency for doctors to abuse the therapeutic effects of the new drugs, using them to keep patients quiet and regimented under conditions of social and physical impoverishment (Barton, 1959). It was all too easy to become disillusioned with the drug revolution, which for some seemed directed more for the benefit of staff and pharmaceutical companies than for patients. Even people who derived no specific benefit from drugs like chlorpromazine were often medicated nonetheless, and the use of the 'chemical straitjacket' sometimes became part of the impersonal institutional regimens (including prisons and penitentiaries) that the introduction of new drug therapy was expected to sweep away.

Drugs and alternative psychiatry

As a reaction to the drug revolution in psychiatry, an alternative move-ment grew up and flourished in the 1960s which rejected the notion that disease processes were the cause of mental disorders. It was argued that mental illness is a myth, perpetrated by doctors in order to silence what amounts to a form of protest by the individual faced with intolerable problems of adaptation and conformity to a 'sick society' (Szasz, 1961). The new drugs used by psychiatrists were viewed at best as palliative treatments for socially unacceptable thoughts, feelings and behaviour, and at worst as instruments of social repression. Interestingly, as well as proposing that psychotic mental disorders might represent for the individual an expansion of consciousness and experience, the use of psychotomimetic drugs such as lysergic acid diethylamide (LSD) and mescaline was advocated in a similar vein. Thus alternative psychiatry did not reject drug use, only that purporting to have a 'therapeutic' effect in suppressing mental illness.

These alternative ideas represented in part a reaction against the threatening dominance of 'biological' or 'mindless' psychiatry, which it was argued had a tendency to reduce human experience to the level of chemical reactions. Today most of these arguments seem overinflated and rhetorical, and particularly with regard to psychotic conditions such as schizophrenia, frankly misguided and naïve. One of the beliefs of alternative psychiatry was that if psychotic patients were allowed to act out their delusions and strange ideas, their mental disturbance would improve after they had resolved their struggles with themselves and with society (Laing, 1967; Laing and Esterson, 1970). So when the advocates of alternative psychiatry looked on with approval at psychotic patients smearing their room with faeces and baying abuse at all authority figures, they innocently expected their behaviour to come to an end once strictures of society had been removed. In reality, most mentally ill people 'treated' in this way continued to deteriorate, and tended to become more rather than less out of touch with reality. The alternative psychiatry movement was also antiscientific, in that it was reluctant to subject its theories to any form of independent testing. When these studies were carried out by others, they found no evidence for the view that abnormalities of communication or control within families, or society at large, were the cause of serious mental illnesses such as schizophrenia (Hirsch and Leff, 1975).

It came to be widely accepted that when used appropriately, psychotherapeutic drugs can be instruments of liberation rather than repression, freeing the person with severe mental illness from the crushing tyranny of disordered thought and feeling. However, the controversy which raged in the 1960s and 1970s was valuable in that it ensured that psychosocial factors relevant to the causes and management of mental disorders were not neglected at a time when an upsurge of new knowledge about the brain might otherwise have resulted in an overly materialistic view. It also helped to focus attention on the many ethical problems surrounding the use of psychotherapeutic drugs, problems which are still very much with us today.

Interestingly, a new school of antipsychiatry has now emerged which once again is highly critical of the use of drugs in mental health care (e.g. Breggin, 1993). However, over the 40 years or so that psychotherapeutic drugs have been widely used, the psychiatric establishment has learnt much about the limitations and drawbacks of drug treatment, so many of the arguments of the new antipsychiatrists seem reactionary and out of date. Nonetheless, there is still a tendency for psychiatrists and pharmaceutical companies to overestimate the value of drug treatments in mental illness (Eisenberg, 1986), undoubtedly in some cases because of the tunnel vision that vested interest can cause. For this reason alone, the new school of antipsychiatry is useful for stimulating dissent and debate, although it is a shame that its principal exponents tend to adopt such an haranguing tone, with arguments that are sufficiently misinformed to qualify as 'brainless psychiatry'. The sophisticated arguments of the old school of antipsychiatry as represented in the works of Thomas Szasz and R. D. Laing can in hindsight seem less strident and unbalanced than their modern counterparts.

The justification for psychiatric drug treatment – the disease model

The main aim and justification for psychiatric drug treatment is the relief of suffering and distress. When faced with a deluded and hallucinating person who is tormented and preoccupied by their mental experiences whilst neglecting virtually every other aspect of their life, the clinician who believes that medication will help, may find many of the arguments against drug treatment at best irrelevant or misguided, and at worse dangerous and inhumane. The more extreme arguments against medication for serious mental health problems often seem to be held with most conviction by those who are rarely if ever faced with such suffering humanity. However, caution is needed in making the case for medication, as it has to be recognized that psychiatric drug treatment is largely empirical and pragmatic, and is based less on scientific and medical theories and proofs than on the demands of expediency and society's expectations. Furthermore, probably the majority of people with mental health problems do not like to take drug treatment.

The fundamental pillar on which drug treatment for mental disorders rests is the *disease model*. The premise of the disease model is that defining features of mental disorders are the reflection of brain processes which are maladaptive in that they cause impairment of fundamental biological functions (sleep, appetite, libido, mood, and in some cases, perception and thinking), and that these impairments threaten the individual's survival. However, although thoughts, feelings or behaviour may be deviant or undesirable, unlike parts of the body, they cannot be 'diseased' in any literal sense.

The definition and diagnosis of mental illness and the related issues of 'illness behaviour' and 'sick roles' involve concepts that are as much social as medical, and the same applies to treatment with drugs when this is advocated. In many conditions treated with mind-altering drugs by psychiatrists, it is likely that there is nothing actually wrong with the brain, either in structure or function. Mental pain and distress, and behavioural disturbance, can be explained without having to evoke concepts of illness or disease (e.g. the suffering of bereavement). The practice of prescribing mind-altering drugs under such circumstances may be questionable, although this is a very common occurrence, as with the use of alcohol, nicotine or illicit drugs. In the short term, the use of drugs in these situations can be justified if the goal is the relief of intolerable distress and suffering. That there may be more appropriate, safe or effective means of help is another matter.

Taking drugs in order to solve problems may create its own problems, and sometimes can undermine a person's ability to resolve their initial difficulties. Drug addiction and physical ill-health caused by drug-taking are obvious examples of this, and it is a common belief that over-reliance on help from drug treatment may prevent people developing skills, strategies or understanding which would otherwise allow them to cope when drugs are no longer available or advisable. When people feel that they are no longer in control of their lives and rely excessively on others to make all important decisions for them, unnecessary and inappropriately prolonged use of drugs can create a state of 'learned helplessness'. This negative aspect of drug treatment can result in people passively waiting for the drugs to take effect rather than doing anything themselves to promote a return to health.

Particular ethical and practical problems arise when the distress and disturbance targeted by drug treatment appear to reflect the individual's response to unfavourable circumstances in their lives. Not only may drug treatment take away people's incentive or ability to solve their own problems, sometimes a person's distress and mental disturbance may reflect a 'healthy' response to unfavourable or malign social influences, ranging from conflicts at the level of the family, to political protest and dissent. Under these conditions, treatment with mind-altering drugs, particularly if given without the person's consent, can be seen as an instrument of repression with the purpose of silencing protest. Drug treatment cannot be justified solely on the grounds that the dissenting person is 'sick' or 'ill', unless one accepts the circular argument that those who are deemed to 'need' powerful mind-altering drugs must be mentally ill by definition.

Defining mental illness

Although 'illness' is often thought of as an exclusive preoccupation of the 'disease' or 'medical model' of mental health disorder, in fact many therapists or mental health workers share the same premise that the patient/client is suffering from a problem or disorder having certain characteristic features which need to be defined and understood in order to deliver individually tailored treatment, regardless of whether this is in the form of drugs, various forms of psychotherapy, or social help and support. It may therefore be possible to come up with a definition of mental illness which would be acceptable even to those mental health workers who have grave doubts and misgivings about a 'disease model' of mental health problems. Any such definition would have to be highly pragmatic, and represent the 'bottom line' which could be applied to most people who come for help from mental health services. Using these guidelines, here are some suggested criteria by which mental illness can be defined and measured:

- A sudden or insidious *change* occurs in a person's thoughts, perceptions or feelings (symptoms) and/or their behaviour and functioning (signs) which is distinct from the characteristics of their personality.
- The condition usually involves distress and suffering to the affected person, and very often to those close to them.
- The condition always impairs social functioning to some extent and results in a variable degree of disability and disadvantage (handicap).
- The pattern and time course of change in symptoms and signs are sufficiently consistent across individuals to represent defining characteristics of illness, although there is often much variation, so that the boundaries between illness and health, and between different categories of illness, are often blurred and dependent on culturally determined norms and conventions.
- Bodily changes and physical malfunctioning may accompany mental illness, but evidence for disease of the brain or body is often lacking.

Depending on the conceptual models used by different mental health workers, the symptoms and signs referred to in these criteria can have different meanings. For those using the disease model, symptoms and signs indicate underlying disturbances in brain and body structure and physiological mechanisms, even though these may not be apparent using current diagnostic and investigational techniques. The more 'biological' the symptoms (for example, impairments in energy, sleep, appetite, weight, biorhythms, levels of arousal and drive), the greater is the expectation that biological treatments such as drugs will help, and this is usually borne out in practice. Alternatively, the symptoms may be seen as disorders in their own right if a behavioural model is the guiding principle, or consequences of irrational thinking in the case of a cognitive model. If symptoms are seen as the products of adverse social forces, as in the social model, or diversionary tactics or 'smokescreens' that obscure underlying psychic conflict, as in the psychodynamic model, this will have profound implications for the different kinds of treatment that are offered to the client.

Although the general illness model outlined above may be applied to most people presenting with mental health problems, one of the specific models mentioned above may be more appropriate for treating particular kinds of problems (Tyrer and Steinberg, 1993). For example, the disease model, in which an abnormality of brain structure or function is assumed, may be more appropriate for treating psychoses such as schizophrenia, or for organic conditions that produce psychiatric symptoms and in which identifiable brain disease is known to exist. The behavioural model may be most helpful for explaining and treating 'neurotic illness' at least with respect to abnormal patterns of behaviour, whereas the cognitive model can be particularly helpful in developing treatments for the irrational thinking that underlies so many mental health problems. The psychodynamic model may be helpful in understanding aspects of both normal behaviour and symptomatology that might otherwise seem obscure or without meaning, although psychodynamic treatment may only be suitable for a selected group of people with mental health problems. Finally, the social model may especially apply to situations in which people's symptoms spring from adverse circumstances in their life, which hopefully can be directly attended to and improved.

Hierarchy of models of mental illness

If a mental illness is 'caused' by a known dysfunction or disease of the brain, this will tend to take precedence over other conceptual frameworks in which the person's problems can be viewed. This is justified because although brain disease may cause problems (impairments, disabilities and handicaps) conceived of in terms of behavioural, cognitive, psychodynamic and social models, directing treatment at the root cause and finding a 'cure' would automatically solve all the other problems. In this sense, the disease model is at the top level of a hierarchy of illness models (Figure 1.1). It also follows that if a 'cure' cannot be found or is not available, then as well as providing palliative physical treatment for the underlying brain disease, it will help to give treatments aimed at all the problems lower down in the hierarchy. Even in conditions such as schizophrenia where the disease model can be applied with some conviction, drugs may not always be effective (see Chapter 6), and treatment strategies derived from and aimed at lower level models may be equally or more useful in practice. Indeed it may well be that

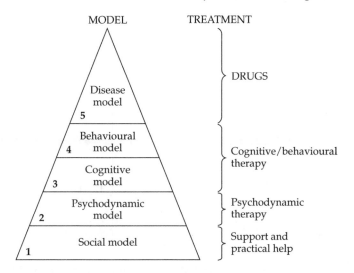

Figure 1.1   *Hierarchical models of mental illness: in the hierarchical organization of mental illness models, the disease model takes precedence. As well as having its own unique features, it incorporates all the features of lower-level models. The supposedly unique feature of the disease model is the effectiveness of drugs (and other physical) treatments. However, problems and treatments associated with models lower in the hierarchy (e.g. various forms of psychotherapy and social support) will also apply to the disease model*

'social therapy' in the form of financial aid and practical help with daily living may be the most valuable service that can be offered to somebody who is suffering mental illness resulting from an incurable brain disease (Tyrer and Steinberg, 1993).

By the nature of the hierarchy principle, this 'top-down' approach to treatment does not apply in reverse. Where illness results from problems at a lower level in the hierarchy, e.g. in the behavioural, cognitive, psychodynamic or social spheres, treatment aimed at non-existent brain disease would be irrelevant. In theory this should apply to drug treatment of any mental disorders that cannot be encompassed by the disease model, but as we shall see, it is actually very rare for psychotherapeutic drugs to be targeted specifically at known brain diseases. In practice, drugs may still be useful as adjuncts to more specific treatments aimed at problems principally located at the behavioural level or even further down in the hierarchy of illness models (Figure 1.2). However, if we go to the lowest level of the illness model hierarchy, i.e. the social level, it is fairly obvious that someone who is 'ill' only in a social sense (e.g. 'off sick' from work because of dissatisfaction with their job) will be best helped by addressing these social difficulties directly. To give drug treatment in this situation might be unhelpful or wrong, and it would be a waste of time to try to discover disturbed brain mechanisms in order to justify using medication. If medication is used regardless, this may compound the problems by encouraging drug abuse or addiction.

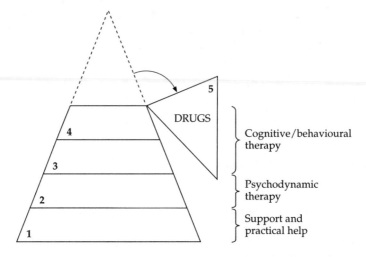

Figure 1.2   *The modified hierarchical structure topples the disease model from its pinnacle and allows for the fact that drug treatment may be useful in the absence of demonstrable brain disease. Drug treatment may facilitate and enhance treatments based on behavioural, cognitive and psychodynamic models. Problems occurring in the sphere of the social illness model are less likely to be helped by drugs*

Case vignette 1.1

Fred was a young man aged 22 years who had just failed his final examinations in zoology. He was not expecting this, and in order to take the examination again, he would either have to take a year without a grant or work part-time in order to finance an extra year of study. He had led all his friends and relatives to believe that he was going to succeed without any problems, and he felt humiliated when he failed. He was advised to see a psychiatrist by his parents and attended a well-known teaching hospital for assessment. He was presented to a group of students by a psychiatrist who was a great believer in drug therapy and was prescribed the monoamine oxidase inhibitor phenelzine (Nardil) in a dose of 15 mg three times daily. The interview took place in front of medical students and lasted about 12 minutes. He was presented as a 'typical example' of some-one who would respond to phenelzine, and no discussion took place about his personal or social circumstances. He was so shocked and affronted by this experience that he decided he would never see a psychiatrist again, and decided not to have his prescription dispensed. However, this unpleasant experience of psychiatry was possibly helpful inasmuch as he decided he would have to help himself in future. Subsequently he enrolled for another year on his zoology course, and he passed one year later with a good second class degree. Whether his 'flight into health' and unresolved psychological problems left him vulnerable to depression later in life is another question.

Where professionals are trained exclusively at one particular level of the illness model, there is an understandable desire to restrict action to that level. For example, a psychotherapist trained exclusively in psycho-dynamic psychotherapy may find it hard to think of people's problems in any other framework, or to apply any other type of treatment. One difficulty about this has already been referred to: even though a particular model may be appropriate for understanding and talking about the disorder in question, treatment stemming from this conceptual level may not be appropriate, feasible or effective. Instead, treatment based on a lower-level model might be the best option in practice. The other difficulty is that whatever the level at which a person's problems arose originally, with time problems may spread both up and down in the hierarchy. For example, what might have started as a problem arising from unconscious psychological conflicts may lead to serious social difficulties on the one hand, and even to the risk of a psychotic break-down on the other, with the possible development of abnormal brain functioning, qualifying as mental disease.

What is wrong with the disease model?

Many psychiatrists seem to believe that to justify their use of drug and other physical treatments in helping people with mental illness, they have to adhere rigidly to a disease model. This is unfortunate, because the disease model may have serious negative implications for the way in which people are treated generally. For example, if someone's problems are assumed to be all due to 'something wrong with their brain', then it may not seem worthwhile trying to understand them as a person or getting to know much about their personal and social circumstances. Of course, all those interested in helping people with mental illness need to apply what knowledge they possess concerning brain sciences, psycho-logy, social sciences, etc., but treating the patient or client as a unique individual must always be paramount (Eisenberg, 1986). This means that any kind of treatment, whatever the conceptual framework that guides it, has to be devised and communicated in a way that takes full account of the person's wishes, feelings and experiences, and the meaning that they themselves give to their problems. In this sense, every therapeutic plan is as individual as the person being helped.

Perhaps too many psychiatrists find it more convenient to prescribe a drug than to get to know their patients, and maybe much the same can be said about other professionals delivering their own specialist services or treatments. More often than we would like to admit, patients are fitted to treatments rather than vice versa. However, these difficulties do apply particularly to the application of the disease model, which is usually practised exclusively by doctors or psychiatrists. Psychiatrists are often criticized for regarding people as collections of symptoms due to chemical disturbances of the brain, with personal meaning and subjective feelings and experiences pushed into the background. This highly materialistic attitude is usually described as 'reductionism'. There is a danger that patients may be regarded almost as a race apart from healthy people, and this tendency to alienate and marginalize patients may be combined with an overbearing and authoritarian attitude towards diagnosis and treatment. From the patient's point of view, personal suffering may seem to be parcelled up and dismissed as mere symptoms of disease, with no sense being conveyed of the need to understand and give meaning to what the patient is going through.

When drug treatments are proposed, it may seem to the patient that the intention is to negate and devalue their personal experience of suffering. For some people, these negative connotations of illness and drug treatment may extend to a feeling of being denigrated or persecuted by all offers of help and treatment from psychiatrists. Other people may be unduly attached to their symptoms and to the 'sick role' they bestow (e.g. the hypochondriac), so that offers of treatment represent a threat to take away something of hidden value. However, everyone who has experienced illness and distress will appreciate the desire to be treated as a 'person who is ill' rather than as a 'case of illness'.

Rehabilitating the disease model

In defence of the disease model, it has to be said that for the most serious mental disorders such as schizophrenia and manic-depressive psychosis, it is likely that causal abnormal ('pathogenic') brain mechanisms will one day be discovered and confirmed. This is supported by a number of lines of argument. Firstly, conditions like schizophrenia and manic-depressive illness often have a family history, due in large extent to the inheritance of genetic factors which increase an individual's susceptibility to the disorder. Secondly, abnormal mental states resembling schizophrenia and manic depression sometimes accompany physical diseases that involve the brain – either directly, as in temporal lobe epilepsy, multiple sclerosis and disseminated lupus erythematosus, or indirectly, as for example in diseases of the thyroid gland. Thirdly, a number of drugs such as those used to treat high blood pressure, appetite suppressants and corticosteroids sometimes precipitate severe disturbances of mood and thinking which qualify as mental illness, and it is well known that prolonged use of drugs such as amphetamines ('speed') can produce an illness very similar to paranoid schizophrenia. Fourthly, and probably most important of all, drugs can cause a specific reduction in symptoms of mental illness, even though so far no drug has been found to bring about a cure. Once the drug is stopped, the mental illness is likely to return, until such time as the condition would have got better on its own.

The disease model therefore still has much to recommend it in terms of understanding and helping people with mental disorders (Table 1.1). However, the aspects of the disease model that result in a dismissive attitude towards patients' personal experience of illness and towards other kinds of treatment 'lower down' in the illness model hierarchy are indefensible. It could be argued that for the purposes of guiding treatment, the disease model should be toppled from its position at the summit of the illness model hierarchy until such time as treatments based on it result in mental illnesses being 'cured' once and for all. In the

Table 1.1 *Pros and cons of the disease model of mental illness*

Pros	Cons
Collects symptoms and signs into meaningful categories, so giving order to diverse clinical observations and phenomena	For most mental illness, there is little or no clear evidence for brain pathophysiology or disease
Attempts to specify the causes and limits of abnormality using pathophysiological rather than sociocultural criteria, with the hope of being more objective and less overinclusive and pejorative	Labelling or diagnosing people as 'cases of disease' may be pejorative or dismissive of their subjective experience and feelings about their predicament and the meaning it has for them
Predicts and specifies physical or chemical treatments aimed at bringing about a cure, or at least a significant alleviation of suffering	Playing down the continuum between normality and mental ill-health may create a 'them and us' attitude towards people who are ill, and encourage stigma and handicap
Encourages humane treatment of some socially undesirable deviant or criminal behaviours which are explained and excused on the grounds of illness rather than badness or personality disorder	May encourage or demand people to be passive recipients of treatment administered by authoritarian experts who 'always know best'
	May be unacceptable to many people who would rather forgo help than be labelled as ill and pressured into accepting treatment which feels frightening, irrelevant or deprecatory

meantime, the disease model could be used as a framework to guide the use of physical treatments like drugs to facilitate and enhance treatment at so-called lower levels of intervention, i.e. the behavioural, cognitive and psychodynamic treatments (Figure 1.2).

Drugs and the mind

Everyone knows of the existence of mind-altering drugs, and indeed most of us consume them every day in the form of alcohol, caffeine and nicotine. It is also common knowledge that these drugs affect the mind through their action on the brain. Since the 1950s a great deal has been learnt about how drugs work within the brain, and some of this knowledge is outlined in Chapter 2; but how exactly are the brain and the mind related so that the effects of drugs on the brain can be translated into effects on the mind and on mental illness?

Straight away it must be said that there is no simple answer to this question, and an attempt to give anything like a comprehensive treatment of the subject is beyond the scope of this book and the knowledge and understanding of the authors. However, if one is prepared to accept some gross oversimplifications, we can try to explain mind-brain relationships in terms that may help a better understanding of drug effects in mental illness.

To put the matter bluntly, the mind can be equated with consciousness, and with one aspect of consciousness in particular, which concerns self-awareness, or the ability to think about thinking. This aspect is termed the *reflexive* nature of consciousness, or in the jargon of cognitive neuropsychology, the ability to make *meta-representations*. Modern cognitive neuropsychology attempts to understand consciousness in terms of information processing, and to link these mechanisms to underlying brain function (Frith, 1992). Since information processing is also the function of a computer, understanding consciousness (and by implication 'mind') and the link with brain function, is rather like trying to understand how a computer program (*software*) depends on, and arises from, the electronic functioning of a computer (*hardware*). Although a few years ago it was thought that the brain might function rather like a modern-day computer in being a very complex interconnection of basic units (electrical switches or transistors), this now seems oversimplistic, and explanations of brain function in terms of 'neural networks' and other mysteries are currently proposed.

However, the information processing mechanisms on which consciousness depends must be rather like a computer program in the sense that the link with brain function is not obvious or direct, even though we may know a great deal about how the brain (and the computer) works. The information generated by the running of a computer program, and the conclusions that can be drawn from it, are in some sense *emergent properties* of the computer itself. By this we mean that the results of the program are dependent on the operation of the computer, but are not entirely explainable by, or reducible to, the known properties of the computer.

Mind can therefore be conceptualized as an emergent property of brain function, just as the computer program is an emergent property of the computer. To use an alternative and more homely metaphor for this emergent property idea, one may say that the sound of a tree rustling in the wind is an emergent property of the tree's structure and the environment in which it exists. The rustling that we hear depends on physical properties of the tree and of the wind, but cannot be explained easily or entirely by these physical realities. The fact that we need a listener (ourselves) to appreciate the particular qualities of the emergent property, and to some extent define it, draws a further analogy with the concept of mind, in the sense that minds are difficult to conceptualize without the existence of other minds to give them meaning.

Drugs, consciousness and information processing

In order not to drift away too far from our original intention to show the link between brain mechanisms and mind, we must return to recent ideas about the nature of consciousness. The type of information processing by the brain that relates to conscious experience is of a high intensity and quality. High-level information processing occurs when we are wide awake and fully alert, and high-quality processing applies when we are carrying out complex, flexible activities which cannot be achieved without focused attention. This will apply to activities that have not yet been learned, or that by their very nature cannot be learned. Many inter-personal social interactions have this feature. Conscious as opposed to unconscious processes have a number of defining features. The first of these is the impression of *continuity of experience* which is achieved in spite of the fact that the sensory input we receive is highly discontinuous at the level of nerve impulses and other basic neurophysiological processes. The second characteristic of consciousness is the ability to *attend selectively* to particular aspects of the many different kinds of infor-mation that are reaching us. Thus we are only aware of what we are focusing our attention on. Other information appears to fade into the background, although it is still being processed by our brains, and is still accessible should it develop any novel or surprising features. The third feature of consciousness is its *limited capacity*, shown by the fact that we can only attend to, or process in detail, a very small amount of material at any one time. Finally, the most important property which was referred to earlier is the *reflexive nature* of consciousness which allows us to be aware of being aware, or to think about thinking (Frith, 1992).

Psychologists have begun to study these different aspects of conscious-ness in the context of different types of memory impairments (amnesias), selective attention experiments and in studies of self-awareness. In this last respect, modern psychology is attempting what was previously thought to be impossible, that is, an experimental scientific approach to introspection. In general, the experimental approach to consciousness concentrates mainly on studying people who have various kinds of brain damage or disease in which different patterns of impairment in consciousness are observed. From this kind of research, it is possible to draw conclusions about the brain systems which underlie consciousness. An example is the phenomenon of 'blind sight' in which people with damage to the visual cerebral cortex are no longer consciously aware of certain visual stimuli, but are still able to respond to them. This tells us that there is a type of information about the outside world that can guide our behaviour but of which we are not conscious, and that this informa-tion is normally processed in parallel with information of which we are aware. Freud's view of the unconscious mind now has parallels in exper-imental neuropsychology.

Other impairments of consciousness are more relevant to the effects of drugs. The first example involves a specific defect in the *continuity of consciousness*, causing a particular kind of amnesia in which people show a loss of memory for specific episodes from the past. This *episodic memory* is in contrast to *procedural memories* which underlie basic skills, and *semantic memories* which concern 'the way things are done' without our actually being aware of how or when we first learnt to do them. Impairments of episodic memory are associated with damage to the medial temporal lobes of the brain including the hippocampus, and similar memory impairments can be produced by anticholinergic drugs such as hyoscine, and by benzodiazepines such as diazepam. Both these types of drug have major effects on neurotransmission in the temporal lobes, as well as in many other parts of the nervous system.

The second abnormality of consciousness that can be affected by drugs concerns impaired control over the *contents of consciousness*, as seen in difficulties in attending to particular things going on around us. Drugs that interfere with neurotransmission in the noradrenergic systems of the brain seem to affect this control of the contents of consciousness, just as may occur in cases of dementia. Dementing brain disease is also associated with a reduction in the *capacity of consciousness*, resulting in difficulty in thinking about and performing complex tasks. Drugs that interfere with the cholinergic systems of the brain appear to mimic this particular aspect of dementia.

Finally, the most interesting aspect of consciousness in relation to mental illness is the loss of reflexivity or self-awareness (being unaware of being aware). This may be the fundamental abnormality of consciousness that occurs in schizophrenia, and may result from specific impairments in the function of the prefrontal and medial temporal cortex. Prolonged use of certain psychotomimetic drugs may also produce this defect. These are just some of the ways in which drugs may affect 'mind' through specific actions on brain systems concerned with information processing and conscious experience. Other examples include the perceptual changes resulting from psychotomimetic drugs such as LSD, and the changes in mood (depression or elation) produced by a wide range of drugs including alcohol.

Many of these theories are speculative and need further testing. It is not necessary to know about them in order to be experienced in administering drugs and monitoring their effects. However, anyone involved with the prescribing and monitoring of drugs that act on the brain should realize that they are acting on the most complex organ in the body, and there are likely to be many subtle effects of drug treatment which may have disproportionately profound effects on people's feelings and behaviour.

Animal models of mood disorder

Perhaps mood is a more 'primitive' aspect of mind, with closer parallels to animal behaviour than other aspects of human mental experience. Mood is closely associated with systems in the brain that are concerned with arousal, drive and motor activity, which are fundamental aspects of behaviour in all animals.

Recent animal work on the effects of maternal and social deprivation in the rearing of rhesus monkeys has indicated that behavioural and brain development may be adversely affected by abnormal experiences in infancy (Kraemer, 1992). This in turn is reflected in persistent changes in brain structure and neurotransmitter levels in the brain (reduced levels of noradrenaline). These biochemical changes appear to lead to subsequent problems in adult life in dealing with loss and separation, and may account for 'despair-like' behaviour in monkeys which closely resembles depressive illness in humans. This may provide a link between the social origins of depression as revealed by a large body of work carried out since the 1970s by workers such as Brown and Harris (1978), and biochemical theories of mood disorders which argue that deficiencies in brain amines such as noradrenaline account for many features of depressive illness.

Experiments suggest that attempts to 'rehabilitate' animals who have been subjected to early maternal deprivation are unsuccessful, whereas antidepressant drug treatment which increases noradrenaline levels in the brain may be more effective. However, this finding should not be extrapolated to suggest that psychological treatments in humans are likely to be inferior to drug therapy in making good the psychological and biochemical damage produced by early traumatic experiences such as maternal separation or loss. After all, the higher intelligence and more sophisticated cognitive functions of human beings may well have a more powerful restorative influence on memories of traumatic experiences and underlying brain chemistry, provided that this is guided by appropriate psychotherapy. However, these developments in brain neuroscience do indicate that the use of drugs to help psychological and mental problems that may have psychosocial origins is a valid approach, even though at present we are largely ignorant about the underlying brain mechanisms involved in mental disorder and 'dis-ease'.

A computer analogy

Returning to the computer as an analogy for the mind-brain relationship, it is quite possible to conceptualize mental problems arising as 'software faults', with no abnormalities at all in the 'hardware' representing brain structure or biochemistry (Figure 1.3). Thus a computer program can go wrong because of faulty program information or incorrect data input, even though the electronics of the computer are functioning perfectly. Although simplistic, this computer analogy would support a 'reprogramming' model of treatment, e.g. some form of psychotherapy, particularly cognitive behavioural therapy. In these circumstances, drug treatment can be conceptualized as physical interventions that indirectly facilitate the process of reprogramming, e.g. analogous to switching off parts of the computer while the program is rewritten. It is also easy to imagine how repeated program (software) malfunctions may lead to a hardware fault such as a blown fuse: a possible model for changes in brain structure or function resulting from prolonged stress or life difficulties.

Computer analogy	Clinical classification		Treatment model	Practical implications
Software malfunction only	Reactive/psychogenic function disorder		Alter input condition, and/or reprogram, with or without partial circuit shutdown	Await spontaneous recovery; alter life circumstances; increase insight; remove psychic conflicts; identify and modify maladaptive thoughts and behaviour. Use drugs to improve person's receptiveness and accessibility to other forms of help and treatment
Software malfunction and secondary hardware defect	Reactive/psychogenic with neurogenic (*biological*) features	OTHER ILLNESS MODELS / DISEASE MODEL	Treat as above to allow eventual self-correction of hardware defect, and/or intervene more directly to repair defect	If possible use drugs which target specific mental dysfunctions arising out of putative *'lesions'* in brain structure or functions; drugs with other selective effects on mental processes may help patient recovery and rehabilitation by reducing symptoms and behavioural disturbance arising from active or residual mental illness
Primary hardware defect and secondary program faults	Neurogenic (endogenous or biological) features predominate (covert organic brain dysfunction)		Repair hardware defect, if possible, and reprogram; otherwise isolate malfunctioning circuits, and reprogram for less demanding tasks	

Figure 1.3 Computer program faults can provide analogies for mental disorders and their management, including the use of psychotherapeutic drugs. The 'disease model' corresponds mainly to 'hardware' faults and 'other illness models' correspond mainly to 'software' malfunctions, although there is likely to be much overlapping

However attractive the idea, it seems unlikely that drugs currently used in psychiatry can correct or repair specific but as yet unidentified abnormalities in brain biochemistry which are directly responsible for mental disorders. It seems much more likely that drugs act on brain processes which, in concert with other factors, lead indirectly to improvements in mental disorder. Some of these delayed actions may be biochemical, or they may depend on external (environmental) influences. One important implication of this is that following drug action on the brain, improvement in the mental disorder may not be immediate or inevitable, but will depend on 'reprogramming' the mental and behavioural abnormalities that have developed around the basic biological lesion or defect. In other words, drugs used to help mental disorders may only create or restore the physicochemical conditions in the brain that are necessary before a return to normal mental state can begin. This may resemble the process of recovering from a stroke, where physical recovery in the brain has to take place before undamaged brain tissue can be re-educated to take over some of the function of brain cells that have been irretrievably damaged. Thus the actual improvement in mental symptoms following drug treatment may rely on environmental and social circumstances affecting psychological and brain processes in the same way that controlled exercises and physiotherapy are necessary in order to optimize recovery of physical function in a stroke patient.

It is hoped that this oversimplified account of mind-brain relationships and the role of drugs may help to support the notion of combined therapeutic approaches for mental conditions, i.e. drugs *and* psychotherapy, rather than a sterile *either/or* debate which sometimes divides opinion amongst mental health workers from different professional backgrounds.

Further reading

Breggin, P. (1993). *Toxic Psychiatry, Drugs and Electroconvulsive Therapy: The Truth and the Better Alternatives*. London: Harper Collins.

Brown, G. W. and Harris, T. (1978). *The Social Origins of Depression*. London: Tavistock.

Eisenberg, L. (1986). Mindlessness and brainlessness in psychiatry. *British Journal of Psychiatry*, **148**, 497–508.

Frith, C. D. (1992). Consciousness, information processing and the brain. *Journal of Psychopharmacology*, **6**, 436–440.

Kraemer, G. W. (1992). A psychobiological theory of attachment. *Behavioural and Brain Sciences*, **15**, 493–541.

Laing, R. D. (1967). *The Politics of Experience*. London: Penguin.

Szasz, T. (1961). *The myth of mental illness*. New York: Harper & Row.

Tyrer, P. and Steinberg, D. (1993). *Models for Mental Disorder*. Chichester: John Wiley.

2

Psychopharmacology – drugs and the brain

The term 'psychopharmacology' refers to the study of drug effects on the mind, but this chapter is mostly concerned with the question of how drugs reach and affect the brain. This will help us understand better the clinical applications of drug treatments for helping mental state disorders, the general principles of which are discussed in Chapter 3. This chapter is not essential reading if you are only concerned with the practicalities of drug treatment of mental health disorders, but it will help you to understand more about how drugs produce their therapeutic effects. It will also help to explain terms that mental health workers often encounter in discussions about medication, even though doctors themselves sometimes seem vague about their exact meaning.

The wide spectrum of psychotherapeutic drug actions

Although drugs used in psychiatry are usually classified as (for example) antidepressant, antipsychotic, antianxiety (anxiolytic), or antiobsessional, in practice most drugs have more than one therapeutic application (Lader and Herrington, 1990). There are probably three reasons for this wide spectrum of action of psychotherapeutic drugs. Firstly, most drugs have several or many pharmacological actions in the brain as best exemplified by chlorpromazine (Largactil, 'large actions'). Secondly, even drugs that have selective or restricted pharmacological actions often affect a wide range of brain functions, presumably because the principal brain mechanism on which the drugs act has a similarly wide spectrum of function and influence within the brain. Probably the best example of this is a relatively new class of drugs called the selective serotonin reuptake inhibitors (SSRIs) which have important effects in depressive illness, anxiety states, obsessive-compulsive disorders and eating and sleep disorders, as well as in conduct disorders characterized by impulsivity and aggression. On the basis of other independent evidence, it is likely that all these conditions involve the serotonergic systems of the brain on which the SSRIs selectively act.

The third reason for the wide spectrum of action of psychotherapeutic drugs is that similar beneficial effects can probably be achieved by influencing a number of different brain mechanisms. Even where there might be evidence for a 'disease process' underlying a particular mental disorder, psychotherapeutic drugs are unlikely to act directly on this, but instead will affect other brain systems and processes that have an indirect influence on the brain mechanisms bringing about the mental disorder. This means that the 'cause' or biological mechanism underlying the psychiatric illness will probably remain operative despite treatment with drugs. Drugs therefore act only to suppress the signs and symptoms of mental illness, and if they are stopped before the natural history of the disease process has run its course, the original problems will return.

The complexity and plasticity of brain cells and their connections

It is estimated that the human brain contains at least ten thousand million nerve cells or neurons, all interconnected to form systems of incredible complexity and intricacy. This has been nicely summarized by the physiologist Sherrington as 'an enchanted loom weaving a myriad of dissolving patterns, always a meaningful pattern, though never an abiding one'. Each nerve cell is like a miniature microchip or mini-computer, although the complex processes that go on within the nerve cells are chemical rather than electrical. These internal chemical reactions are controlled by the flow into the neuron of certain ions (electrically charged molecules) such as calcium, and by enzymes which are produced and regulated under the influence of special genes. Different chemical processes going on within neurons result in varying properties of the cell membrane and internal cell structures, and in the production of chemicals which carry messages from one part of a cell to another, and between one neuron and its many neighbours.

This is where electrical processes play a part in the function of nerve cells. The membrane of each nerve cell is like a chemical battery which is capable of producing waves of electrical current that pass along the main projection pathway of the cell body, called the axon (Figure 2.1). The axon of one nerve cell branches out and makes connections with many thousands of other nerve cells in the brain. The connections are not direct, but rely on the electrically triggered release of chemical messengers or neurotransmitters. These chemicals are released in minute measured amounts from the axon nerve ending, and then flow onto the twig-like processes or dendrites surrounding each neighbouring nerve cell. Contact with another neuron's receptors may bring about changes in the electrical charge across the membrane of adjoining cells, which if the change in voltage exceeds a threshold level, may also fire waves of electrical current down their axons. In order for the nerve cell's threshold voltage to be reached, and for the cell to be stimulated to fire off an electrical wave (action potential) of its own, there may have to be a critical pattern of electrical signals arriving via chemical transmitters from other cells. Although some neurotransmitters stimulate the receiving nerve cells and make them more ready to fire, other trans-mitters damp down or inhibit the electrical activity of cells with which they make contact. Still other transmitters change the response character-istics of the receiving cells in other ways.

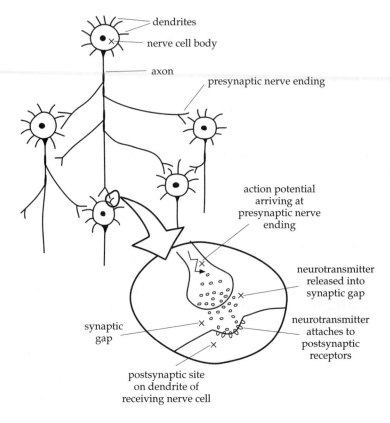

dendrites

nerve cell body

axon

presynaptic nerve ending

action potential
arriving at
presynaptic nerve
ending

neurotransmitter
released into
synaptic gap

neurotransmitter
attaches to
postsynaptic
receptors

synaptic
gap

postsynaptic site
on dendrite of
receiving nerve cell

Figure 2.1   *Nerve cells in the brain showing their synaptic interconnections. Minute waves of electrical current (action potentials) arriving at presynaptic nerve endings cause the release of chemical neurotransmitter into the synaptic gap. Neurotransmitter molecules interact with receptor molecules on the postsynaptic membrane of dendrites of adjoining nerve cells, causing further electrical changes or other chemical reactions which constitute the transfer and processing of information between nerve cells*

Thus the pattern of brain cell activity, and the communication and interconnection between cells, is highly complex, and forms the basis for the brain's capacity to process information. In this sense, the brain resembles a modern computer which also comprises relatively simple electrochemical building blocks or components, linked up into highly complex circuits. Apart from the fact that the human brain is infinitely more complex and subtle than the most powerful computer, the other main difference is that the brain can constantly change and modify its circuits by altering the way individual neurons respond and are connected to other brain cells via chemical transmitters. This is called neuronal *plasticity* and explains the brain's capacity to adapt and change in accordance with past and present influences on it. In other words the brain can learn and remember, and develop new capabilities in response to changing circumstances.

Drugs, synapses and neurotransmitters

The gap between one nerve ending and another nerve cell is called a synapse, and the peptide structures in the postsynaptic membrane of the neighbouring cell onto which the chemical neurotransmitters bind are called receptors. A receptor is rather like a lock, and the chemical neuro-transmitter that binds to it is like a master key. When the master key neurotransmitter enters the lock of the receptor, a 'door' is opened and a large range of chemical and electrical processes begin. In fact, the opening of the 'door' resulting from the neurotransmitter binding to the postsynaptic receptors either involves the activation of enzymes or the opening of ionic channels in the cell membrane. The latter produces electrical currents across the cell membrane, and as we have mentioned, may trigger action potentials which travel down the axon to reach other parts of the brain circuits. In the case of neurotransmitter-triggered enzyme activation in the membrane adjoining the synapse, this is the 'message' for increased or decreased production of various chemicals which in turn will alter the cell's receptivity to incoming messages and the chemical messages it puts out.

When a neurotransmitter, or another chemical that resembles it, fits into the receptor, and 'opens a door', this is called an *agonist action*. Many drugs act as neurotransmitter mimics or agonists, but usually an agonist will only fit one of the several locks or receptors which the master key neurotransmitter can open. Thus when a particular neurotransmitter opens many different but similar receptor locks. it is usually the case that several agonist drugs will need to be found to selectively open each of these different locks. If a drug acts like a key which enters the receptor lock but will not turn, this will effectively prevent or block the door being opened by other agonists, and this will represent an *antagonist action* of the drug at the receptor. More unusually, some drugs fit the lock of a receptor, but instead of turning it and opening the door, the drug key may for example trigger off the equivalent of a fire alarm. This represents an opposite or *inverse agonist* effect of a drug. There are many different neurotransmitter chemicals in the brain, and new ones are regularly being discovered (Table 2.1). Neurotransmitters are manufactured in the cell body or in the nerve ending using simple chemicals as building blocks, before being stored in special packages or vesicles within the nerve endings. The contents of the vesicles are released into the synaptic gap when an electrical charge or action potential passes over the membrane of the nerve ending.

There appear to be two main types of synapse in the brain. In the first type, there is a close link between the nerve ending and the receptor site on the adjoining cell. The communication between cells that is produced is rather like a one-to-one telephone conversation. The other type of synapse involves a wide gap between nerve endings and adjoining cells,

Table 2.1 *Neurotransmitter effects on brain cell activity (excitation or inhibition) are not related in any simple way to their behavioural actions or to possible involvement in clinical syndromes. For example, neurotransmitters causing nerve cell inhibition are not necessarily associated with behavioural inhibition or with states of clinical depression*

Neurotransmitter	Effect on brain cell activity and behavioural actions	Possible changes in neurotransmitter function in mental disorders	Effect of psychotherapeutic drugs
Acetylcholine	*Excitation:* important in learning and memory	Decreased in dementia and in mania	Increased by lithium; decreased by anticholinergic drugs
Bioamines			
Dopamine	*Inhibition:* involved in voluntary movement, emotional arousal, memory and learning	Increased in schizophrenia and mania; decreased in Parkinson's disease and in some types of depression	Increased by cocaine, amphetamine and L-dopa; decreased by antipsychotic drugs
Noradrenaline	*Inhibition:* involved in emotional arousal, selective attention, memory and learning	Decreased in depression; possibly increased in mania	Increased by antidepressants; decreased by lithium
Serotonin (5-HT)	*Inhibition or excitation:* found in brain regions that regulate sleep and appetite, and influence emotional arousal and pain sensitivity	Decreased in depression and mania; possibly increased in anxiety and in schizophrenia	Increased by antidepressants and lithium; decreased by some antipsychotic drugs

Table 2.1 (*continued*)

Amino acids			
Glutamic acid	*Excitation:* may be involved in learning and memory	Increased in some types of epilepsy; possibly decreased in schizophrenia	Decreased by anticonvulsants
Gamma-aminobutyric acid (GABA)	*Inhibition:* appears to be the primary inhibitory neurotransmitter in the brain	Decreased in anxiety, and possibly in schizophrenia	Increased by benzodiazepines
Neuropeptides			
Small chains of amino acids which may be involved in neurotransmission, or in modulating the effects of other neurotransmitters; examples: melatonin, oxytocin and many others	*Mostly inhibitory:* believed to influence eating, drinking, sexual and maternal behaviour, sleep, temperature regulation, pain reduction and responses to stress	Uncertain	Morphine and other opiates mimic endorphins Some antipsychotic drugs block opiate receptors

and many cells may be exposed to the neurotransmitter chemicals that are released. This is more like a public address system playing background music, because the information that is conveyed is of a general, controlling or background type, as opposed to the specific detailed conversation of the first type of synapse. Drugs can affect the transfer of information at both types of synapse, but the drug actions that tend to be useful therapeutically in mental health disorders are those affecting the second type of synapse. Drug-induced changes in chemical neurotransmission in the first type of synapse will tend to disrupt the transfer of information that normally occurs, just as electrical interference on the line will disturb the conversation of two people speaking on the telephone. By contrast, drug-induced changes in neurotransmission at the second type of synapse might have an effect analogous to increasing the volume of background music broadcast by a public address system, or changing the music from something soothing to something lively and alerting.

As far as drug effects on the brain are concerned, particularly in relation to the treatment of mental disorders, by far the most important chemical neurotransmitters are the *bioamines*, principally noradrenaline, dopamine, and serotonin or 5-hydroxytryptamine (5-HT). The two other important neurotransmitters affected by mind-altering drugs are acetylcholine and gamma-aminobutyric acid (GABA). Some of the drugs that interact with these chemical neurotransmitters, and their possible effects on brain function, are summarized in Table 2.1; the interested reader is also referred to other texts (Leonard, 1992; Cookson *et al.*, 1993).

How drugs affect neurotransmission in the brain

In Table 2.1, the effects of psychotherapeutic drugs on the function of various neurotransmitters are described merely as 'increased' or 'decreased'. What do these terms mean exactly in this context, what mechanisms are involved, and how can these be detected and studied?

The simplest way to describe the mechanisms of action of drugs affecting neurotransmission in the brain is to consider the whole process in four stages (Figure 2.2). In *stage one*, neurotransmitter chemicals are synthesized from simpler building blocks which flow or are drawn into the nerve cell from the fluid outside, and are then stored in small packages or synaptic vesicles concentrated in the axon terminals or nerve endings. Levodopa (L-dopa) is one of the building blocks for dopamine, a neurotransmitter which is decreased in Parkinson's disease. When taken by mouth, L-dopa enters the blood stream and then the brain, where it increases the production of dopamine and helps treat the symptoms of Parkinson's disease. This mainly happens in nerve endings where dopamine is normally manufactured and used as a neurotransmitter because it is at these sites that L-dopa can easily be taken up and where the enzyme that is necessary to bring about the conversion of L-dopa to dopamine is also located. So L-dopa tablets taken by mouth end up as increased dopamine neurotransmitter just where it is needed to make up for the deficiency causing the symptoms of Parkinson's disease.

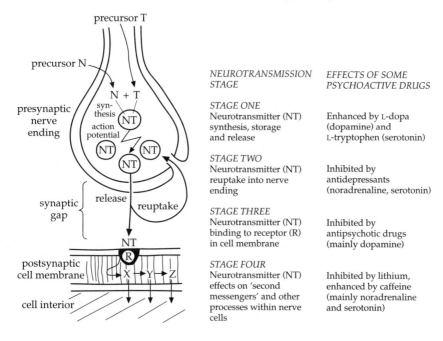

NEUROTRANSMISSION STAGE	EFFECTS OF SOME PSYCHOACTIVE DRUGS
STAGE ONE Neurotransmitter (NT) synthesis, storage and release	Enhanced by L-dopa (dopamine) and L-tryptophen (serotonin)
STAGE TWO Neurotransmitter (NT) reuptake into nerve ending	Inhibited by antidepressants (noradrenaline, serotonin)
STAGE THREE Neurotransmitter (NT) binding to receptor (R) in cell membrane	Inhibited by antipsychotic drugs (mainly dopamine)
STAGE FOUR Neurotransmitter (NT) effects on 'second messengers' and other processes within nerve cells	Inhibited by lithium, enhanced by caffeine (mainly noradrenaline and serotonin)

Figure 2.2   *Stages in neurotransmission and the mechanisms of action of some psychoactive drugs at presynaptic and postsynaptic sites*

Other drugs act at this stage to increase levels of neurotransmitters within nerve endings, not by increasing synthesis of neurotransmitters, but by reducing their metabolic breakdown. The monoamine oxidase inhibitor (MAOI) drugs are good examples of this. These drugs attack and destroy the enzymes that normally break down and inactivate neurotransmitters such as noradrenaline, dopamine and serotonin. These neurotransmitters are continually leaking from their storage sites into the fluid within the nerve cell, where they are broken down. If this inactivation is prevented by an MAOI, there is more neurotransmitter available to be released onto other nerve cells. Furthermore, the same enzymes that inactivate the neurotransmitters are also used by the body to break down certain chemicals from the diet (e.g. tyramine). If following MAOI administration these chemicals are taken by mouth and allowed to reach the brain, they will cause even more neurotransmitter to spill out onto other nerve cells and profoundly affect their activity. Not surprisingly in view of all this, MAOI drugs can have important effects on mental functions and are useful in treating depression and various types of anxiety disorder. However, if taken with other drugs or certain foods (e.g. ripe cheese containing tyramine), dangerous adverse effects may result.

Stage two involves the release of neurotransmitter into the synaptic gap when an action potential or electrical signal reaches the nerve ending.

The amount of free neurotransmitter in the synaptic gap will depend on how much is released, but also on how quickly it is inactivated by enzymes in the region of the synapse. An even more important factor is how effectively neurotransmitter is drawn back into the nerve ending to be stored for future use. The reuptake of free neurotransmitter back into the nerve ending where it is stored is the most effective mechanism for limiting the action of neurotransmitter on neighbouring nerve cells. It is an active process, involving a special transport pathway through the membrane of the nerve ending which would otherwise be impervious to the neurotransmitter molecules.

Several types of antidepressant drugs inhibit the active reuptake of neurotransmitters such as noradrenaline and serotonin (5-HT) and so increase the amount of free transmitter which can interact with other cells. The original tricyclic antidepressant drugs inhibit noradrenaline and 5-HT reuptake to approximately the same extent, whereas the new selective serotonin reuptake inhibitors, as their name implies, have their effect almost exclusively on the serotonin or 5-HT system. Interestingly, SSRIs have properties not shared by most of the older antidepressants, e.g. powerful suppressant effects on appetite and on symptoms of obsessive-compulsive disorder. These effects are therefore most probably due to selective actions on the serotonin systems of the brain. In contrast, although their side-effect profile is different, the antidepressant effect of the SSRIs appears to be similar to that of the older tricyclic drugs. This implies that an antidepressant effect can result *either* from an increase in noradrenaline neurotransmission *or* from a similar increase in the effectiveness of serotonin neurotransmitters.

It might be expected from this understanding of the mechanism of action of antidepressant drugs that it would be easy to demonstrate that people suffering from depressive illness have a deficiency in the brain of either noradrenaline or serotonin or both. There are various ways of looking for abnormalities of this sort. For example, measuring the concentration of these amines or their breakdown products (metabolites) in the fluid that bathes the brain and spinal cord (cerebrospinal fluid, CSF) should give an idea of the amount of neurotransmitter free to act at synapses within the brain. The CSF can be sampled reasonably easily by performing a 'spinal tap' or lumbar puncture. Although some evidence has been found for reduced levels of noradrenaline and serotonin in the CSF of some depressed patients, the results have been inconsistent and difficult to evaluate. However, less direct evidence, mainly based on measuring the levels of circulating hormones which are controlled by noradrenaline or serotonin in the brain, supports the idea that the activity of these neurotransmitters is reduced in depressive disorders.

An interesting clinical experiment has reawoken interest in an earlier idea about the biochemical basis of depression called the *permissive amine theory*. This postulates that a serotonin system keeps a check on a brain noradrenaline system concerned with mood regulation, which may be abnormally over- or underactive in various mood disorders. As we have said, there is a lack of direct evidence for abnormalities in brain noradrenaline in depression, but experimenters have shown that if the serotonin systems of the brain are suddenly 'switched off' in people who have recently recovered from severe depressive illnesses with the aid of antidepressant drugs, their depressive symptoms will return suddenly and as severely as before. The 'serotonin switch-off' is achieved by exploiting a 'stage one' neurotransmitter mechanism as described above. Patients are given an amino acid drink lacking the one amino acid – L-tryptophan – essential for the synthesis of serotonin in the brain and for neurotransmission at 5-HT synapses. The excess of non-serotonin amino acids causes the flow of L-tryptophan into the brain to be completely cut off, and within a relatively short time (24 hours or less) it is likely that the brain stores of serotonin become depleted and 5-HT neurotransmission reduces or ceases.

The observation that the symptoms of depressive illness can return so dramatically after 'serotonin switch-off' in people who have recently recovered, strongly suggests that antidepressant drug treatment works by boosting a serotonin mechanism in the brain. Perhaps this indirectly compensates for or corrects a faulty noradrenaline system without having any marked action on mood states by itself. This is confirmed by other experiments in which healthy people who are subjected to the same 'serotonin switch-off' treatment only experience trivial changes in mood and feeling.

These studies illustrate two important general principles. Firstly, that drugs or other procedures with known effects on neurotransmission in the brain can be used as tools to discover more about biological mechanisms of mental health disorders and how drug treatments work. Secondly, that psychotherapeutic drugs often seem to act on biological processes or mechanisms which are not themselves the cause of mental health problems but which are capable of affecting those processes which are.

The *third stage* of neurotransmission at which drugs can act involves the effect of the neurotransmitter on receptors located within and on the outside of the cell membrane in the region of the synapse. We have already mentioned the properties of agonists and antagonists, which are substances capable of binding to the receptor and mimicking and blocking respectively the actions of the normally occurring neurotransmitter. We did not mention earlier the fact that, as well as being located on the postsynaptic membrane of a cell adjoining a nerve ending, receptors for a neurotransmitter can also be found on the nerve ending itself. When free neurotransmitter in the synaptic gap binds to these *autoreceptors*, the effect is usually to inhibit further release of neurotransmitter from its own nerve ending. In other words, this acts as a negative feedback mechanism to limit the release of neurotransmitter.

Many different types of psychotherapeutic drug act as antagonists at receptors and block the effect of the naturally occurring neurotransmitters. The best examples are the antipsychotic drugs which bind to dopamine receptors and prevent their activation by dopamine. This effectively interrupts normal dopaminergic neurotransmission, but the effect may be limited initially by the fact that the drugs also 'block' the autoreceptors. As a result, a brake on the release of dopamine is removed and the levels of dopamine in the synaptic cleft will rise and help to drive off the receptor-blocking drugs. Other examples of receptor antagonists are the beta-blockers which bind to some of the postsynaptic receptors normally activated by noradrenaline and prevent some of its effects, many of which are important in bringing about the bodily symptoms of anxiety. Other receptors that are activated by noradrenaline are called alpha-receptors and those in the brain are particularly important in systems concerned with arousal and activity. Alpha-blockers therefore tend to cause drowsiness and sedation. Substances like alcohol may affect receptor mechanisms indirectly by a general disruptive effect on the cell membrane in which receptors are embedded.

The *fourth stage* of neurotransmission at which drugs may act concerns all the processes that go on *inside* the nerve cell as a result of the neurotransmitter binding to the receptors on the *outside* of the cell. These processes involve chemicals called *secondary messengers* and these may in turn trigger off electrical changes in the cell owing to the flow of electrically charged ions and/or other chemical reactions which affect and determine the function of the nerve cell and its ability to influence other nerve cells. The best example of drugs acting at this stage is lithium, which has complex, mostly inhibitory effects on the secondary messengers for a number of neurotransmitters. Other examples are the xanthine drugs which include caffeine. In contrast to lithium, these substances enhance the effects of secondary messengers activated by receptors responsive to adrenaline and noradrenaline. This explains why a cup of coffee has a similar arousing effect to the pumping out of a little natural adrenaline.

The four stages of neurotransmission and some drugs acting on them are summarized in Figure 2.2.

Receptor adaptation

When a receptor antagonist fits into the 'lock' of the receptor, the effect can usually be reversed by the neurotransmitter or by other agonist chemicals which will compete for the same receptor sites and push out the obstructing substance. However, sometimes chemicals bind to receptors permanently, rather like a key getting stuck in a lock. Then the only way of getting rid of the blocked receptors is to manufacture new ones, just as a jammed lock will need to be replaced. Many receptors need to be occupied by a neurotransmitter or a drug in order to produce a useful effect on the receiving cell, but usually the total number of occupied receptors necessary for a maximum response is small compared with the total number available. Furthermore, a nerve cell may react to an agonist drug stimulating its receptors by withdrawing receptors from the cell membrane (*downregulation*) which will tend to cause desensitization or tolerance to the effects of the agonist drug. By contrast, if an antagonist occupies the receptors, the cell may respond by increasing the number of receptors (*upregulation*), which will tend to limit the antagonist effect and again restore the 'status quo'. Thus the brain adapts and adjusts to the presence of drugs, and does its best to carry on regardless.

Drug effects on faulty neurotransmission and mental illness

There has been an enormous growth of knowledge about how drugs alter neurotransmission and other processes within the brain. For many drugs that are used in treating mental illness, we have a very good idea of how they affect brain processes. This has led scientists to speculate that these effects may be crucial for therapeutic actions in mental disorders, possibly by restoring a biochemical imbalance or correcting a faulty brain mechanism. Unfortunately, in most cases this is just guesswork, and it is quite possible that the drugs help mental disorders by entirely different means which are yet to be discovered. Even when we are fairly sure that we have identified and understood the action in the brain which is responsible for a drug's helpful therapeutic effect (see Table 2.1), it is still by no means certain that this drug effect is directly relevant to the cause of the psychiatric condition under treatment.

Since therapeutic drug effects in mental illness are usually slow to develop, scientists have looked for drug actions in the brain that have a comparably delayed time course in order to help understand the mechanisms of the therapeutic actions. This is a promising approach, but it still does not guarantee that the effects of drugs that we can observe and measure are necessarily the ones that are crucial for their therapeutic actions. This is particularly important if we wish to improve on drugs that were discovered by chance, in order to develop new, more effective and safer drugs. Perhaps the best example of this dilemma is given by the atypical antipsychotic drug clozapine. Clozapine has a unique ability to reduce schizophrenic symptoms that have not responded to other drugs (*British Journal of Psychiatry*, 1992) (see Chapter 6). Unfortunately clozapine is quite a toxic substance, and if we knew for sure how it worked therapeutically, safe alternatives might be produced. Clozapine is known to have a wide range of effects on the brain, but so far it has proved impossible to identify which of these actions, if any, is responsible for the drug's unique clinical spectrum of action.

Pharmacodynamics and pharmacokinetics

The exotic sound of these terms may conjure up images of weird and wonderful treatments or practices. In fact the term 'pharmacodynamics' simply refers to the processes by which drugs affect the body, and 'pharmacokinetics' describes the processes of absorption, distribution, metabolism (breakdown) and disposal (excretion) of drugs.

The dose-response relationship

We have already dealt with the important matter of how drugs interact with receptors on nerve cell membranes. The number of receptors on which a drug acts will depend on the concentration of the drug in the vicinity of the nerve cell. The increase or change in effect of a drug that occurs as its concentration is raised is called the dose-response relationship. Usually the effectiveness of a drug increases rapidly as its concentration rises above a certain threshold point, and soon reaches a plateau or maximum beyond which no further improvement in response can occur, even though the drug concentration is further increased. However, with further increases in drug concentration, other systems of the body are likely to be affected, sometimes having effects which will oppose the first action of the drug. If so, and if the initial drug effect was the therapeutic action for which the drug was given, then the effectiveness of the drug will tend to decline as its concentration exceeds a critical level. On the other hand, if the initial effect constitutes an unwanted action of the drug, this may, somewhat paradoxically, first increase and then decrease as the drug concentration goes up and brings into play a secondary action which serves as an antidote to the first (Figure 2.3). More usually, there is simply an increase in the number and severity of unwanted or adverse effects as the concentration of a drug is increased. The aim is to achieve the optimal therapeutic effect of the drug at drug concentrations that cause no (or only minimal) adverse effects.

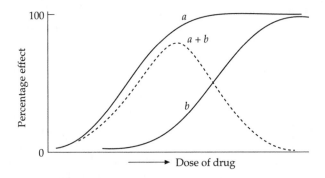

Figure 2.3   *Dose-response curves for two opposing effects, a and b, shared by the same drug. Effect b develops at higher doses than effect a, and will act to limit the overall effect (a + b) of the drug obtained in practice. In the case of neuroleptic drugs, a and b may be antipsychotic and psychotomimetic effects of the same drug, or parkinsonian and antiparkinsonian actions due to dopamine receptor blockade and anticholinergic effects respectively*

Although there are many examples of drugs that have therapeutic actions only at concentrations well above those already causing troublesome unwanted effects, fortunately for most of the drugs used to treat mental health disorders, therapeutic effects can be achieved in the majority of patients without too many unwanted side-effects. More recently developed drugs tend to be much better in this respect than the older ones, although even with these new medications, in some people unacceptable side-effects may limit the possibilities of drug treatment. There are two aspects to this. Firstly, some people appear to be extremely intolerant to *any* effects of medication, and secondly, with most psycho-therapeutic drugs, unwanted effects at a particular drug concentration tend to wane over a period of continued administration, whereas beneficial actions tend to build up over days and weeks (see Chapter 3).

The therapeutic index

For some old-fashioned drugs, the difference between the amount of drug needed for a useful effect and the amount that will produce an unacceptable quota of harmful or toxic effects may be quite small. For example, with the older type of barbiturate sedatives, only two or three times the dose used to produce sedation or sleepiness may cause a dangerous suppression of vital body functions such as respiration. In contrast, most of the drugs used in psychiatry nowadays are safe in the sense that drug concentrations that produce dangerous effects are many times those necessary for a therapeutic action. Such drugs are said to have a *high therapeutic index*. However, it is not always appreciated that although modern psychotherapeutic drugs may have a high therapeutic index with regard to toxic adverse affects, more subtle counter-therapeutic effects can occur at concentrations only a little higher than those that are useful for treatment.

For all these reasons, it is important to try to get dosages right, and to use the lowest effective doses possible. However, for many drugs, the relationship between the dose of drug administered and the concentra-tion in the brain is likely to be extremely variable from person to person. With one or two exceptions (e.g. lithium, carbamazepine), measuring the amount of drug in the blood is not often very useful, as equivalent therapeutic results may be obtained in different people having widely different blood levels of the drug. The level of a drug in the blood may vary a great deal from time to time in the same person, and may not bear any simple relationship to how much drug is actually reaching the important sites in the brain. In practice this means that there is often a wide variation in the dosages of a particular drug that are needed for a therapeutic effect in different people. Often the only practical way to find the right dose of a drug for any individual seems to be by trial and error. It is also helpful to follow the basic rule that persistent side-effects usually mean that the optimal dose has been exceeded, or is not achiev-able in the particular person being treated with that particular drug.

Pharmacokinetics

Pharmacokinetics is a rather daunting term which refers to all the factors determining how much drug there will be at the relevant site of action within the brain. It is concerned therefore with how much of a drug dose reaches the brain, what happens to the drug once it gets there, and how its effect is limited or switched off.

The brain consists of a complex collection of neurons, grouped into clumps or nuclei and surrounded by many other supporting cells (glial cells), the whole structure protected and excluded from the rest of the body's fluids by a special barrier membrane (blood-brain barrier) which only allows certain chemicals through. The brain is a particularly avid consumer of glucose, which is its only energy fuel, and because the brain is largely made up of lipid or fatty tissue, it also provides easy access to fat-soluble chemicals. Other chemicals, however, have limited access to the brain. The brain has a rich blood supply, and apart from lipid solubility, the other main factor determining how much drug gets to the brain is the amount of drug in the blood stream.

Before reaching the blood, a drug taken by mouth must be absorbed from the gastrointestinal system. This may be an erratic process, assuming of course that the patient swallows the medication in the first place! Liquids tend to be absorbed from the gut better than tablets, and are much less easily held in the mouth and spat out later, if patients wish to conceal their non-compliance. Less well known is the fact that a heavy intake of tea and coffee can reduce the absorption of many psychotherapeutic drugs. Since the 'teapot' and 'coffee-cup' syndromes are occupational hazards for many people with mental health problems, poor response to medication may be unfairly blamed on their not taking their tablets, when in fact it is their drinking habits that are causing the problem.

When drugs reach the blood stream after being absorbed from the gastrointestinal system, their first port of call is the liver, which is a very effective chemical recycling plant capable of removing many of the chemical substances, including drugs, which pass through it. If instead a drug is introduced directly into the blood stream by intravenous injection, or is allowed to initially bypass the liver, as happens after intramuscular injection or when the drug is absorbed under the tongue or via the rectum, this will also result in more of the administered drug reaching the brain.

However, in all cases, as soon as a drug enters the body the process of its breakdown and elimination will start, with the liver and kidneys leading the field in this waste-disposal and recycling race. For many drugs, the rate at which they are eliminated from the body depends on how much is administered in the first place (*first order kinetics*), but for a few drugs (e.g. alcohol) the body can only get rid of the drug at a relatively slow, fixed rate, regardless of how much drug is present (*zero order kinetics*).

For many drugs, the initial stages of breakdown in the tissues or in the liver result in products that are active and effective drugs in their own right, albeit sometimes with different properties from the 'parent' drug. The breakdown of the administered drug may be essential in order for it to have an effect on the patient. This is the case where 'depot' injections of antipsychotic drugs are given as an inactive (precursor) form dissolved in vegetable oil. The oil is administered by deep intramuscular injection and rests inertly within the muscle tissue. The drug precursor gradually and steadily enters the blood which circulates through the muscle. In the blood it is converted into the active form of the drug which then passes into the brain. In this way, the patient's brain receives a steady 'dose' of medication over long periods, with the option of increasing the dose either by increasing the amount of oil injected (up to a limit of 2 ml at any one site) or by reducing the interval between injections (usually once or twice per month).

When a drug is given repeatedly, the final concentration of drug that is achieved in the blood and in the brain will depend on the balance between the amount and frequency of drug administered and on the rate of elimination. When the movement of a drug into the body is balanced by its elimination from the body, it is said to be in a *steady state*. For drugs that are eliminated quickly from the body, steady state conditions will be achieved relatively quickly, whereas for slowly eliminated drugs, the steady state may take many days to be achieved. The *plasma half-life* is a measure of how long it takes for the concentration of drug in the plasma to fall to half its initial level. This measure can be used to estimate how long steady state conditions will take to be achieved. Thus when a drug is being administered regularly, after a period equivalent to approximately five times the plasma half-life, the drug level in the body will be nearly at a steady state. For a drug with a plasma half-life of 24 hours, the steady state will therefore not be achieved until about 5 days, and for a 'depot' drug with a half-life of about 3 weeks, nearly 4 months will be required before steady state levels are reached. Steady state conditions cannot be speeded up by increasing the frequency of administration. However, this will obviously increase the amount of drug in the body, so that concentrations equivalent to the steady state level can be reached early by using *loading doses* or more frequent administration in the initial stages of treatment. Since most psychoactive drugs have long half-lives, oral medication may only need to be taken once a day, making it easier for the patients to remember.

When a drug is taken over a long period, the ability of the body to break it down and get rid of it is usually increased, and this will tend to limit the effect of the drug if the dose is not increased to compensate. Other drugs administered at the same time may also increase the ability of the body to eliminate drugs generally, so that two drugs given together may result in both being less effective than when given alone. A good example of this is when the anticonvulsant drug carbamazepine is given at the same time as the oral contraceptive pill. In combination, both drugs are eliminated from the body more quickly, so the effectiveness of both drugs will be reduced, possibly resulting in an unwanted pregnancy and/or poor control of epilepsy. It is not always appreciated that heavy smoking can also stimulate the body's capacity to break down and eliminate other drugs. Occasionally the reverse process takes place: one drug may interfere with the elimination of another, resulting in increased concentrations of that drug even though its dosage remains the same. An example of this is when chlorpromazine is given at the same time as the antidepressant imipramine. This produces a reduction in the metabolism of the latter drug and a rise in the levels of imipramine in the body.

When drugs circulate in the blood, they are bound to a variable extent to plasma proteins such as albumen. Only the fraction of the drug that is *not* bound to plasma proteins is available to enter the brain, so the amount of protein binding will alter the drug's effectiveness. Protein binding will be affected by the amount of protein available, which can change in certain disorders or diseases, and also by the presence of other substances which will occupy the same protein sites. Thus substances that displace the drug from the protein sites will increase the amount available to enter the brain, whereas drugs that increase protein binding will have the opposite effect.

Tolerance, dependence and withdrawal effects

When some drugs are given for long periods, the body develops ways of eliminating them more effectively. This means that the drug will eventually produce less effect than when given initially. This phenomenon is called *tolerance*. However, sometimes tolerance is due to the cells on which the drug works developing compensatory mechanisms that oppose the drug's action, as in the receptor upregulation and downregulation mentioned earlier. The compensatory mechanisms are usually counterbalanced by the presence of the drug, but when this is withdrawn, the compensatory mechanisms are unopposed and the body will be in a different state from how it was before drug administration was started. This may lead to withdrawal symptoms, showing that the body has in some way become physically dependent on the presence of the drug to maintain the status quo. Nearly all drugs when administered for long periods will produce some kind of withdrawal phenomena, and when this is associated with a psychological craving for the drug, it is known as *addiction*. Addiction is most commonly associated with drugs that produce euphoria or other highly pleasurable and sought-after effects which cause in people a strong desire to repeat them. Addiction is therefore relatively uncommon with the drugs that are used to treat mental disorders, because most of these drugs produce neutral or slightly unpleasant subjective effects. The main exceptions are the benzodiazepine antianxiety drugs which can produce a pleasant state of mind, particularly in people who are already anxious. As well as the physical dependence that these drugs can produce, they may also produce a craving for the drug which will constitute drug addiction (see Chapter 9).

However, the physical and psychological dependence associated with benzodiazepines is a mild problem compared with the intense drug addiction that can result from powerful euphoriant drugs such as cocaine, amphetamines or opiates. Surprisingly, strong cravings produced by 'stimulant' drugs such as amphetamines and cocaine are not accompanied by noticeable tolerance or physical withdrawal effects, whereas the addiction produced by 'depressant' drugs such as morphine and heroin (opiates) is associated with dose escalation, tolerance and physical dependence, as revealed by the well-known 'cold turkey' withdrawal reaction. Although highly unpleasant, the opiate 'cold turkey' is not particularly dangerous, in contrast to the physical withdrawal syndrome produced by other depressant drugs such as barbiturates and alcohol. Not only do these latter drugs produce craving and addiction, but in physically dependent people they are also associated with dangerous withdrawal effects, such as epileptic convulsions.

Withdrawal effects can be reduced or rendered less dangerous by the slow reduction and phasing out of drugs that cause dependence, provided the person taking the drugs will co-operate with this. When discontinuing non-addictive drugs such as antidepressants after a long period of administration, it is also important to reduce the dose slowly in order to avoid physical withdrawal effects such as sleep disturbance, nausea and headache.

Further reading

Cookson, J., Crammer, J. and Heine, B. (1993). *The Use of Drugs in Psychiatry.* London: Gaskell/Royal College of Psychiatrists.
Leonard, B. E. (1992). *Fundamentals of Psychopharmacology.* Chichester: John Wiley.

3

Drug treatment in clinical practice

Psychotherapeutic drugs in current use

Psychotherapeutic drugs can be broadly grouped according to their main use for treating mental health disorders. The three main groups are (1) hypnotics and antianxiety drugs, (2) antidepressant and mood stabilizing drugs, and (3) antipsychotic drugs (major tranquillizers or neuroleptic agents). Within the three main groups, there are a number of subclasses based on similarities in chemical structure and pharmacological properties. Within any subclass of medication, there is usually considerable variation in terms of clinical potency (amount of medication needed to produce a particular clinical effect) and the ability to induce certain side-effects, whether adverse or advantageous. These differences in potency and side-effects can often be related to the chemical and other biological properties used to classify the drugs. However, it is usually much less certain whether any particular properties can be directly or indirectly related to the drugs' principal therapeutic actions in mental health disorders.

Hypnotics and antianxiety drugs

Many drugs acting on the brain produce sedation, a term which in the past was strictly used to mean a reduction in anxiety. However, most antianxiety drugs also produce drowsiness and slowing of thought processes, actions which may be an advantage if medication is taken at night in order to induce sleep. Benzodiazepines, which are by far the most widely used antianxiety drugs, are often effective at dosages that do not cause noticeable drowsiness. The term 'minor tranquillizer' is commonly used for drugs with this characteristic. However, the reduced potential for drowsiness with benzodiazepines compared with older sedative drugs such as barbiturates is probably over-rated, as even benzodiazepines can be shown to impair alertness and increase reaction times if sensitive tests are used. Anxious people tend to prefer benzodiazepines to the older drugs because a more normal mood is attained, even in the presence of drowsiness.

The most striking advantage of benzodiazepines over older sedative drugs is their much greater safety. Even in overdose, benzodiazepines are relatively non-toxic, whereas two or three times the normal dose of a barbiturate may have fatal effects, mainly by depressing breathing. People who are usually timid and inhibited may become aggressive or self-assertive when they take benzodiazepines, but there is nothing comparable with the striking release (*disinhibition*) of aggression that is often produced by another brain depressant, alcohol. Similarly, the euphoric sensations associated with low doses of alcohol and barbiturates are mostly lacking with benzodiazepines, and this partly explains why benzodiazepines are much less likely to be deliberately abused than barbiturates and alcohol. However, there is no doubt that people can get addicted to the antianxiety effects that benzodiazepines produce, and tolerance and physical dependence have often been demonstrated when benzodiazepines are given for more than a few months. This can produce troublesome withdrawal symptoms in a proportion of people who suddenly stop the drugs. This is particularly likely if they have been taking benzodiazepines which have a short duration of action, since the direct effects of the drugs will wear off rapidly once the medication is stopped.

Some benzodiazepines are useful anticonvulsants, and all cause a reduction in muscle tone owing to an enhancement of physiological inhibition in the spinal cord. A reduction in muscle spasm associated with anxiety may contribute indirectly to the helpful effects of these drugs on anxious mood. The antianxiety properties of benzodiazepines are frequently and effectively exploited for treating insomnia, since anxiety is a common reason for problems in falling asleep. In high doses, benzodiazepines produce noticeable drowsiness, but for hypnotic drugs this is an advantage.

Most hypnotic drugs produce an abnormal pattern of sleep as gauged by neurophysiological measures such as the electroencephalogram (EEG) which records the minute electrical waves that pass through the skull from the brain. However, the normal sleep pattern is less markedly disturbed by benzodiazepines than by the older hypnotic drugs. Hangovers can still be a problem with benzodiazepines, and this is linked to the duration of action of the particular drug used. Many benzodiazepines have active metabolites with a long duration of action which act like drugs in their own right, and this needs to be borne in mind when choosing a suitable benzodiazepine. A rapid onset of action and a duration of action of 8 hours or less are likely to be useful properties for a hypnotic drug. Temazepam is probably the best example of a useful hypnotic benzodiazepine; other examples are given in Table 3.1.

Anxiety, agitation and insomnia may be prominent symptoms in other mental health disorders, especially depressive illness. The best way of relieving these secondary symptoms is to treat the underlying disorder rather than to use hypnotic or anxiolytic drugs such as benzodiazepines. Some antidepressant drugs also cause drowsiness in their own right, particularly early on in treatment, and this may be an additional advantage in depressed people who are agitated and unable to sleep. Most antidepressant drugs have antianxiety effects independent of their main action in helping depressed mood or of their ability to induce drowsiness. Patients who have anxiety disorders without any depressive features will therefore be helped by these drugs. Thus phobic anxiety and panic attacks – disorders that are associated with depressive illness but are quite distinct from it – are helped by a number of antidepressant drug

Table 3.1   *Formulary of drugs for use in mental health disorders. Allocation of drugs to the following suggested groups or categories is provisional and discretionary, and not all prescribers will agree with the choices made. Group A (first-line drugs) are well-established drugs which should be regarded as first-line treatments in their particular applications. All have clear value and advantages which outweigh considerations of cost and adverse effect potential for most applications. Group B (second-line drugs) are drugs with clear value for particular applications, or with advantages over similar drugs or preparations sufficient to warrant availability to all prescribers. However, owing to considerations of high cost and/or relative novelty and/or high potential for adverse effects, all in relation to probable therapeutic value, prescribers are advised to consider first-line drugs in preference. Group C (restricted drugs) are drugs with clear value for particular applications or with advantages over similar drugs or preparations, but owing to very high cost and/or potential for very serious adverse effects, availability is restricted for use in registered patients, with prescriptions by consultants only. (Examples are clozapine, cyproterone acetate, remoxipride and tryptophan.) Group D (new drugs and non-recommended older drugs) are drugs of uncertain, unproved or dubious value, or whose advantages over better-established or cheaper alternatives are in doubt or lacking. This category includes most newly introduced drugs awaiting review following the publication of further information from clinical studies*

Group A (first line)	Group B (second line)	Group C (restricted)	Group D (new and non-recommended)
Tricyclic and related antidepressants			
amitriptyline	dothiepin		amoxapine
clomipramine	trimipramine		iprindole
imipramine	mianserin		butriptyline
doxepin	desipramine		protriptyline
lofepramine			maprotiline
			viloxazine
			nortriptyline
Monoamine oxidase inhibitors			
	phenelzine		tranylcypromine
	isocarboxazid		
	moclobemide[1]		
Compound antidepressant preparations			
			Limbitrol
			Motipress
			Motival
			Parstelin
			Triptafen

Table 3.1 *(continued)*

Other antidepressants – selective serotonin reuptake inhibitors etc.

fluoxetine[2]	fluvoxamine tryptophan[4]	venlafaxine[5]
	sertraline	nefazodone[5]
	paroxetine[2, 3]	citalopram[5]
	trazodone	
	flupenthixol	

Antimanic and related substances

all lithium carbonate	all lithium citrate
preparations	preparations
carbamazepine	sodium valproate
droperidol	lorazepam injection
	diazepam injection

CNS stimulants and appetite suppressants

dexamphetamine[6]	fenfluramine
methylphenidate[7]	dexfenfluramine
pemoline[7]	diethylpropion
	phentermine

Antipsychotic drugs – oral

chlorpromazine	flupenthixol	clozapine	loxapine
haloperidol	fluphenazine	remoxipride[8]	pericyazine
trifluoperazine	pimozide[9]		perphenazine
thioridazine	sulpiride		oxypertine
	zuclopenthixol		trifluperidol
	risperidone		sertindole[10]
			olanzapine[10]

Antipsychotic drugs – depot injections

fluphenazine	zuclopenthixol acetate
decanoate	zuclopenthixol decanoate
	pipothiazine palmitate
	flupenthixol decanoate
	haloperidol decanoate
	fluspirilene

Hypnotics, anxiolytics, etc.[11]

temazepam[12]	loprazolam[12]	zolpidem[14]
diazepam	lormetazepam	nitrazepam
	chlormethiazole[13]	flunitrazepam
	chlordiazepoxide[13]	medazepam
	chloral hydrate[12]	bromazepam
	zopiclone[12]	clobazam
	oxazepam	clorazepate
	lorazepam	meprobamate
	buspirone[15]	hydroxyzine
	promethazine[12]	chlormezanone
		alprazolam
		all barbiturates

Table 3.1 *(continued)*

Antimuscarinic drugs for parkinsonism[16]

procyclidine[17]	orphenadrine	biperiden
benzhexol	benztropine[17]	methixene

Miscellaneous substances

propranolol[18, 19]	promazine	cyproterone	benperidol[21]
atenolol[18]	tetrabenazine[20]	acetate	donepezil[23]
	cyproheptadine	(Androcur)[21]	
	bromocriptine		
	disulfiram		
	(Antabuse)[22]		

[1]Safe, short-acting and well tolerated, with few side-effects. High cost.
[2]Also licensed for panic states and obsessive-compulsive disorders.
[3]Paroxetine may be preferred to fluoxetine in elderly.
[4]Named patient only. Consultant and pharmacist to register with manufacturer.
[5]New drugs. Side-effects similar to SSRIs such as fluoxetine.
[6]For use in narcolepsy and in hyperkinetic children over the age of 6 years.
[7]For use in hyperkinetic children over the age of 6 years.
[8]Risk of aplastic anaemia. Withdrawn from general use. Named patient only.
[9]ECG advised before starting treatment: observe dose restrictions, as can be cardiotoxic.
[10]New drug – indications similar to risperidone; better tolerated than other antipsychotic drugs, and possibly more effective against negative symptoms; high cost.
[11]Preferably for short-term use only. For long-term use, all antidepressants have anti-anxiety effects independent of their sedative properties.
[12]Especially for use as a hypnotic.
[13]For alcohol withdrawal states.
[14]New drug, a non-benzodiazepine similar to zopiclone.
[15]Has similar delayed anxiolytic effect to that of most antidepressants except that it is relatively ineffective in panic disorder.
[16]May exacerbate psychosis and tardive dyskinesia.
[17]For administration by mouth and by injection.
[18]For somatic symptoms of anxiety.
[19]For akathisia due to neuroleptics.
[20]For tardive dyskinesia, may exacerbate depression (clozapine may be preferable alternative).
[21]Sometimes used to reduce libido in men with psychological or behavioural problems due to hypersexuality.
[22]Used as an aid to alcohol abstinence.
[23]For use in mild to moderate Alzheimer's disease.

types, including monoamine oxidase inhibitors, tricyclic antidepressants, and especially the selective serotonin reuptake inhibitors. The SSRIs are also especially helpful in a particular type of anxiety state called obsessive-compulsive disorder.

Neuroleptic drugs or 'major tranquillizers', which in higher doses are used as antipsychotic drugs, are sometimes used for treating anxiety, their chief advantage being the avoidance of drug dependence and addiction. However, even in low doses, major tranquillizers carry the risk of producing movement disorders. A long-term drug-induced movement disorder called *tardive dyskinesia* may be very disabling and is sometimes irreversible.

Many of the unpleasant bodily sensations associated with anxiety are produced by the effects of noradrenaline and adrenaline on various systems outside the brain (e.g. tremor, flushing, faintness and dizziness). These somatic symptoms often make people even more anxious but can sometimes be reduced by beta-blocking drugs such as propranolol which directly interfere with the actions of noradrenaline and adrenaline on the blood vessels, heart and muscles. Some beta-blockers may also help anxiety by an action on the brain, although the mechanisms are not well understood.

Antidepressant drugs

The most important antidepressant drugs currently in use belong to the class called monoamine reuptake inhibitors (sometimes abbreviated to MARI). The original members of this group (e.g. imipramine, amitripty-line) have a tricyclic chemical structure and a wide spectrum of pharmacological properties similar to those of the phenothiazine major tranquillizers. Newer MARI drugs such as the SSRIs are chemically distinct from the tricyclic antidepressants and are different clinically in many important respects, mostly relating to the spectrum of side-effects produced. Whereas the older drugs tend to produce drowsiness, dry mouth, blurred vision, constipation, urinary retention and weight gain, the SSRIs have nausea, anorgasmia, headaches and anorexia as their main side-effects. The most important difference between the SSRIs and the other drugs is their improved safety, mainly because of their fewer adverse effects on the heart and circulation. Whereas SSRIs mainly affect brain serotonin or 5-hydroxytryptamine, tricyclic antidepressants affect other biological amines as well, particularly the noradrenaline and cholinergic systems. It is this major difference that probably accounts for the different side-effect profiles of the two drug types, but interestingly, in terms of antidepressant effectiveness, the SSRIs are no better than the older drugs, with 20–30% of depressed people not being helped by either type. In contrast, the SSRIs have been shown to have definite advantages when it comes to treating anxiety disorders, particularly obsessive-compulsive disorder.

The first antidepressant drugs to be introduced into clinical practice in the 1950s were the monoamine oxidase inhibitors (MAOIs). Originally these were not thought to be as effective as the tricyclic antidepressants which were introduced a little later. After the discovery that MAOIs could produce potentially dangerous interactions with some foods (e.g. ripe cheese containing tyramine) and with other drugs such as opiate painkillers, they were much less often used. However, these drugs may have special advantages for treating certain kinds of mood disorder (e.g. 'dysthymia' or chronic mild depression, panic attacks and social phobias), and interest in them has recently been rekindled since the introduction of a new short-acting MAOI (moclobemide) which has little risk of harmful interactions with foodstuffs or other drugs (Tyrer and Harrison-Read, 1990).

Some people who have a history of recurrent depressive illnesses are also liable to episodes of elevated mood and speeded thinking (hypomania or mania). Although antipsychotic major tranquillizers are useful for treating mania, a somewhat more specific antimanic drug is lithium, although its effects take time to build up. The most valuable use of lithium is probably in the preventive treatment (or prophylaxis) of manic-depressive mood disorder, especially now that worries about lithium's long-term safety have been largely put to rest. However, it is probably necessary for lithium to be taken consistently for 2 years or more to have any impact. Alternative drugs for people who do not like or respond well to lithium are carbamazepine and valproate, drugs that are also used as anticonvulsants. Lithium has important effects on the serotonin or 5-HT system in the brain, and it was this real-ization that gave an impetus to the development of other 5-HT drugs such as the SSRIs which have useful effects in mood disorders. However, apart from carbamazepine and valproate, no other drugs have been found that share lithium's unique antimanic and prophylactic effects in manic-depressive disorders.

Antipsychotic drugs

Antipsychotic drugs have the ability to improve psychotic states, the central feature of which is a distorted perception of reality. When given in doses that tend to be higher than necessary for an antipsychotic action, a striking reduction of movement and emotional reactions is produced which is termed a *major tranquillizing action*. These drugs characteristically produce a range of movement disorders, especially parkinsonian side-effects, which can severely limit their use. Some antipsychotic drugs such as chlorpromazine, which has low clinical potency, also have a wide range of other actions on the brain and the body. Many of these actions are unrelated to the effects on the dopamine systems of the brain which are thought to underlie the antipsychotic action. Among these many other effects of low potency major tranquillizers or neuroleptics are sedation and drowsiness, postural hypotension, anticholinergic autonomic effects, weight gain, hormonal disturbances, photosensitivity and skin pigmentation, eczema, increased risk of convulsions, and very rarely, impaired immunity due to a dramatic fall in white blood cell count. Movement disorders are the most striking side effects of high potency drugs such as haloperidol with the slowly developing abnormal involuntary move-ment disorder called tardive dyskinesia causing the most concern because it is socially handicapping and potentially irreversible. Tardive dyskinesia is believed to result from degenerative changes in the brain which can also occur as part of the normal aging process, and may be more common in people suffering from psychotic mental illnesses, regardless of the use of neuroleptic drugs. However, taking neuroleptic drugs appears to greatly increase the risk of developing this type of movement disorder at a younger age.

Aims and stages of drug treatment for helping mental health disorders

There are four main aims of drug treatment for mental health disorders, which roughly coincide with four overlapping stages in the course of treatment. These stages are the acute and subacute treatment phases, continuation treatment and maintenance treatment. The acute phase of treatment refers to attempts to reduce distress and disturbed behaviour, whereas the subacute phase covers the period of treatment necessary to promote a remission of symptoms, to improve coping and to reduce the associated disturbance in social functioning that results from mental health breakdown. The continuation phase refers to a period when the illness appears to have gone into remission or has disappeared, but when it can be assumed that underlying neurobiological 'causes' or 'pathogenic processes' are still in operation. Drug treatment is aimed at keeping symptoms at bay during this phase (relapse prevention) and promoting spontaneous recovery of the underlying biological disorder. The maintenance phase of drug treatment is intended to minimize the frequency and severity of recurrences of mental illness, which may occur out of the blue, or in response to life stresses following previous full recovery.

Acute drug treatment

Acute drug treatment usually involves drug effects that occur within minutes or hours of drug administration. The drug effects produced in people with mental health problems are *qualitatively* similar to those that would occur in otherwise healthy people, although in people who are ill or disturbed, acute drug effects are often *quantitatively* more marked. Most of the drug actions in this category can be broadly divided into those stimulating the nervous system and those causing depressant or sedative effects. It should be noted that in low doses, drugs that depress the activity of the nervous system cause *disinhibition* or release of behaviours and thought processes that are normally kept in check. This is most commonly seen after small amounts of alcohol. Larger doses of central nervous system depressant drugs produce inhibition of brain functions, as shown by a reduction in most mental processes and behaviour. However, this is not the same thing as 'clinical depression' which refers to a specific clinical syndrome of low mood and negative thinking.

Some acute psychoactive drug effects are usually associated with pleasant subjective sensations, and therefore these drugs are all too readily abused or misused. The relief of anxiety produced by anxiolytic drugs, although not necessarily associated with a euphoriant effect, may still lead to drug-seeking behaviour or addiction. Inappropriate or excessive reliance by the prescriber or the patient on short-term relief produced by anxiolytic drugs may be at the expense of learning how to cope with problems. If the drug continues to be prescribed, then physical dependence may follow, with a cascade of further psychological difficulties.

Even the acute, tranquillizing effects of antipsychotic drugs can be used inappropriately, as sometimes happens when trying to control aggressive or confused patients. Over-reliance on drugs as 'chemical straitjackets', in preference to personal contact, reassurance and reality orientation, is likely to alienate patients, possibly impede their recovery, and certainly reduce their trust in mental health services.

Normal unhappiness, problems and handicaps resulting from certain personality traits, and the ordinary ups and downs of life, are not usually regarded as proper indications for the prescription of psychoactive drugs. The fact that many people prescribe themselves mind-altering drugs such as alcohol, nicotine and cannabis indicates that there is nonetheless a powerful drive to change the experience of unpleasant reality by ingested substances. As far as 'official' prescribing is concerned, the presence of 'illness' is often seen as a necessary if not the sole condition for initiating drug treatment. If there are clear-cut symptoms present, then confidence in the justification and likely effectiveness of drug treatment is increased, especially if the symptoms (or signs) have a psychosomatic character (for example weight loss, reduced appetite and altered biorhythms in depressive illness). However, this is not to say that physical signs and symptoms always require physical or chemical treatment. Psychological measures (psychotherapy or placebo) may be just as effective, and in any case psychological mechanisms may be the clear cause of physical symptoms, as seen in certain types of hysterical disorder (dissociative and conversion states).

Syndrome-specificity of subacute drug actions on mental health disorders

Here we define subacute drug effects as those that develop gradually or after a delay, taking several weeks or even months to reach their full effect. Syndrome-specificity indicates that the drug effects are relatively specific to people with certain mental health disorders and cannot be fully replicated in people with normal mental health.

Subacute drug actions tend to work against mental syndromes, which are collections of different symptoms and signs occurring with a characteristic course and outcome. Although similar syndromes may occur in people with different mental illness diagnoses, for the most part, drug effects are syndrome-specific, irrespective of the overall diagnosis. For example, antipsychotic neuroleptic drugs produce a therapeutic effect across the full range of 'positive' psychotic symptoms (hallucinations, delusions, thought disorder, catatonic behaviour, etc.), regardless of diagnostic labels such as schizophrenia, paranoid state, delusional depression, mania, etc. (Johnstone et al., 1988). The same can probably be said regarding the mood-normalizing properties of lithium, which in this respect may be just as effective in people with schizophrenia as in patients with mania or severe depression.

When more than one mental syndrome is present in the same patient, it is usually helpful to decide whether one is secondary to the other, because it is usually best to aim drug treatment at the primary condition.

For example, patients with severe depression often develop secondary obsessional symptoms (Gittleson, 1966), which will usually respond quite well to drug treatment of the underlying depressive illness. However, where obsessional symptoms are primary, specific antiobsessional drug treatment has to be used. In practice this is with drugs (e.g. SSRIs) that also have antidepressant properties, but higher doses are often needed in order to obtain an effect against primary obsessional symptoms.

It is usually a mistake to use drugs to treat symptoms in isolation from the syndrome to which they belong. For example, insomnia is usually an integral part of some other mental health problem such as depressive illness. Treating the depression will usually help the insomnia, but treatments aimed specifically at the insomnia (e.g. benzodiazepine hypnotics) may sometimes make it worse if it is not the primary disorder, because the underlying condition is either not helped or is allowed to deteriorate.

Just to confuse everything, many people presenting with similar psychiatric syndromes often respond very differently to particular drug treatments. On most occasions the reason for this is unclear, but sometimes it may be related to individual differences in the way people's metabolism works on the particular drugs they are taking (i.e. a pharmacokinetic explanation, see Chapter 2). The more fundamental reason for individual differences in responsiveness to drugs may be that the brain processes or mechanisms underlying related syndromes are possibly quite different, despite superficial similarities at the clinical level. The ways in which illness can be expressed may be restricted and may belie the diversity of the underlying mechanisms. Also of great importance are the patient's personality and previous experience of drug treatment. A history of prior responsiveness to a particular drug may help in predicting whether the same drug is likely to help now (Pare, 1985). However, the usefulness of such predictions is limited because response to drug treatment seems to vary both with the state of the illness and with the person's age. Unfortunately, there are no special tests or indicators to help us choose an effective drug. The choice of drug treatment still has some of the elements of a lottery, and whilst we may all congratulate ourselves when we hit the jackpot, we should not delude ourselves that this is a triumph of science.

Continuation and prophylactic drug treatment

Once medication has allowed symptoms of mental ill-health to be brought under control, the risk of relapse may be reduced by continuing treatment until the underlying (presumed biochemical) disturbance has settled down spontaneously. In general, the continuation phase of medication treatment will last for 4–12 months after symptoms have settled. Deciding exactly when the continuation phase of medication is over and when it is safe to start phasing out medication is largely a matter of guesswork, based on what knowledge exists about the natural history of the mental illness in question. The aim of maintenance treatment is to prevent a new episode of mental illness. In this context a new episode is called a 'recurrence'. In chronic conditions such as schizophrenia, where full recovery is uncommon, long-term drug treatment is really an extension of continuation therapy. To avoid confusion about the terms *continuation* and *maintenance* treatment, it may be best to stick to the term *prophylactic* treatment which applies to prevention of both relapses and recurrences of illness.

Severity and chronicity of mental ill-health and underlying physical disease as determinants of drug treatment

It is commonly found that the benefit resulting from drug treatment is correlated with the severity of the initial mental health disorder. Mild conditions tend to get better on their own, or with simple support and reassurance. In these situations, drug treatment may be no more or no less than a placebo. However, in some mild conditions, particularly those of long duration, the placebo response may be low, whereas the specific response to drug treatment may be clear-cut, although not necessarily marked in degree. In general, mental health conditions that have persisted for a long time usually reflect previous treatment failures, either because of inadequate doses or inappropriate medication, or because of adverse psychosocial factors, all of which may have contributed to a state of 'treatment refractoriness' which may then persist despite improved circumstances. Only when a mental health disorder has become chronic through neglect or omission of treatment is there likely to be good response when treatment is at last begun. Usually there is no alternative but to make a trial of treatment and see what happens, despite low expectations of a good outcome.

A moderate degree of symptom severity usually predicts a favourable outcome with drug treatment. Thus moderately severe forms of depressive illness tend to show a low placebo response and only protracted spontaneous recovery, and yet usually respond very well to drug treatment. Very severe forms of depression, in contrast, may respond poorly to antidepressant drugs, although the reasons for this are not clear. Since these conditions are often associated with extreme distress and risk to life due to self-neglect or suicide, the alternative effective and rapid-onset treatment, electroconvulsive therapy (ECT), may be invaluable (Avery and Winokur, 1977).

Medical or physical illnesses are often associated with mental health problems. If so, psychotherapeutic drugs can be just as helpful in these conditions as in cases where physical health is not impaired. However, sensitivity to drug treatment may be changed by the underlying physical disease. Psychiatric conditions due to clear-cut brain disease are often associated with oversensitivity to psychoactive drug effects, so great caution must be observed. In contrast, where a person is feeling and behaving 'as though' mentally ill (as seen in certain culture-bound syndromes or cases of hysteria), drug treatments may be surprisingly ineffective. In these situations, the symptoms appear to have a special symbolic meaning or purpose, even though the person may not be consciously aware of this. Trying to remove the symptoms with drug treatments may not only be ineffective because the wrong underlying mechanisms are being addressed, but also because consciously or unconsciously, the affected person may hang on to the symptoms until the real underlying causes are recognized and helped. This way of looking at symptoms, and the lack of response to drug treatment, is particularly important where people are identified as having severe hypochondriasis (abnormal preoccupation with bodily complaints or illness). For those unusual people with primary hypochondriasis, which may be intrinsic to their personality (see Chapter 10), their marked preoccupation with being ill often'seems to give their life meaning, and attempts to remove these so-called problems by drug treatment will only be resisted or undermined.

Drug dosages and duration of treatment

For most drugs it is advisable to start at a low dose and build up gradually towards an effective level. Side-effects are usually dose-related, and are most prominent early on in treatment, but tend to get better as the treatment is continued. Under steady state conditions, most people show a good therapeutic response to most drugs at dosage levels below those causing troublesome side-effects.

Predicting drug responsiveness

If a patient is eventually going to show a favourable response to a drug, in most cases some indication of this should be detectable early on in treatment, even though the full benefit of treatment is likely to take weeks or even months to build up. If no early sign of improvement is detected, it may mean that the initial dose was pitched too low, and the dosage should be cautiously increased. On the other hand, if an initial beneficial effect disappears with continuing treatment, and if this does not seem to be a reflection of a short-lived placebo response, then perhaps the dose was increased too rapidly, and a dose reduction should be considered before proceeding further.

   In the absence of any detectable early improvement in clinical state, or if there is a worsening in the patient's condition, it is unlikely that the eventual outcome will be favourable. In most situations, dogged perseverance with a drug that has shown no early benefit at all is probably a waste of time. However, there are always exceptions to this rule, particularly when considering persistent disorders that have proved resistant to other treatments. Perhaps the best example of this is treatment-resistant schizophrenia which may respond to the atypical antipsychotic drug clozapine, but sometimes only when treatment is persevered with for a year or more.

Drug dosage

With most drugs and with most patients, there are marked individual differences in how much drug is required for an optimal effect. The best dose for a given person can only be worked out by painstaking trial and error. As with adverse effects, most treatment failures with psycho-therapeutic drugs can be explained by pharmacokinetic rather than pharmacodynamic factors (see Chapter 2). Different people when given the same dose of a particular drug will show widely different concentra-tions of the drug in body fluids such as the blood, whilst in the brain, drug levels are likely to vary even more. This takes no account of the fact that even when exposed to the same concentration of drug, brain cells are likely to respond differently in different people. For these reasons, measuring the blood levels of a drug is rarely helpful. The only important exception to this is lithium, for which there is a well worked-out range of therapeutic blood levels, beyond which benefit is severely compromised by the onset of adverse effects.

For most drugs, the basic principle is to use doses that are just below those producing noticeable side-effects. This begs the question of whether we should give precedence to side-effects noticeable to the patient (subjective) over those noticeable to the clinician (objective). Some people seem to be exquisitely sensitive to some unpleasant side-effects of drugs, and even tiny doses of medication are objectionable to them. The situation is complicated by the fact that some drugs have different thera-peutic applications requiring a different range of doses for each applica-tion. The best example of this is seen with the SSRI drugs in which the dose-response 'ceiling' is lowest for conditions such as panic disorder, intermediate for depressive illness, and highest for obsessive-compulsive disorders and eating disorders. Interestingly, the usual clinical impres-sion is that in each of these three different applications, troublesome side-effects may come into play at doses just beyond the particular dose-response ceiling in each case. Thus people being treated for panic disorder with low doses of SSRIs usually experience troublesome adverse effects at low to medium doses, whereas patients being treated with high doses for obsessive-compulsive disorder can usually tolerate these intermediate doses without any adverse effects.

The question of what is the maximum safe dose for a drug often arises when dealing with treatment-refractory patients. There is probably never a simple answer to this question since the appearance of – and tolerance of – adverse and toxic drug effects is dependent on so many variables. Guidelines, provided for example by the *British National Formulary*, are not always clear or helpful, although increasingly prescribers are becoming very cautious about exceeding these advisory maximum dose limits, even when the scientific basis for such limits may be shaky. (The *British National Formulary* is published twice a year, and is sent to every practising doctor in the UK.) In deciding on maximum dose limits, there is often a confusion between what is safe and what is effective, and this is particularly seen with the antipsychotic drugs. In the *British National Formulary* it is suggested that some antipsychotic drugs can be used in exceedingly high doses which are likely to be far in excess of the maximum effective dose. The principal consideration here appears to be how far doses can be increased whilst still keeping within the bounds of reasonable safety. For other antipsychotic drugs, the advisory maximum doses relate more to the limits of what is considered effective for treating psychosis, and these doses are likely to be well below the upper limits of safety.

As with subacute drug treatment intended to bring symptoms of mental illness under control, the dosage of medication is also important for the success of prophylactic medication. Research has suggested that the maintenance dose of antidepressant medication is best kept at the level used to bring about the initial improvement in symptoms (Frank et al., 1990). In the past, doctors probably reduced the maintenance dose of antidepressants too far, thus undermining the protection against recurrences that medication might afford. In schizophrenia, there has been an opposite tendency, with a trend towards lower doses of antipsychotic medication for maintenance treatment. This is a reflection of a general trend towards the use of lower doses of antipsychotic drugs in the management of serious mental illnesses (Johnson, 1988).

Treatment refractoriness

Once an 'adequate' dose of a drug has been tried for a 'reasonable' period without therapeutic success, the next step is usually to try a different drug. It is often best to try a drug from a different chemical class. This is in case the first drug failed because the patient's metabolism dealt with it in a particular way which led to an unfavourable therapeutic response. Since drugs from the same chemical class are likely to be metabolized in a similar way by the same person, there is probably a high chance that another drug of the same chemical type will be ineffective likewise.

After trying two drugs without success, it is then probably worth trying some form of *augmentation treatment*. This means adding a different type of agent to the one that was ineffective, or only partially effective, on its own. Although the effectiveness of combined treatments may also sometimes have a pharmacokinetic explanation (e.g. one drug may increase or decrease the levels of the other drug in body fluids and thereby improve its effectiveness), for most well-established combination or augmentation therapies the mechanism appears to be pharmacodynamic: in other words, the effect of the combined treatments is qualitatively different from that achievable by either drug alone. Perhaps the best example is the use of lithium as an adjunct or booster to antidepressants and neuroleptics in refractory cases of depression and schizophrenia respectively (Cookson et al., 1993).

The third phase in dealing with refractory cases of mental disorder involves the use of more radical and possibly hazardous treatments; examples include ECT for affective disorders and clozapine for schizophrenia. However, this rather unsatisfactory situation is likely to improve as more is understood about the nature of drug refractoriness in different psychiatric disorders.

The fourth phase in this process may involve abandoning drug treatment altogether as part of a complete reconsideration of the whole basis for the person's problems. For example, a person with unremitting depression, resistant to all drug treatments, may benefit from focusing therapy on previously unconsidered marital difficulties; and a person who is labelled as schizophrenic may in fact be in the throes of a 'culture-bound' syndrome which masquerades as psychosis, but may improve when drug treatment is stopped and the appropriate healing or ritual attended to. Finally, if all else fails, it may be necessary to start again from the beginning, on the assumption that treatment responsiveness is likely to change over the course of an illness, and treatments that were ineffective at the start may now work.

Dissatisfaction and non-compliance with prescribed medication

Patients in general, and psychiatric patients in particular, are very likely not to take their medication as prescribed. Probably more than half the patients prescribed medication by psychiatrists will express dissatisfaction about and not co-operate with the treatment plan proposed by the prescribing doctor. Some doctors seem to find it difficult to come to terms with this, and may be reluctant to accept that the consumer should have at least as much say in treatment issues as the prescriber. Some doctors do not take enough account of the not unreasonable belief, held by many people, that drugs are as likely to do harm as bring benefit. Doctors prescribing medication often fail to convince the patient that the treatment is worthwhile and necessary. It is an unfortunate fact that some psychiatrists appear to take a perfunctory view of people's personal difficulties before prescribing medication. This will not inspire confidence that the doctor really understands the nature of the problem from the patient's point of view. Interestingly, it may not always be necessary for the patient to agree with the prescriber about the cause of the problem in order to ensure good co-operation with taking medication. On the other hand, people with 'full insight' into the nature of their psychological problems may not necessarily be reliable in taking medication. The prescriber's ability to convince the patient of their concern and goodwill and their receptiveness to the patient's point of view, without necessarily sharing it, seems to be the most important consideration here.

As well as rejecting the prescription of a particular medication, patients may sometimes insist on other treatments, for example other drugs, psychotherapy or 'alternative' medicine such as hypnotherapy or acupuncture. Sometimes a battle of wills ensues, and the prescriber may lose sight of what the patient is objecting to about their prescription. Of the many possible factors involved, perhaps the most important is that the person may have had previous unfavourable experiences of drug treatment, either due to unpleasant side-effects, or because there was no apparent benefit from treatment. Some of the most objectionable side-effects of medication are the least well understood and appreciated by doctors. Examples include physical restlessness (akathisia) and a subjectively unpleasant state of mood (dysphoria) associated with antipsychotic neuroleptic drugs; tremulousness and sexual dysfunction, which occur with some antidepressants; and weight gain, which is a side-effect of many psychiatric medications. There is a case to be made for doctors having to 'taste their own medicine' at some stage in their career in order to sharpen their appreciation of the so-called 'harmless' but highly undesirable side-effects of the medications that they prescribe. After all, if these side-effects really are harmless, why should not doctors experience them, if this is likely to make them more sensitive and understanding prescribers?

Whether people will accept and take their medication is also influenced by their personality traits. There are many ways of defining and classifying personality, and when personality traits are extreme and cause problems to the individual or to others, they are usually regarded as 'disorders' by the psychiatric profession (see Chapter 10). *Antisocial* and *dependent* personality traits tend to lead to overuse or misuse of certain mind-altering drugs, whereas *withdrawn* and *inhibited* personalities tend to reject or be intolerant of prescribed medication. The antisocial personality is often impulsive, easily bored, and prone to sensation-seeking; such people have the propensity to overuse any mind-altering drug for 'kicks'. If overuse or abuse of medication is prolonged, it may produce physical dependence or addiction, or occasionally cause serious mental state changes (for example the paranoid psychosis that sometimes occurs in amphetamine addicts). A dependent personality is timid and anxious, and may easily become addicted to sedative-anxiolytic drugs like the benzodiazepines. Although such people may not take more than the prescribed amount, they are likely to be resistant to any change in their medication, especially attempts to reduce it or discontinue it altogether. Problems in discontinuing these drugs will be exacerbated if there are withdrawal effects due to physical dependence, because people with dependent personalities are much more likely to be distressed by these withdrawal effects and will soon give up the attempt to phase out their medication. For all these reasons, it is often best to avoid prescribing mind-altering drugs to people with antisocial and dependent personality traits, unless it is absolutely essential.

Withdrawn (paranoid) and *inhibited* (obsessional and hypochondriacal) personalities are in contrast resistant to the idea of starting drug treatment. Paranoid patients may be particularly sensitive to the feeling that they are being fobbed off, or not taken seriously, by the offer of drug treatment. In more extreme situations, the offer of drug treatment may be experienced as something intrusive and threatening, especially if the medication is to be administered by injection. A person with this kind of personality may find any offer of help threatening, if it obliges them to acknowledge and accept their need and vulnerability. People with withdrawn, hypochondriacal or depressive personality traits may resist offers of treatment which are aimed at 'curing' them, because despite appearances, this would threaten to reduce or eliminate the very things (their problems and complaints) which may give their life a richer meaning, and which provide a means to rewarding contact and communication with professional helpers.

Irrespective of the person's personality trait, there are other factors related to the nature of drug treatment that may undermine a person's willingness or ability to co-operate with it. A long delay before full benefit of medication is felt by the patient is a common experience, and this may very often shake people's confidence in the treatment, especially if side-effects are troublesome at an early stage. It is a great help if mental health carers involved in the prescribing contract are able to see the patient frequently in order to offer support and encouragement. This is particularly important because in many conditions such as depressive illness an objective improvement may occur before the person receiving the medication notices any change for the better. A trusted mental health carer may notice the improvement first and be able to convince the patient that progress is being made, and that this will soon be felt by them as well. A similar degree of trust is required in order to convince people of the need to continue with medication long after their symptoms and complaints have settled. It is a common and not unreasonable assumption that when you are feeling well, there is no need for medication. People are very likely to need full and careful explanations of why prophylactic treatment is advisable in order for them to stay well, if there is to be even a reasonable chance that they will comply with medication in the long term.

Prescribing combinations of drugs

Regardless of people's personality, side-effects of medication, or the phase of treatment, complicated drug plans reduce the reliability of drug consumption. 'More drugs means less compliance' should be a motto for all drugs prescribed in community settings. For this reason, every effort should be made to keep the number of different drugs and the frequency of administration to a minimum. Not every symptom has to be treated, and usually the best strategy is to focus on drug treatment of the major mental health syndrome that is troubling the patient. It is usually advisable to choose only well-established medications, and to keep to a maximum of three mind-altering drugs except under exceptional circumstances.

However, there are sometimes good reasons for prescribing a patient several drugs from different groups or chemical classes of medication. For example, there may be more than one major mental health disorder or syndrome to treat, or a particular syndrome may already have failed to respond adequately to a single treatment applied as intensively and as expertly as possible. The use of two different classes of medication to treat the same condition (for example, antipsychotic neuroleptics combined with benzodiazepines in severe states of acute psychotic break-down) may allow the use of lower and better tolerated doses of each drug. This will better allow the benefits of both to be exploited, which may add up to more than the sum of their parts (therapeutic synergism). Most commonly of all, side-effects of the main therapeutic medication may require the use of another drug in order to give relief, assuming that withdrawing or reducing the dose of the main drug is not feasible

Drug treatment in clinical practice 55

because of fears of a relapse (Table 3.2). However, when combinations of drugs are used, there is always an increased risk of adverse effects due to interactions which may be worse than the side-effects for which the additional drug was prescribed. For this reason, the best strategy for dealing with adverse effects of medication is always dose reduction if and when possible.

Table 3.2 *Drug treatments for adverse side-effects of psychotherapeutic medication*

Psychotherapeutic medication	Side-effect	Remedial drug treatment
Neuroleptic	Parkinsonism	Anticholinergic (e.g. procyclidine)
	Akathisia	Beta-blocker (e.g. propranolol)
SSRI	Akathisia	Beta-blocker
	Anorgasmia	5-HT blocker (e.g. cyproheptadine)
Tricyclic antidepressant	Erectile impotence	Parasympathomimetic (e.g. bethanechol)
	Urinary retention	Parasympathomimetic
	Reduced libido	Anticholinesterase (e.g. neostigmine)
	Impaired ejaculation	Anticholinesterase
	Excess sweating	Alpha-1-blocker (e.g. terazocin)
Lithium	Tremor	Beta-blocker (e.g. propranolol)
	Polyuria (increased urine)	ADH sensitizer (e.g. carbamazepine)
	Hypothyroidism	Thyroxine
Carbamazepine	Leucopenia	Lithium (increases white cell count)
	Inappropriate ADH (low plasma sodium)	ADH desensitizer (e.g. lithium, demeclocycline) (causes diuresis)

ADH, antidiuretic hormone 5-HT, 5-hydroxytryptamine (serotonin) SSRI, selective serotonin reuptake inhibitor

There is rarely any rationale for prescribing together more than one drug from the same general class (e.g. two antidepressants or two antipsychotic drugs). This type of polypharmacy may be just as likely to produce adverse drug reactions, and is usually objected to on the grounds of waste or unnecessary complexity. It may also obscure the fact that the overall dose of a particular type of medication may exceed the recommended maximum. Prescribing at the same time two antipsychotic drugs at doses corresponding to 75% of the advisory maximum dose limit for each may obscure the fact that the patient is receiving a combination which is 50% over the maximum dose limit for that type of medication. However, sometimes patients may only be willing to accept a dose of medication which is thought to be suboptimal for a therapeutic effect. The addition of another similar drug may be acceptable to the patient, allowing the net equivalent dose to reach a therapeutic level. Sometimes a 'two-drugs strategy' needs to be adopted because troublesome side-effects with one drug have developed before an optimal dose has been reached. Supplementing the initial drug with another from the same general class, but with a different side-effect profile, may solve the problem.

A particular reason for avoiding 'same class' polypharmacy has arisen with the introduction of atypical antipsychotic drugs such as clozapine and risperidone. The clinical advantages of these drugs appear to result from the fact that they have a particular combination or profile of effects on different symptoms in the brain (see Chapter 6). The addition of another conventional or typical antipsychotic drug is likely to obscure or obliterate the precise profile of pharmacological effects on which the atypical drugs' special clinical advantages crucially depend.

Perhaps the most common example of the use of two drugs from the same general class is when oral and depot antipsychotic drugs are prescribed together. This can often be justified early on in treatment, or for dealing with short-term exacerbations of a long-term illness, since the oral component of medication can easily be changed and adjusted to suit the patient's fluctuating mental state. Once the situation has settled down, the medication is best switched to either all oral or all depot, and the long-term use of an oral-depot combination is often a reflection of sloppy prescribing. However, it may also reflect the fact that the patient is reluctant to switch to more sensible 'monodrug' therapy, because they have confidence in the combination that made them well, and do not wish to change.

Sometimes a person taking prescribed medication will claim that an oral antipsychotic drug has special properties which cannot be matched by a depot injection. There may appear to be little pharmacological rationale to support their argument, although it is sometimes difficult to be sure of this. However, more often than not the patient receiving the medication likes to have some of their antipsychotic drug quota in a form that will allow them to adjust their intake according to their own rules and choices, even though they may be reluctant to admit this to the prescriber.

Thus, although polypharmacy is often regarded as a mark of poor prescribing, this is not always the case. On the contrary, if at all possible, and provided abuse and dependence can be avoided, it is much better to give the patients (the consumers) what they want and prefer, even if this does not conform to strict rules of logic and scientific nicety. Prescribing potentially hazardous drug combinations is another matter, and it may be better to prescribe no drugs at all rather than risk a compromise involving a drug combination that could prove a danger to the patient.

Rational prescribing

As an illustration of the contrast between sloppy (some might say soppy) prescribing and sensible, well-considered schedules of medication, take the example of two alternative drug prescriptions for a 60-year-old man suffering from a severe depressive illness. He feels 'irrationally' guilty and pessimistic, and complains of severe insomnia, anxiety and agitation. He also has mild urinary symptoms due to an enlarged prostate gland.

It is decided that the patient would benefit from a tricyclic anti-depressant drug in full dosage and a relatively low dose of a major tranquillizing drug to provide extra help for his agitation and anxiety.

Prescription 1

- dothiepin
    two 25 mg capsules in the morning
    one 75 mg tablet in the evening
- thioridazine
    one 10 mg tablet in the morning
    one 25 mg tablet at bedtime
- haloperidol
    four 0.5 mg capsules three times daily
- procyclidine
    one 5 mg tablet three times daily

This prescription is much too complicated, involves unnecessary 'divided doses' and includes inappropriate medications and 'same-class polypharmacy'. Dothiepin, a long-acting sedative tricyclic antidepressant, could be given in a single dose at night, which would also help insomnia, but it may not be the best choice of tricyclic antidepressant because its anticholinergic effects are likely to exacerbate the patient's urinary problems.

Two major tranquillizers (thioridazine and haloperidol) are used when one would suffice, and at such low doses, the addition of procyclidine, an anticholinergic drug, is not likely to be necessary to counteract parkinsonian side-effects. In any case, the combined anticholinergic effects of dothiepin and procyclidine are likely to cause significant urinary problems (e.g. urinary retention) and may even precipitate mental confusion in an elderly person owing to a toxic effect on the brain.

Prescription 2

- lofepramine
    one 70 mg tablet morning and evening
- thioridazine
    one 100 mg tablet at bedtime

The greater simplicity of this prescription is obvious, and the patient is therefore much more likely to take it reliably. Although lofepramine is a short-acting, relatively non-sedative tricyclic antidepressant, it has fewer side-effects than dothiepin, and insomnia should improve within days as the depressive illness starts to be successfully treated. Thioridazine does have sedative and anxiolytic properties, can be given as a single night-time dose with major tranquillizing effects lasting a full 24 hours, and is unlikely to cause extrapyramidal (parkinsonian) side-effects at this dose.

Psychotherapy and subacute drug treatment for mental health disorders

Although the relief of symptoms and encouraging the illness to go into remission are the main aims of subacute drug treatment, it is hoped (and usually found) that there are additional benefits for the person's ability to cope and function in their everyday life. This is important because social functioning is usually, if not invariably, impaired in most psychiatric disorders for which drug treatment is considered.

Research has shown that psychological and social treatment can produce definite and measurable benefits in psychiatric disorders. This applies not only to conditions such as depression and anxiety, but also to serious mental illnesses such as schizophrenia (e.g. Kingdon et al., 1994). To make a rather obvious generalization, whereas drug treatments have most beneficial effect in reducing symptoms of mental illness, psychotherapy and social treatments have more impact in improving problems in social functioning and interpersonal relationships.

Psychosocial treatments therefore appear to be especially indicated where the severity of mental health symptoms is mild, but where personal or psychosocial problems are marked. Under these circumstances, treatment with powerful psychoactive drugs may benefit the patient merely through a placebo effect, whereas psychotherapy may achieve at least this, and often much more. The question of whether particular types of psychotherapy have a specific effect above and beyond the non-specific benefit of a caring therapeutic relationship is a complex one. Most people would agree that the relationship and alliance between patient and therapist, which is fundamental to many forms of psychotherapy, is equally if not more important than any specific component of treatment, at least in relatively mild disorders.

These generalizations have been demonstrated by an impressive amount of research. For example, one large multicentre study carried out by the National Institute of Mental Health in the USA compared supportive management and medication with placebo with two forms of focused psychotherapy and with antidepressant drug treatment in patients with major depressive illness. All treatments were approximately equally effective over the period of study when *mildly ill* people were assessed; however, with *more severely ill* patients, drug treatment was clearly superior to either form of psychotherapy and to placebo (Elkin et al., 1989). The psychotherapies used (interpersonal therapy and cognitive behavioural therapy) were only a little better than placebo in these severely ill patients, and again there were no differences in effectiveness between the two types of psychotherapy.

The question of whether it is a good idea to combine drug treatment with psychotherapy has often been asked in the past, but it is only recently that studies have looked at this question in any detail. The potential objections to a combined approach can be viewed from two polarized perspectives. Firstly, does drug treatment undermine the benefits of psychotherapy? This may happen if there are negative attitudes and expectations towards drug treatment on the part of the patient and sometimes of the mental health worker or therapist as well. For example, either the patient or the mental health worker (or both) may feel that to prescribe medication is equivalent to labelling the person as a 'biological deviant'. Also, by relieving symptoms of mental stress 'artificially', drugs may be thought to reduce motivation for more difficult, but more enduring psychological change. By 'sweeping symptoms under the carpet' by using drugs, it may be argued that psychotherapy may become more difficult or impossible.

The second and contrasting perspective is that psychotherapy may undermine drug treatment. It may be argued that psychotherapy is a waste of time in the context of drug treatment, or worse, that stress related to psychological treatment may cause the patient to drop out of treatment altogether, or interfere in other ways with the beneficial response to drug treatment.

However, in all the studies that have taken place since the 1980s, there has been little or no evidence for any negative interaction between drug treatment and psychotherapy. This is not to say that negative interactions can never occur under some circumstances. Perhaps the most likely example of a possible negative interaction between drug and psychological treatment is where benzodiazepines are given to patients undergoing cognitive behavioural therapy for phobic disorders such as agoraphobia. If anxiety is banished prematurely, albeit temporarily, by anxiolytic drugs, this may preclude the experience of relief of anxiety which comes when exposure to the feared situation is successfully weathered. As a result, drug treatment may interfere with the successful resolution of the problem through psychological treatment.

In mild psychological disorders, psychotherapy alone may be highly effective, and drug treatment relatively ineffective, so combining both treatments may confer little additional advantage. On the other hand, in severe psychological disorders, especially those that constitute major mental illnesses or psychoses, drug treatment may be more effective than psychotherapy, but again with no additional benefits from the combined treatment. In situations where both forms of treatment are less than optimal, for whatever reason, combining the two is often likely to confer an additional advantage (Falloon and Fadden, 1993). Some of this combined advantage comes from better compliance with medication in patients who are also being supported and helped in ways which perhaps they find more relevant to their own perception of their problems. Conversely, drug treatment may be more effective against symptoms such as insomnia or anorexia, which may particularly trouble the patient and distract them from attempts to help them with other, more psychological, approaches.

Placebo and nocebo effects

It is not enough for the prescriber and other mental health team workers to agree on appropriate indications for medication, even when this has been part of a comprehensive assessment of someone's problems, including their personality and previous experiences. It is also crucial to agree on the terms and conditions of the treatment to be undertaken, or in other words to make a contract with the patient which is sometimes called a therapeutic alliance. This is just as important in prescribing and administrating medication as it is in psychotherapy, or for that matter in any business transaction. In all cases, the patient or client must have confidence in the therapist and in the treatment on offer before being willing to 'sign on the dotted line' in order for therapy to proceed. As any salesman knows, the first step in winning the trust and contract of an apprehensive and doubtful client is to bolster firstly their self-esteem, and secondly their confidence in a decision to accept the treatment on offer. Even if this is impossible, at the very least, the mental health prescriber must ensure that the patient's doubts do not polarize into strong negative attitudes towards treatment. The risk of this is greatest if the patient already feels that in coming for help they have somehow failed to deal properly with their difficulties and have lost something of their self-respect and individuality. An offer of drug treatment may feel to them like being coerced into a frightening 'Dr Frankenstein' type of scientific experiment. Alternatively, people who admit that they feel ill and unable to cope, may respond to the offer of drug treatment in an overanxious, child-like state of mind. This may result in their either being passively overcompliant in the expectation of a 'miracle cure', or reacting with procrastination and niggling objections to every detail of the proposed treatment plan.

Overcoming these negative attitudes to the drug treatment plan, and making the person feel as much at ease as possible with it, constitutes an important part of what is sometimes called a *placebo* ('I will please'). Conversely, increasing negative attitudes and expectations of treatment represents a *nocebo* ('I will harm') aspect of treatment which can take several forms (Tyrer, 1991). For example, unrealistic and therefore unfulfillable expectations of treatment may lead to disappointment and disillusionment with the prescriber or mental health professional involved. On the other hand, suggesting to the patient that they need drug treatment because they are too sick to help themselves, may increase their feelings of helplessness and overdependency, which could undermine their successful recovery. A particular form of nocebo effect is where a change in the presentation of a medication occurs without alteration of the active ingredient. This may be interpreted by the patient as a reduction in or withdrawal of medication that was previously benefiting them. Under the influence of this belief, patients may actually experience adverse 'withdrawal effects' which are clearly 'all in the mind', but no less troublesome for that (Tyrer *et al.*, 1983).

Case vignette 3.1

Beryl was 48 years old and had been taking diazepam (Valium) for 10 years. She had read newspaper reports about the dangers of dependence on Valium and became extremely concerned. She was only taking 5 mg daily but thought she ought to reduce as soon as possible. She consulted her general practitioner who helped her by prescribing her tablets in the 2 mg form so that she was able to reduce more slowly and easily. Unfortunately, whenever she reduced her dose by even half a tablet (1 mg) she experienced extreme anxiety and panic. This convinced her that she was dependent on the drug and she became even more alarmed. She was then seen by a psychiatrist to establish the degree of dependency. In fact it was far from clear that she was dependent on the drug. For example, she experienced her symptoms of panic only a few hours after reducing the dose of tablets, whereas one would have expected the withdrawal symptoms to have been delayed by at least a few days because the effects of diazepam are long-lasting. Beryl agreed to take part in an experiment in which she took 'active' 2 mg tablets of Valium on some occasions but on others these would be replaced by placebo tablets of identical appearance. A pharmacist was responsible for providing the tablets, and neither the psychiatrist nor Beryl knew which were which (i.e. the experiment was 'double-blind'). It was found that every time that Beryl received a new supply of tablets she experienced the same apparent withdrawal symptoms. This happened on six occasions, but on breaking the code, it was found that on three of these occasions the tablets had not been replaced by placebo but had continued in the same dosage as before. This demonstrated to Beryl that she was not having genuine withdrawal symptoms, but was clearly showing a 'nocebo' effect. This reassured her greatly, and in the next few months she was able to reduce her Valium without significant problems. One year later she remains without any medication and is virtually symptom-free.

Judging how best to work with the patient, and how to enhance the placebo component of the medication and other forms of treatment, depends on a careful assessment of the patient as a person, including not only their current mental state, but also their personality, past experiences, and social and cultural background. This may take time and trouble, but it always pays dividends, because ultimately the factors that lead to a favourable placebo response will also enhance the benefits of active medication.

What may be a good formula for a therapeutic alliance and a favourable placebo response in one patient may not apply to another person. For example, taking care to probe deeply into a person's past and present difficulties, and underplaying the role of mental illness in these, may make some people feel that they are being understood sympathetically and taken seriously, whereas in others, the same approach may cause much distress and increase feelings of guilt and inadequacy for a state of helplessness which they are unable to change. It is necessary to try to predict and understand the patient's reaction and point of view, and as far as possible, to share these feelings (empathize) so long as this does not undermine the very basis of the drug treatment that is proposed. For example, agreeing with a paranoid patient that the medicine they are to be given is poisonous is unlikely to be helpful!

Although every patient will require an individually tailored approach, there are several basic strategies to enhance the placebo response of treatment. It is usually helpful to frame the person's distress in terms of an illness or 'nervous breakdown', whatever the actual diagnosis or the person's own perception of the causes and events leading up to their problems. For many distressed people, confirmation that they are 'ill' confers status and meaning to what can otherwise appear a disadvantaged and humiliating position. At the same time, frightening experiences can be brought into the realm of the everyday and familiar, so reassuring people who feel alienated by their mental state that their experiences are in fact due to an illness that is known about and understood. If time and trouble is taken to explain how and why medication may help, this will not only be reassuring, but it will also help to ensure compliance with treatment and contribute to its success. It pays to be frank in telling the patient that it is not known how medication which is being prescribed works exactly, other than to suggest perhaps that it compensates for 'chemical imbalances' in the nervous system which, directly or indirectly, are contributing to their distress. Sometimes it may be helpful to focus more on particular symptoms that are troubling the person, e.g. insomnia, as this may make it easier for them to accept the idea that an illness is the cause of their difficulties. Although the person is being offered a 'sick role', it should be stressed that this is likely to be only a temporary state of affairs, and that once treatment has got under way, patients will want and be able to do more to help themselves.

In the same way that it is often helpful to stress to people that their symptoms and experiences are well understood and not at all 'freakish', so it can be more reassuring than alarming to mention expected side-effects of medication, and to point out that in the early stages of treatment, these may be more noticeable than the therapeutic effect which can be delayed by days or weeks. This frankness will help people to have confidence in the prescriber's experience and expertise with treatment.

As well as advising about the likely delay in benefit from medication, it is usually a good strategy to warn people in advance that sometimes treatments prove unsuitable or ineffective, and because everybody is different, finding what is right for them may take time. It pays to be honest about the empirical nature of drug treatment in mental health problems, whilst at the same time emphasizing that there are many treatment choices available which are tested and safe, one of which will no doubt be right for them.

For people who feel threatened by the idea of ingesting a powerful foreign substance (which after all is a good definition of a drug), it may be helpful for the first tablet or injection to be taken in the presence of a trusted mental health worker who may also be the prescriber or the patient's key worker. In this way the person's reaction to the medication can be monitored carefully over a few hours, and if necessary, checked against objective tests, for example pulse and blood pressure. Witnessing the patient go through any subjective reaction and taking it seriously is likely to greatly improve mutual credibility and understanding.

Alternatives to long-term medication

Since benefits from long-term drug treatment do not seem to outlast its administration, this implies that for maximum protection against recurrences and relapses of illness, drug treatment may have to be continued indefinitely. However, for people who have had only one or perhaps two episodes of serious illness, it is usually worth the risk of gradually reducing and stopping prophylactic medication at some stage in an attempt to discover whether long-term treatment is really necessary. Unfortunately there are no reliable ways of predicting the outcome of this, although clinical experience has shown that people who are still experiencing low-grade symptoms of their mental illness while still on medication are most likely to get worse when the medication is reduced and stopped. Thus for people who have recovered from an episode of severe depression, a slight but definite awareness of reduced vitality and interest in life, or persistent, albeit mild, sleep disturbance, may indicate that the outcome of stopping prophylactic medication would be unfavourable.

If people are set against carrying on with full-dose prophylactic medication indefinitely, it is usually worth recommending a compromise position of lowering the dose of maintenance medication, even though this may not afford full protection against recurrences or relapses of illness. With suboptimal prophylactic drug treatment, the risk of further illness is likely to be less than with no medication at all, and any recurrences or relapses of illness are likely to be less severe while some medication is being taken, compared with none at all.

Nonetheless, many people are very discouraged by the prospect of long-term medication, and there is usually a strong incentive to come up with other forms of help which will reduce people's risk of further episodes of illness. This is an important area of research and clinical study, which has already had a major impact on the long-term management of a number of psychiatric conditions. Thus the likelihood of relapse may be greatly reduced by psychosocial therapies aimed at reducing the levels of 'expressed emotion' in the domestic environment of people who have suffered a schizophrenic breakdown (Kuipers et al., 1992). The impact of these non-medication approaches can be as great as medication itself, and what is more, medication and psychosocial therapy appear to have additive effects, each boosting and benefiting the other. In mood disorders, cognitive behavioural techniques are not only useful in bringing acute symptoms of mental illness under control but may also be helpful in preventing further episodes (Clark, 1990). Cognitive behavioural techniques can be applied by patients themselves as part of a self-help strategy which they can use at the earliest stages of a threatened relapse of illness. For conditions such as obsessive-compulsive disorder which tend to be chronic in nature, patients themselves can deliver their own 'maintenance psychotherapy', perhaps with occasional refresher courses in therapy from a professional mental health worker.

Thus, as with subacute drug treatment for mental health problems, combining drug treatment with psychotherapy or other psychosocial help appears to be the best strategy initially. In this way symptom control can be consolidated, allowing the affected person a breathing space for psychological treatments and coping mechanisms to be learned and practised effectively. Subsequently, drug treatment may be withdrawn if long-term maintenance medication is unacceptable or undesirable for whatever reason, allowing the psychological treatments and techniques to work alone. In this way, drugs may be seen as part of a combined strategy, but with the emphasis on short-term use for many people. At the same time it is important to encourage the motivation and commitment to take part and complete psychological treatment programmes.

Treatment discontinuation and withdrawal effects

Where people have their hearts and minds set against continuing drug treatment, it is nearly always best to try to accommodate their wishes and work with them to set up the best alternative management strategies. Of course, if it is considered that stopping medication may lead to serious mental deterioration and possible harm to the person or others, every effort should be made to keep the drug treatment going. Thinking about and discussing the possible discontinuation of treatment should probably begin from the outset of treatment, and if at all possible, the patient should be given some idea of the likely duration of treatment. This may be as vague as 'for the foreseeable future' with drugs such as antipsychotic maintenance medication, or as definite as 'two weeks or less' with anxiolytic benzodiazepines. It is ironic that the people who most need to continue with medication are the ones who usually press most strongly for a trial of discontinuation. In contrast, pressure for the phasing out of 'addictive' drugs such as benzodiazepines usually comes from the prescriber who perceives a negative risk/benefit balance for the patient with continued treatment.

The key to any medication withdrawal programme is gradual dose reduction combined with careful control and monitoring. For most drugs, and most people, the slower and more flexible the withdrawal process the better. If the patient is taking short-acting drugs, it may help to switch to longer-acting medications which are less likely to produce noticeable and possibly distressing withdrawal symptoms. Thus in the case of benzodiazepine withdrawal, it is usually best to switch to diazepam which is a very long-acting drug.

Withdrawal syndromes have been described for all the major classes of drugs used in mental health treatment, and sometimes it is difficult to distinguish the features of these withdrawal symptoms from a recurrence of the original disorder for which medication was prescribed. However, if the withdrawal syndrome has clinical features that are qualitatively different from those associated with the original condition, it can reasonably be considered to be a valid withdrawal phenomenon rather than a simple recurrence of the original condition.

Assessing the effectiveness of drug treatment

For the individual patient, it is usually difficult to be certain how helpful drug treatment is or has been. Drug treatment is invariably only one part of a more-or-less comprehensive package of care, so the relative contribution of each component of treatment is difficult or impossible to tease out. With medication, there is the option of being able to withdraw the treatment in order to assess how well the patient can do without it; however, this does not strictly provide evidence for its previous effectiveness, but is only a test of whether medication is still required. The withdrawal of effective medication will only result in a rapid return of symptoms if the underlying drug-sensitive processes are still operative. Since one of the theoretical functions of medication is to help such processes resolve spontaneously, the failure of symptoms to reappear when medication is withdrawn does not mean that the medication had no beneficial effect at some earlier stage of treatment.

Clinical trials

The only reliable way of building up knowledge about effectiveness of medications used for mental health problems comes from conducting controlled clinical trials. This involves a careful selection of volunteers who are suffering from the mental condition under study, as defined by applying various rules and guidelines for identification and diagnosis. Although it is important to define the condition to be treated as reliably as possible, it is also important to scientifically test treatments against conditions that are likely to be seen in everyday practice. This will usually entail a fairly broad definition of the type and severity of mental health problem to be subjected to tests in a clinical trial. However, it is usually important to exclude from the clinical trial people who might not be considered for treatment in the ordinary way of things. For example, people with mild or very severe forms of the disorder in question might be excluded on the grounds that their specific response to treatment is likely to be low. Similarly, people with coexisting physical ill-health or other psychiatric problems might not be eligible for a clinical trial, if under normal circumstances, these other conditions would make treatment with the medication in question difficult, complicated or hazardous.

To establish that medications are effective, it is important to take account of the fact that spontaneous improvement can occur, and that wishful thinking on the part of the patients or the observers can have a powerful effect on the outcome. These problems are overcome by participants in the trial being assigned at random either to treatment with the medication under consideration, or to treatment with a placebo, which all parties should be unable to distinguish from the real thing.

Although placebo-controlled trials are obligatory at some stage in the assessment of new medications, once effectiveness has been proved it is often difficult to justify further placebo-controlled trials, because withholding active treatment may be regarded as unethical. The trouble is that although the treatment has been shown to be effective in one clinical trial involving, say, a small group of patients in a particular context, it may not be possible to generalize the findings to other situations which are superficially similar. An alternative approach is to compare a new treatment with a standard treatment which is already well established. This will allow all participants in the clinical trial to receive active treatment. However, if the condition under study has the potential to improve spontaneously, or if there is doubt about the effectiveness of the standard treatment in this particular context, showing that the new treatment is similar to the established treatment is not necessarily a demonstration of its effectiveness. Furthermore, when two treatments of similar effectiveness are compared, unless very large numbers of subjects are used in the trial, failure to find a statistically significant difference between the treatments does not necessarily prove that they are the same ('absence of proof is not proof of absence'). Small but clinically important differences between a new and a standard treatment may be easily missed, or conversely, the new treatment may be erroneously judged to be as good as the standard, when in this particular setting, the standard treatment would have had no advantage over a placebo.

The complexities of clinical trials have to be faced for new medications that are being introduced by the pharmaceutical companies. However, medications that have been available for years have not usually been subjected to the same rigorous testing. This means that the established treatments may not be as well established as we think. Once again, we have to consider whether results can be generalized from one situation to another. Just because a treatment is known to work in one setting, it cannot be assumed to work in another situation that may be superficially similar. In one respect, however, older treatments do have an advantage. Medications that have been around for many years will have a 'track record' regarding their adverse effects. This is a great advantage even though their safety profiles may be relatively unfavourable. If a newly developed medication proved to have some of the known drawbacks of some older drugs, it might well be kept off the market. Take the example of aspirin, which has many potentially serious adverse effects, but is freely available with few restrictions on its use: if aspirin were introduced on the market today, almost certainly it would become a 'prescription-only medication', with carefully laid down rules about how and when it should be prescribed.

Nonetheless, knowing about the potential adverse effects of medications is tremendously important for assessing the risks and benefits of treatment, and this is certainly the area where the largest question marks hang over new treatments. With some rare, but potentially serious, adverse effects of medication, there may be a lag of several years before these effects become clearly associated with the drug in question. There have been quite a few examples of apparently safe drugs later being shown to have rare but potentially catastrophic adverse effects associated with them. For this reason, many doctors are cautious about prescribing new drugs until they have been available for a number of years. Obviously some risks have to be taken, because unless promising new treatments are prescribed to sufficient patients, potential problems will never emerge.

Once it is established that a new treatment has significant advantages over previously available treatments, it makes sense to prescribe the medication to all the patients who are likely to benefit from it. Only then can a track record of safety be established. For a new treatment where early clinical trials indicate only marginal benefits over better-established drugs, it is questionable whether the new treatment should be prescribed at all. Although the therapeutic advantages of a new drug may be definite, albeit marginal, there is always the risk of a dramatic and unexpected adverse effect emerging with time. If a newly introduced drug is not prescribed, it will soon fall by the wayside and be withdrawn by the manufacturer as an unprofitable item.

Conclusions

It has to be borne in mind that for most mental health conditions, even well-established psychotherapeutic drugs are likely to show little more than a 30% specific effect. Thus in conditions such as schizophrenia which if untreated have a poor outcome, the advantage of active and established medication over placebo or other general management strategies is rarely more than about 30%, however this is measured or assessed. To put it another way, for most mental health problems, a quarter or more of people fail to respond to whatever medication is tried, and of the remaining 75% who do respond, about a half would do quite well on placebo or some other non-drug treatment. This is not to say that the extra benefit conferred by medication may not be considerable, but it does mean that the benefits of medication have to be kept in perspective. Highly trained practitioners have a tendency to overvalue treatments in which they are expert, and this applies to psychiatrists as much as to any other therapists. This tendency has to be guarded against if it is not to cause problems within the multiprofessional mental health team. A healthy scepticism about one's own professional methods, provided this does not degenerate into cynicism or therapeutic nihilism, is likely to improve respect for other therapeutic disciplines and approaches. This will hopefully lead to better co-ordinated and more comprehensive treatment plans in which the patient or client receives the most appropriate and most acceptable treatment package for their particular problems. It should also help avoid the drawbacks of restrictive practices resulting from mental health professionals working in effective if not actual isolation.

Further reading

British National Formulary (revised twice yearly). London: BMA/Royal Pharmaceutical Society of Great Britain.

Cookson, J., Crammer, J. and Heine, B. (1993). *The Use of Drugs in Psychiatry*. London: Gaskell.

Lader, M. and Herrington, R. (1990). *Biological Treatments in Psychiatry*. Oxford University Press.

4

Drug treatment and multidisciplinary teamwork

'We don't need to know anything about the details of drug treatment. If a patient is receiving drug treatment we just call in a doctor and continue to deal with the other problems.'

'We try to do everything we can to avoid drug treatment. If this does not work we transfer the patient to the psychiatrist.'

'Drug treatment is the responsibility of the doctor and it is not for us to interfere with this.'

These are all statements that have been made to the authors at different times by members of teams who often refer to themselves proudly as 'multidisciplinary'. The reason for this is perhaps most clear from the third quotation. Only doctors (at present) are commonly allowed to prescribe drugs, although this is increasingly being challenged in many settings in which emergency treatment is necessary and in which there are established treatments to be given in response to the emergency. Nevertheless, the selection of drugs for treatment, the dose to be administered, planned duration of treatment and a full understanding of both the positive effects of drugs and their possible adverse effects (benefit/risk ratio) are part of the specialized training of the doctor and not of other disciplines in mental health. It is therefore to be expected that whenever drug treatment is contemplated the doctor will be called, will arrive quickly in a suit of shining impenetrable medical armour, and then depart, leaving others to deal with the less specialized (and some would say the more personal) forms of care.

This assumption begs several questions. Is a doctor an integral member of a multidisciplinary team? If not, why should he or she be excluded? If a doctor is included, to what extent should the doctor's skills and knowledge be available to all members of the team? If these skills are not made available, how will the team know whether drug treatment is indicated or, indeed, whether existing drug treatment should be continued?

It seems clear to us that unless a doctor is part of the multidisciplinary team then it cannot regard itself as being comprehensive in its mental health responsibilities – unless it has a clear remit for a population that would never take drug therapy. The quotations at the beginning of this chapter are out of date; they come from individuals who worked in teams which only provided community care oriented to the less severely ill. In such teams, drug treatments are given less often and the referral of a patient to a doctor for drug treatment is often construed as a sign of failure, best summarized as 'you were too ill to be helped by us; you will have to see the psychiatrist'. Most multidisciplinary teams benefit from having a psychiatrist involved, but only if attention is paid to the essential elements of team working (Onyett, 1992). A comprehensive service that takes all types of referral (Marriott *et al.*, 1993) also must have a doctor included.

If we accept that the doctor has to be a member of the multidisciplinary team (even if not always as fully active as other members), it follows that, as drug treatment is so common in psychiatry, all members of the team should have a working knowledge of the common drugs used in psychiatry. This should include an understanding of the classification of psychiatric disorders and the rationale behind drug treatment. If teams are not to become bogged down by controversy over the relative place of drug treatment for mental health disorders there also needs to be a common philosophy of care which applies to all forms of treatment. This does not mean that all practitioners are going to be equally skilled in giving all treatments. It merely means that a theoretical framework exists that allows each treatment an appropriate place, which a good multidisciplinary team can identify more or less consistently without excessive rancour and debate (Ovreteit, 1993).

Philosophy of drug treatment in community psychiatry

The six elements underpinning the philosophy of drug treatment are shown in Table 4.1. The same six elements are true of drug treatment in any setting, although they could be expressed differently in a hospital setting. It is worthwhile discussing each of these elements in more depth, as they are fundamental to our argument. They have already had an airing in Chapter 1 but can bear repetition.

Drug treatments used appropriately in psychiatry have a positive benefit/risk ratio. In other words, they help to relieve suffering rather

Table 4.1 *Philosophy of drug treatment in community psychiatry*

Effective drug treatment reduces distressing mental symptoms

Drug treatment requires no motivation beyond compliance

People with severe mental illness may only respond to drug treatment

Many mental illnesses have an organic component that can be helped by drug treatment

Drug treatments act rapidly

Drug treatment can be combined effectively with other types of treatment than create it. Drugs rarely cure; but when you come to think about it, few treatments in general medicine are curative either. Psychotropic drugs suppress unpleasant mental symptoms, sometimes entirely, often to a significant degree, and rarely by a trivial amount. If one could be confident that symptoms can be improved greatly by a treatment which has no special associated risks, then to deny the patient the benefit of that treatment would be at best unnecessarily puritanical and at worst inhumane. Of course there are always problems in treating mental health disorders, because patients are often not aware of the significance and seriousness of their symptoms when they have the most severe forms of mental illness such as schizophrenia and manic-depressive (bipolar affective) psychosis. However, it is usually obvious to all experienced mental health workers when such people require help. Nonetheless there is some argument in the borderline cases about the most appropriate way forward. The *first and essential point* is that effective treatment, whether it be drugs, counselling, in-depth psychotherapy or behaviour therapy, should be part of a multidisciplinary team's comprehensive treatment programme, specifically tailored to meet the needs of particular patients or clients. The important thing is not the mode of the treatment or treatments; it is whether there is evidence that the therapy is effective when given to the person with the problem in question.

The *second element*, that drug treatment requires no motivation from the patient beyond compliance, is often used as a criticism of drug treatment. If a patient is a passive recipient of treatment and plays no active role in its success then this may be alleged to be counterproductive. Again, this criticism comes from a mistaken premise. If the treatment is effective it does not matter if the patient is passive or active in its administration. Kidney surgeons do not ruminate for days because their patients have played no active part in receiving their kidney transplants.

The *third element* follows from the second. For a drug treatment to be effective it has to enter the body, and then ultimately reach the brain in most instances (a very few drug treatments affect mental states indirectly by working on the body tissues and organs). This may be perceived as a disadvantage, since many things can go wrong along the way. This does not mean the patient is totally uninvolved in treatment – one of the ways in which a community mental health team can be most effective is by improving compliance with treatment, so that an effective dose of medication is given for the right length of time. Sometimes when therapists boast that they are able to treat all their patients without the need for drug treatment, they disclose more about their clientele than about their clinical skills. It is perfectly possible to treat a wide range of disorders without drugs, but one of the major advances of psychiatry has been the introduction of effective drug treatments which have had an impact on the whole of therapy for mental illness. Sometimes, as mentioned in Chapters 1 and 2, the benefits of drug treatment can be overstated, and for a period in the 1950s and 1960s we were so seduced by the idea of 'wonder drugs' that we often lost our more critical faculties and expected too much of them; but even discounting this, we have now a number of valuable therapies that are particularly useful in the most severe forms of mental illness. Although there are arguments over the exact contribution of drug treatment in reducing the mental hospital population in the UK by over 70% since the 1950s, there is little doubt that the introduction of effective drug treatment has had a major impact on the most severe mental illnesses.

The *fourth element* is a pragmatic one; we give people treatments that are effective even though we do not always know how they work. One of the less cogent criticisms of drug treatment is that as doctors do not know how drugs work in mental illness, their readiness to give them so frequently to patients is irresponsible. 'We pour drugs, of which we know little, into people of whom we know less' is one of the antidrug slogans of the age. It is certainly true that the adverse effects of drugs are not all known and recognized immediately, and it may take many years to obtain a full profile of a drug that enables its place in therapy to be defined exactly. However, the detection of adverse effects has become much more sophisticated, and few drugs are now marketed without adequate checks on their safety. Of course, knowledge of safety is not the same as knowledge of mechanism of action; however, it would be excessively pedantic to delay the use of a treatment until its mechanism of action was completely understood. Aspirin has been available for over a century and only now are we beginning to understand exactly how it works in reducing pain and, more recently, in reducing the coagulability of the blood. We now have much greater knowledge of the changes that occur in the body during mental illness and which may be affected by drug treatment. These are discussed more fully in Chapter 2 and will not be repeated, but they provide a rational basis for most drug treatment of mental health disorders. Underlying the symptoms and disturbances described in Figure 1.2 are sometimes biochemical, anatomical, physiological and hormonal changes that may all justify drug treatment.

The *fifth element* of drug treatment is speed of action. An intravenous injection of a drug such as chlorpromazine or diazepam begins its therapeutic effect within seconds, and even the slowest-acting group of drugs, the antidepressants, normally begin to show benefit within the first 3 weeks of treatment. This is sometimes used as a criticism against drug treatment, but it is really its main advantage over other forms of treatment. Just as the orthopaedic surgeon will put a broken bone in plaster, so that repair and restitution can go on without interruption and allow the plaster to be removed several weeks later, drug treatment can be similarly used to effect speedy repairs while the more slowly paced natural processes of psychological repair are taking place.

The *sixth element* of drug treatment is its flexibility. It goes well with almost every other form of treatment. Drug and psychological treatments are not in conflict; it is only competitive therapists that have made them so. With rare exceptions, drug treatment combines extremely successfully with psychological, behavioural and other non-pharmacological treatments. All these treatments work in different ways, but the differences reinforce their therapeutic value and allow each to have its proper place (see Chapter 3).

One of the most important tasks of a multidisciplinary community team is to make sure that drugs are neither given excessive importance nor regarded as a 'last resort'. All members of the team can help in contributing to a proper balance in their discussions about the value of drug treatment with patients. If drug treatment is overemphasized there is a danger that far too much improvement is attributed to the drug treatment alone. This can lead to unnecessary dependence on the drug (which although mainly psychological at first, could easily become physical if treatment is prolonged). It can also limit the amount of independent initiative that the patient might otherwise show. On the other hand, if drug treatment is dismissed as irrelevant or unimportant it is likely to be taken inappropriately, and may be stopped prematurely. All members of the team must give the same message to the patient, otherwise the combination of drug and psychological treatment is unlikely to be followed correctly (Falloon and Fadden, 1993).

This process must be started early in management. There is a phenomenon described as the avoidance of cognitive dissonance which can be paraphrased as 'when a person makes a choice he or she will then find reasons to justify it subsequently'. Just as therapists will attempt to resolve any cognitive dissonance after they have chosen a course of treatment, patients will act likewise after they have accepted an offer of treatment. If the proper place of all the treatments likely to be given during the course of a problem is explained to the patient at the beginning of treatment, inappropriate cognitive dissonance is unlikely to develop. If a prescription for say, diazepam, is given with the clear instruction that it will not be represcribed after 2 weeks, the patient will hopefully obtain benefit from the drug while realizing throughout that the drug will not be renewed. This in itself is liable to make consumption of the drug more prudent. If it is then clear that another treatment is likely to take over after that time, the patient is prepared for it in advance, and will often adjust accordingly. On the other hand, if the patient is unprepared for these changes, stopping one drug and replacing it with another will create cognitive dissonance, and a possible adverse psychological reaction.

Diagnosis

Diagnosis in community mental health practice – and indeed in the world of the psychiatric patient – does not have a good name. For many years it was critically reworded as 'labelling', which implies that the process was devoid of any scientific merit and merely carried out for administrative reasons with the risk of stigmatizing the person so labelled. It is also an activity that has been linked to the 'disease model' discussed earlier, which is sometimes considered to be an out-dated approach for use in multiprofessional mental health teams.

In fact, diagnosis is another word for a system of classification and, whether we admit it to ourselves or not, we all classify to make our lives more ordered and organized. Classification is a system of order; nothing more, nothing less. There can be dozens of classifications depending on the use to which they are put, and a fundamental question to be asked for all classifications is, does this classification serve the purpose for which it is being used? For example, I classify the objects in my kitchen according to whether they are edible or not. The crockery goes in one cupboard, the cutlery in another and the food is further separated (tinned food, perishables, spices, etc.) into other compartments. The placing of these compartments depends on how frequently they are used and whether two or more groups are commonly used together. Although there are bound to be individual ways in which kitchens are organized, there are common characteristics also. Food is not normally mixed indiscriminately with crockery, cutlery is normally stored together, frequently used items such as cups and plates are normally in readily accessible places. Dishwashers and draining boards are also so designed so that cutlery, crockery and cups are placed in different positions.

It is worthwhile comparing a kitchen classification with a mental health classification to illustrate their similarities (Table 4.2). The first stage of classification is to separate the major conditions. In the case of diseases, mental disorders have to be separated from other disorders, mainly physical ones. There is a special section in the International Classification of Disease (ICD-10) for mental disorders (World Health Organization, 1992). Similarly, in the kitchen it is reasonable to separate food in its many forms from items of equipment used in preparing food. Table 4.2 therefore illustrates the second phase of classification, items of equipment in the kitchen and psychiatric disorders in ICD-10.

Because there are so many individual groups it is important at first to establish a major classification to allow all the individual elements to be grouped together. Thus crockery, pans, cutlery, bakery and cookware, storage items and special utensils are all used as the major groups in the kitchen, and organic conditions, substance abuse, schizophrenia, mood, neurotic and personality disorders are major groupings in ICD-10. The individual categories within each group are also listed; each has a common characteristic that gives it membership of the main group but also some individual differences that allow it to be classified separately. The process of subclassification can continue. For example, spoons could be classified together as one category or subclassified into table, tea, soup, dessert or fruit spoons.

In the kitchen, the tendency would be to put most of the main groups in the same part of the kitchen; similarly, each of the individual psychiatric disorders are normally kept together with their main group. A good classification separates the conditions cleanly from each other, an activity nicely summarized as 'carving nature at its joints'. Such a classification brooks no argument; there is no difficulty in allocating every item to the groups concerned and no argument over this allocation subsequently. In the kitchen it is difficult to mistake crockery for cutlery, and any new items of equipment within these categories would automatically be classified appropriately. In mental health classifications there is much more overlap and the same applies with some items of kitchen equipment. This overlap can be resolved in two ways; either there are strict rules which

Table 4.2 A comparison of kitchen and (ICD-10) classifications

Main classification	Group 1		Group 2		Group 3		Group 4		Group 5		Group 6	
Sub-classification	Kitchen Crockery	ICD-10 Organic disorder	Kitchen Pans	ICD-10 Substance abuse	Kitchen Cutlery	ICD-10 Schizophrenias	Kitchen Bakery and Cookware	ICD-10 Mood disorders	Kitchen Storage Items	ICD-10 Neurotic and stress related disorders	Kitchen Special utensil	ICD-10 Personality disorders
Individual members	Plate Bowls Cups Saucers Gravy boats Teapots	Alzheimer's dementia Vascular dementia Delirium Other organic mental disorders	Saucepans Frying pans Lids Poachers Steamers Wok	Alcohol Opioids Sedative/hypnotics Cocaine Solvents	Knives Forks Spoons Teaspoons	Schizophrenia Schizotypal disorder Acute psychotic disorder Schizoaffective disorder	Food mixers Casserole dishes Baking trays	Depressive and manic episodes Bipolar affective disorder Recurrent depressive disorder Persistent mood disorder	Jars Plastic containers Freezer bags Storage bowls	Phobias Panic Generalized anxiety disorder Obsessive compulsive disorder Adjustment disorder Conversion disorder Somatoform disorder	Fish slice Egg whisk Melon corer Potato peeler Cherry stoner Cheese grater Egg slicer	Paranoid Schizoid Dissocial Unstable Histrionic Anankastic Anxious Dependent Habit/impulsive Gender identity

make it clear to which main category the new items should be allocated or, if the problem occurs repeatedly, a new classification system can emerge which better fits the items needing to be classified.

Often one item may be classified in one category but have common associations with another one, and this leads to arguments about where the item belongs. Thus the humble potato peeler is classified under special utensils and kitchen equipment because it is specially made for one major task, that of peeling potatoes (and also other foods with skins such as carrots and kiwi fruits). However, it could also be regarded as an item of cutlery in group 3, and indeed in many households the potato peeler will be found nestling with other items of cutlery. The rules for allocating potato peelers could therefore be adjusted to allow them to be placed in group 3 (cutlery classification) by grouping them together with knives (e.g. in an appropriate definition all manually operated instruments for cutting food in any form will henceforth be called cutting utensils and classified in the cutlery section). However, this may lead to argument when the cherry stoner is being classified. The cherry stoner acts by squeezing the stone out of a cherry but in doing so cuts through the skin. Should the cherry stoner stay in group 6 or be moved to group 3? (The equivalent dilemma in psychiatry often leads to a series of international conferences before resolution.)

These are the arguments that preoccupy psychiatric classification and sometimes appear unnecessarily trivial. Thus, for example, anxiety and depression are very commonly grouped together as neurotic disorders (group 5 in Table 4.2). However, depression is the major condition in group 4 (mood disorders). Can depression be allowed as a category in the neurotic disorders or should it be entirely placed amongst the mood disorders? This is a hoary debate in psychiatry. In ICD-9 (which was in use between 1968 and 1992) there was a category called 'neurotic depression' or 'depressive neurosis' that allowed depression to stay within the neurotic group of disorders. However, it has now been decided that any significant depression within this group should be reclassified as a mood disorder (mild, moderate or brief depressive episode, apart from one condition, mixed anxiety-depressive disorder, which is in the neurotic and stress-related disorders).

Although these issues may seem trivial, they are in fact important. A classification has to be comprehensive so that everyone is included, even conditions that are difficult to classify. In the same way that anyone making an inventory of a kitchen's contents has to describe everything in the kitchen in some way or another, every single patient referred to the mental health services needs to be classified somewhere (even if it is in an unsatisfactory group called 'not elsewhere classified'). This exercise is nothing to do with the disease model; it would happen if there were no doctors involved in psychiatry, although the classification might look somewhat different. The disease model is sometimes introduced because of implications that a specific condition in a classification should always be treated with a specific (medical) treatment such as a drug. Under these circumstances there is naturally a suspicion that a doctor is looking for an opportunity to treat a person with a specific drug and therefore manipulates the diagnosis accordingly to justify that treatment. This is nicely summarized in an epigram of Marshall Marinker, formerly a Professor of General Practice, in which a doctor says to a patient, 'you are a case of diazepam, I will prescribe you some anxiety'.

When one uses an integrated model of psychiatry, in which the disease model (a better term than the medical model in this context), psychodynamic, behavioural, cognitive and social models are all combined (see Chapter 1) (Tyrer and Steinberg, 1997), there is still an essential place for a classification system. This will include not only the major mental disorders listed in Table 4.2 but also have a separate axis of classification for social function and disability, precipitating factors and current medical illnesses. Each member of the community mental health team will have a part to play in helping to make this classification a success. Psychiatrists tend to have a major role in classifying the main mental disorders themselves (axis 1), occupational therapists are excellent at classifying axis 2 (social function and disability), social workers and psychologists are good at identifying social factors and other precipitants of mental disorder, and we have found in our practice that community mental health nurses are increasingly suspecting, and subsequently identifying, the presence of other medical illnesses in patients that they are seeing. Thus multiaxial diagnosis is an excellent exercise for the multidisciplinary community mental health team and should not be a reason for conflict.

Multidisciplinary drug treatment

This heading may appear to be an oxymoron (an association of words that are mutually contradictory). Drug treatment, say many people, is unidisciplinary; it can only be given by the doctor. There is no point in repeating the arguments against this, but the reasons why drug treatment in the multidisciplinary team ought to be jointly decided should become clear from the following accounts. These accounts are all derived from the experience of practitioners in community-based mental health teams in areas of west London whose model of care has been demonstrated to be both effective and efficient in reducing the need for hospital treatment (Merson et al., 1992). Although these are discussed under the headings of the separate disciplines involved in community mental health, the teams operate with many fewer boundaries between disciplines, using a model of care which we call the *skill share model*, in which the members of each discipline pool their knowledge to a great extent so that other members of the team are able to take on a greater range of problems than would otherwise be the case. Each section begins with a short case vignette illustrating the advantage of the multidisciplinary approach to drug treatment. We know that examples of things going well are rarely the full story and so we shall also be discussing the drawbacks and problems that need to be overcome before multidisciplinary drug treatment can work well, both in secondary and primary care (Jackson et al., 1993).

Care assistant

Care assistants (or unqualified health care professionals) are becoming much more common in community mental health teams. They do not have special professional qualifications in mental health but can display a wide range of skills and understanding which can be valuable in drug therapy.

> *Case vignette 4.1*
> *A young man, Alan, with a diagnosis of schizophrenia left his family home in the Midlands and came to London. He was unable to find accommodation and slept rough before being identified at a day centre for the homeless as someone who was mentally disturbed. He agreed (somewhat surprisingly in this context) to take medication by depot injection in the same dose that he had received formerly: 40 mg of flupenthixol decanoate (Depixol) every 3 weeks from a community mental health nurse. A care assistant was involved in ensuring that he did not default on his injections and arranged to link up with him at weekly intervals to maintain contact.*
>
> *After 5 months the dosage of medication was increased to 80 mg every 2 weeks because Alan's schizophrenic symptoms appeared to be getting worse. He became more suspicious and was troubled by a constant barrage of auditory hallucinations (voices) of an accusatory nature. It was far from clear why he was getting worse, but then the care assistant noted when he met Alan that he was mixing with other young men who were known to be dependent on drugs. Subsequent investigation revealed that Alan had been buying tablets of LSD from this group and that almost certainly these were responsible for the deterioration in his schizophrenic symptoms. Alan was some-what naïve and did not realize that the tablets were LSD (although he was aware that they were illegal drugs), and as LSD cannot be identified in the body fluids, this abuse could not have been recognized without the help of the care assistant.*

Although care assistants do not have a common set of qualifications, they are normally committed, altruistic and intelligent staff who often pursue a career within the caring services. Because they see patients in a wide variety of settings and are not perceived in quite the same way as other mental health professionals, they can glean information that others would find difficult to obtain.

In community mental health work care assistants are particularly valuable in:

- Helping to assure compliance with treatment by a collaborative approach with patients that emphasizes the importance of taking medication appropriately.
- Ensuring that patients are at the right place at the right time for receipt of drug treatment, whether by injection or by mouth.
- Identifying any unusual attitudes, behaviour or beliefs that may alter attitudes towards drug treatment.

● Helping to establish regimens of treatment that are most likely to be successful with the patient.

There are potential difficulties in linking care assistants with drug treatment, although we have not encountered these in practice. The absence of any specific professional qualifications can sometimes lead to unusual attitudes over drug treatment and fixed beliefs that certain types of treatment are dangerous, inappropriate or ineffective. As we all know, a little learning can be a dangerous thing, and sometimes isolated items of information can assume disproportionate importance as a consequence. However, if the care assistant is fully integrated into the multidisciplinary team this is unlikely to happen. There is also a bonus that sometimes follows from having a non-professionally trained person in the team. Common sense sometimes gets pushed to the margins of our consciousness when we are trained formally to do things in a certain way. Someone who is untrained, and whose opinion is untrammelled by such considerations, may well be best placed to give sensible advice.

Community mental health nurse

The professional title 'community mental health nurse' is being increasingly substituted for the older title 'community psychiatric nurse' (CPN). Although this is partly for historical reasons (CPNs have traditionally been associated with psychiatrists and not independent of them), there is also the realization that these well-trained professionals do much more than give psychiatric care, and are also actively involved in promoting mental health. The abbreviation CMHN will therefore be used throughout this book.

Case vignette 4.2

A 27-year-old woman, Barbara, was referred to the service by a general practitioner in a state of acute depression. She had just left her husband after she found out he had been unfaithful, was in temporary housing and lacked any support. She was seen by a psychiatrist and a CMHN at home and confirmed to have a depressive episode of moderate severity which appeared at first to be almost entirely precipitated by the separation from her husband. She was prescribed lofepramine (one of the safest tricyclic antidepressants) in a dose of 140 mg at night, and the CMHN continued to see her as the key worker and to help in addressing her housing and support needs. In subsequent interviews with the (female) nurse Barbara disclosed – somewhat reluctantly at first – that she had not taken her medication regularly because of the concern that she might put on weight (one of the side-effects that was mentioned when the prescription was first issued). When this was enquired about further it also became clear that Barbara had a long history of concern over her weight, sometimes associated with self-induced vomiting and the taking of laxatives. She had low self-esteem and after she found out that her husband had been unfaithful she no longer felt attractive and believed she should be blamed to some extent for his infidelity.

This problem was discussed further and the patient introduced to a self-help manual for eating disorders. It was felt that a subsidiary diagnosis of bulimia nervosa was probably justified in view of the nature of the patient's symptoms. The CMHN suggested that it would be more appropriate to prescribe one of the newer antidepressants, a selective serotonin reuptake inhibitor (SSRI) as these are associated with anorexia and nausea as side-effects and there is much less likelihood of weight gain when taking them. The psychiatrist therefore saw Barbara again and, with the additional information obtained, agreed to prescribe fluoxetine (Prozac) in a dose of 20 mg daily. The patient continued on fluoxetine for 6 months and both her depression and bulimic symptoms continued to improve. At the same time she was able to discuss more openly her feelings of low self-esteem (which still persisted to some extent, even when she was no longer depressed) and the CMHN suggested the appropriate time for the patient to start reducing fluoxetine. She continued to see Barbara over this period and, when there were no signs of relapse after the drug had been stopped completely the patient was discharged from the service 2 months later.

This example covers many of the issues in which CMHNs can prove to be both instigators and monitors of effective drug treatment. The skills and training of the CMHN are helpful in the following ways:

- Monitoring of treatment can be followed closely and compliance measured.
- Regular assessments (usually more frequent than those of medical staff) allow adverse effects of drugs to be more quickly recognized and identified as drug effects.
- The dual role of drug monitoring and psychological treatment allows the benefits of drug treatment to be integrated with those other psychological approaches.
- Regular monitoring and application of other treatments ensures that drugs are discontinued at the most appropriate time.

Of course, these benefits could be the responsibility of other members of the multidisciplinary team, but the training of the CMHNs, together with the way in which they are regarded by patients (as having special knowledge of both drug and psychological treatments) makes these tasks somewhat easier for the CMHN.

Unfortunately there is a likelihood that in some settings, particularly when multidisciplinary involvement is minimal, CMHNs and (in general practice) practice nurses will administer treatment always as prescribed by the doctor and not question the type, dosage and duration of treatment sufficiently. In far too many centres, depot injections of antipsychotic drugs are given for many years in exactly the same quantities at exactly the same intervals to patients whose needs for these dosages have not been properly reassessed, and in some cases are quite inappropriate (Johnson, 1988). Under these circumstances the CMHN may often develop a good relationship with the patient, but this is independent of the administration of the drug. The drug treatment is regarded as the exclusive province of the doctor, and the nurse is only carrying out the doctor's prescribing orders.

In well-organized multidisciplinary teamwork the nurse is able to monitor the effects of drug treatment and has the knowledge, either pre-existing or derived from discussions at clinical review meetings, of potential adverse effects and how they should be detected. In the instance cited above, the nurse concerned already knew that fluoxetine had been found to be effective in treating bulimia nervosa as well as depression, and recommended this drug for Barbara. This was a reasonable conclusion and could probably have been reached by the psychiatrist in the same way when faced with the same amount of information. Unfortunately, there is a tendency for some psychiatrists to feel that the decision about prescribing should be left entirely to themselves. A suggestion from a nurse that a different antidepressant was indicated – particularly if accompanied by the name of the drug and its dosage – could create irritation, and provoke the contrary reaction of ensuring that whatever antidepressant was prescribed it was certainly not going to be that suggested by the CMHN!

This silly gamesmanship should never be part of community mental health practice; it is reasonable to argue for the merits of different types of treatment, but it is hardly surprising that on many occasions a key worker with detailed knowledge of the patient may be able to suggest a more appropriate drug treatment than the psychiatrist, even allowing for the latter's greater knowledge.

There is sometimes a danger that this could go too far and the doctor then accepts the word of the nurse without ever seeing the patient. Apart from the illegality of writing prescriptions without seeing the patient, it is not good practice. Responsibility for prescriptions has to rest with doctors and, even if the psychiatrist is confident about the ability of the non-medical staff in the multidisciplinary team, it is wrong to permit prescription without contact with the patient. However, a general practitioner may be prepared to prescribe medication for a known patient who has refused to see a psychiatrist, but where problems are sufficiently clear-cut for the psychiatrist to make a recommendation on the basis of other team members' assessments.

Occupational therapist

The occupational therapist is not normally associated with any part of psychotropic drug treatment. In a multidisciplinary team the importance of the occupational therapist is sometimes underestimated, and because they do not have the capacity to administer drugs in the same way as community nurses, they are sometimes regarded as a non-essential luxury in the community mental health team (Joyce, 1993). The following account may help to dispel such notions.

Case vignette 4.3
Colin was a 26-year-old single man who was referred to the community mental health team after five psychiatric admissions in 4 years. Referral details revealed that he was totally lacking in motivation and everything had to be done for him by his mother. The only way in which he could be kept relatively well was by taking large doses of medication – 300 mg flupenthixol decanoate (Depixol) every 2 weeks – and he relapsed if this dosage was reduced.

He was seen by the community occupational therapist who worked out a programme with him after assessing how he spent an average day (Daily Living Assessment). It was decided to test out his abilities to carry out each of the individual elements on the programme and he proved to be much more competent than expected in activities such as cooking for himself, self-care and budgeting. These activities seemed to be associated with a reduction in his psychotic symptoms, particularly his persistent auditory hallucinations which he said were 'much more in the background' when he was actively occupied. After review with the psychiatrist it was suggested that he might have greater motivation and energy if his drug dosage was reduced and so this was done in stages. He continued to improve despite the former predictions of relapse whenever his medication was cut, and achieved much greater independence.

However, further progress was handicapped by his mother continuing to insist on doing things for Colin that he was capable of doing for himself, and in many cases preferred to do so. The occupational therapist therefore had to spend a considerable amount of her time in emphasizing to his mother that he was quite capable of looking after himself and if progress continued at the same rate he would soon be able to live independently. This caused distress in his mother, who in many ways felt more secure and happy with her son at home. When it was agreed that there would be no sudden move away from home and that Colin could continue to live there if he wished, his mother co-operated more with the programme involving a gradual withdrawal of her input into her son's care. This was replaced more by a monitoring role with which she became more satisfied. Nevertheless, there continued to be times in which she did things on her son's behalf unnecessarily and he was taught to be more assertive in refusing his mother's ministrations. By this time his dosage of medication had been reduced to 80 mg of flupenthixol decanoate fortnightly and he had developed a range of new activities in his leisure time, including reading and going to the cinema.

This is not an unusual case; we are convinced that the same could be repeated throughout the length and breadth of the country if there was closer liaison between occupational therapists and psychiatrists, together with other members of the multidisciplinary team. There is some evidence that maintenance dosages of antipsychotic drugs are unnecessarily high in many patients (see Chapter 6) and that by reducing emotional pressures at home, particularly levels of high critical expressed emotion (EE), patients can function well on lower doses of drug treatment. The occupational therapist, with special skills in assessing functional improvement, can:

- Monitor social function and performance which are sensitive indicators of both positive and adverse effects of drugs.
- Assess a patient's state of arousal (a continuum between full wakefulness and coma) more accurately than many other workers, so that sedative effects of drugs can be detected easily.
- Be a major motivator for allegedly unmotivated patients by being able to demonstrate immediate gains from positive behaviour.

Pharmacologists repeatedly talk of benefit/risk ratios when discussing the merits of different drug treatments, but it is important to realize that benefits and risks accompany every type of treatment. The occupational therapist in the case vignette above was engaged in a parallel exercise to the psychiatrist prescribing the flupenthixol decanoate (Figure 4.1). Progress was made by both approaches in improving the patient's functioning and performance (axis 2 in ICD-10), only to be thwarted by the interference of Colin's mother. If the occupational therapist had persisted in following the programme and ignored the mother there could have been a relapse and a return to poor social functioning. Similarly, the psychiatrist, in reducing the dosage of the antipsychotic drugs, had to be aware of the dangers of relapse and a return of serious symptoms.

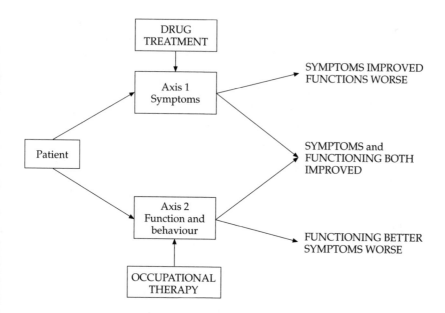

Figure 4.1   *Synthesis of occupational therapy and drug treatment in case vignette 4.3*

There is a danger that when the individual disciplines work alone that symptoms can be improved while functioning slowly becomes more impaired, or, conversely, that functioning improves but the patient develops more severe symptoms. By combining treatments the preferred outcome of both symptoms and functioning improving simultaneously is more likely be achieved.

By working in this way the community occupational therapist has many advantages over hospital occupational therapists who sometimes still work in a unidisciplinary way. No one who has worked in one of the older mental hospitals will forget the groans from the patients as the occupational therapist arrives on the ward to round up her recalcitrant charges and march them off to the occupational therapy department. Similarly, many will have been present at patients' ward meetings in which the only topic that arouses animation is the preferential treatment given to patient X who is excused going to the department while all other patients have been forced to go. This is not the stuff of therapeutic endeavour.

Things are very different when patients are seen at home and have clearly identifiable therapeutic targets which they wish to achieve themselves. By linking these improvements with the minimal effective dose of drugs to control symptoms, one can achieve even greater motivation to get better. Thus the activities of the occupational therapist, psychiatrist and patient are all mutually reinforced and the middle outcome shown in Figure 4.1 is more likely to be achieved.

Psychiatrist

Many community mental health teams do not have a psychiatrist. Others have them at arm's length, available for consultation but not as members of the team. It will be clear from reading the rest of the book that such arrangements are not likely to be efficient.

> ### Case vignette 4.4
> Dorothy was a woman of anxious and dependent personality who had had symptoms of agoraphobia for many years. She was permanently anxious, and when put under additional stress she was reluctant to leave the house and when she did so she was often troubled by attacks of vomiting which made her feel embarrassed and ashamed and led to socially phobic behaviour also. These symptoms extended to psychiatry; she was terrified about any appointments with psychiatrists and would vomit for days before the appointed time. Attempts were made for her to be seen by the community mental health team and the general practitioner. Because of concerns over prescribing benzodiazepines, the doctor treated her with paroxetine (Seroxat) and she also had thioridazine (50 mg twice daily) given as a sedative.
>
> After referral to the community team, Dorothy was seen by a care assistant, a social worker and a psychiatrist. As she was seen at home she was much less nervous and was amazed that she did not feel like

vomiting at all, although she remained somewhat nauseated. After review it was decided that, as paroxetine could cause nausea as one of its main side-effects, it would be better to change this drug. She was therefore treated with clomipramine (which has similar antiphobic properties to paroxetine), and at a dosage of 75 mg daily she was more confident and her vomiting and nausea almost entirely disappeared. However, the psychiatrist remained the key worker because there continued to be problems over her additional medication, and at various times it was felt necessary to treat her symptoms of panic during her acute phobic attacks by giving small doses of benzodiazepines in anticipation of exposure to agoraphobic and social phobic situations. Subsequently Dorothy was referred to a day hospital and was able to attend regularly without any avoidance. However, as she still retained some phobic fears she was referred to a self-help phobia group where she is currently making excellent progress with others who have similar fears.

This vignette illustrates several important aspects of the psychiatrist's role as part of a community mental health team that can only be achieved by active involvement beyond merely administering drug treatment. These functions include:

- Home treatment when necessary.
- The adoption of a key worker role.
- Destigmatization of the psychiatrist.
- Integration with other professional colleagues.

None of these can be achieved by having a psychiatrist at the periphery of the team who is 'only available for consultation', usually at the wrong time and in the wrong place. One of the major criticisms that could be made of psychiatrists until recently was that they were happy to promote community care provided that they were not part of it (Burns *et al.*, 1993). Extra resources were recommended by them for the employment of community nurses and others who could see patients at home and in other community settings, but if direct mental health input was needed the patient needed to be brought the psychiatrist for consultation. The case of Dorothy illustrates how inappropriate this is; her contact with psychiatrists in hospital settings had only aggravated her problems which were therefore, to some extent, iatrogenic (induced by therapy). By placing the psychiatrist in the role of key worker the excessive anxiety that the patient had developed over contact with psychiatry was removed (deconditioned) and treatment could be established on a new footing. This allowed the replacement of one drug, paroxetine, which can lead to nausea and vomiting, with the very similar drug clomipramine, which is much less commonly associated with this adverse effect. The judicious use of benzodiazepines subsequently could also only be achieved by close contact with patient and explanation of the benefits and risks of the treatment.

Perhaps more importantly, the close involvement of the psychiatrist in the community team can act as a support to other workers who otherwise might feel overwhelmed with the problems created by patients and their helplessness in the face of severe adversity. One of the chief advantages of having a psychiatrist available is that when drug treatment is necessary it can be given quickly and in a way that is appropriate in the context of other treatments. It completes important parts of the therapeutic jigsaw that would otherwise remain disconnected.

There used to be an oversimplified notion of drug treatment in psychiatry. When the therapist had found the 'magic bullet' (to use a phrase introduced by Paul Ehrlich, one of the early pioneers of drug treatment in medicine), one only had to sit back and watch the patient get better. Although this may apply to some drugs in medicine, such as penicillin, drug treatment in psychiatry rarely acts in such a simple way, and even when apparent cure is achieved after acute treatment there is still the important decision about how long treatment should be continued for and how it should be monitored. All the workers in the community mental health team can help the psychiatrist to come to the right decisions over these matters.

Psychologist

Psychologists are traditionally thought to have rivalled psychiatrists. They are sometimes (and irritatingly to them) defined as psychiatrists who do not prescribe pills. However, their skills complement rather than conflict with medical ones, as illustrated by vignette 4.5.

Case vignette 4.5
Elizabeth was a 22-year-old woman whose life was full of conflict. She was adopted as a child and had many different carers before being brought up by a doting grandmother. She was unsettled in adolescence and did not do well at school, although she managed to complete sufficient examinations to be accepted for an art and design degree course. She became involved in intense relationships with many students during her first 2 years at college. This only seemed to make her more unsettled. She had frequent mood swings and on three occasions took quite serious overdoses when acutely depressed. She was treated with carbamazepine (Tegretol) in a dose of 200 mg three times a day for her mood swings and appeared to improve. However, after yet another overdose of paracetamol she was referred to the community mental health team. On assessment she was angry and critical of most people in her life, including health professionals. She complained that no treatment she had been given had ever helped, until it was explained to her that she needed carbamazepine for her mood swings but that this had not been working as well as it could.

She was seen by a psychologist and a CMHN initially, and it was felt, on review, that the diagnosis was more likely to be that of an impulsive or borderline personality disorder with no evidence of severe mood disorder. She was taken on by the psychologist as key worker who adopted a multimodal approach (i.e. many combined approaches) in which her symptoms, general functioning, dynamic conflicts and behavioural goals could all be addressed. Good progress was achieved but Elizabeth was extremely reluctant to attribute any significant part of her treatment to anything other than carbamazepine. The psychiatrist also saw the patient with the psychologist at home and felt that the improvement shown by the patient was more likely to be due to the psychological treatment. In particular, carbamazepine seemed to have a marked placebo effect, since when Elizabeth took it she felt better within a matter of 2 minutes. Similarly, when she forgot to take her drug at the appointed time she often felt extremely depressed a few minutes later (an example of the nocebo effect described in Chapter 3). Although it was considered that it might be better to replace the carbamazepine by a placebo tablet eventually, through joint discussion it was agreed that medication would be reduced gradually and more emphasis placed on the gains that had been achieved through psychological treatments. These were clearly related to the patient's improved maturity and reduced tendency to blame others for all her problems. After 8 weeks total reduction of medication was achieved and did not need to be restarted. There were times subsequently when she wanted to return to taking medication but when this was explained to be inappropriate and she subsequently improved the excessive attribution of drug effects was finally overcome.

This vignette illustrates the value of a psychologist in:

- Adopting a systematic approach to learning and unlearning.
- Understanding the non-pharmacological component of drug action and withdrawal.
- Ensuring that attribution of improvement is accorded proper attention in therapy.

Psychologists are among the most highly trained of community health workers, but sometimes they have a tendency to confine their skills to their own discipline and work alone in 'office psychiatry'. They are well trained and able to carry out this work, but in this setting are not easily able to integrate drug treatment with cognitive therapy, behavioural therapy and similar approaches. In the integrated mental health team, they can help to define the true place of drug treatment in a wide range of conditions. This is a necessary antidote to claims made by others (including patients) that either a certain drug is the only possibly remedy for their condition or, alternatively, that it is an absolute poison and should not be given to anybody. To do this effectively the psychologist also has to believe that drug treatment has a place for certain conditions. There will clearly be problems if recourse to drug treatment is perceived as a sign of failure and likely to interfere with psychological treatment. As noted elsewhere in this book, this is rarely a problem and conflict of this sort about treatment is almost always in the minds of the therapists concerned rather than in the nature of the treatments.

Social worker

Social workers rarely get a good word from the public. They are variously seen as interfering busybodies, incompetent practitioners with no satisfactory basic science training, or do-gooders with no knowledge of the real world. All this is unfair and results mainly from the fact that we give social workers a set of extremely trying tasks which is bound to bring them into conflict with the public. Child care and compulsory admissions under the Mental Health Act are the two most obvious examples.

> ### Case vignette 4.6
> Norman, a 27-year-old man, who lived alone, was referred by his general practitioner (under pressure from Norman's mother) for urgent assessment and possible admission to hospital under the Mental Health Act. It looked as though compulsory admission would be essential as Norman was neglecting himself, stealing cans of alcohol from local supermarkets, and would not let his family into the flat.
>
> On assessment with a psychiatrist it became clear that Norman's mother was abnormally overinvolved with her son and also had fixed ideas of how he should be treated. She had worked as an auxiliary nurse in the past and had some knowledge of mental illness which she had elevated into expertise. She considered that her son needed compulsory admission to hospital in order to be given psychotherapy to make him a better motivated, sociable and hard-working individual.
>
> It was decided that compulsory admission was inappropriate and the social worker continued to see Norman together with an occupational therapist and (less frequently) with the psychiatrist, to improve his functioning while living at home. This approach was supported by some members of his family but not his mother, who continued to criticize and make inappropriate demands (e.g. to make visits up to three times a week on a regular basis). Sufficient rapport was established once the social worker had helped in arranging for Norman's rent, gas and electricity arrears to be paid off and for him to accept a small dose of oral medication in the form of sulpiride, 200–400 mg daily. Although Norman was not motivated sufficiently to obtain the drugs from the general practitioner, his father did so on his behalf.
>
> Norman continues to make good progress and at the time of writing this vignette he is expressing interest in employment on the open market. Although this is unlikely to be realized, he is likely to enter some form of sheltered employment for further assessment and training shortly.

Unfortunately the social worker is often placed in a position of potential confrontation with other members of the multidisciplinary team. In fact, when one looks at the role of social workers, it almost seems as though they are set up to be in confrontation with one major group or another. Social workers have to decide whether a mother can look after her newborn baby, whether a child should stay with the family, and whether a patient with psychiatric illness should be deprived of liberty and brought into a psychiatric hospital. Clearly these roles can be carried out in collaboration and without conflict, but the potential is always there and no social worker can survive in the post for long without a thick skin.

The case of Norman was a little easier than most, as both social worker and psychiatrist agreed that admission was not necessary. However, unlike the social worker in this example, and certainly since reforms in the UK National Health Service were introduced in 1993, the opportunities for social workers to work therapeutically with patients on whom they have made assessments under Section 12 of the Mental Health Act are getting fewer. In this instance considerable progress was made, although it took some time to be established. The important step was to develop a therapeutic alliance with the patient; this was aided through a supportive role and, to put it frankly, a financial one. The support by the social worker of the need for antipsychotic drug treatment was also important in helping the patient accept this despite the unpromising start.

The skills of the social worker are extremely helpful to the multi-disciplinary team and are complementary to other members. Knowledge of child protection legislation, a guide to the complexities of benefit provision and a knowledge of social services resources are just a few of the important practical elements of knowledge that a multi-disciplinary team tends to lack without the presence of a social worker. Add to this an understanding of family therapy in its broadest sense, an ability to work with extremely disturbed people over a long period and an understanding of sociology and social structures, and we have a therapist who can reinforce all other professions within the team (Huxley, 1990).

Unfortunately, as is discussed in greater detail below, the history of social workers and psychiatrists working together is one of recurring conflict. Much of this is related to the power and position of the doctor and the perceived use of drug treatment as a means of exercising psychiatric power. If the social worker shows the same philosophy of care, including the use of drug treatment discussed earlier, these conflicts do not arise. In fact, in our services social workers have integrated more effectively than many other disciplines for reasons that appear to be as much due to their professional training and common sense as to their personal characteristics.

This is not say that conflict does not arise and arguments do not ensue. There can be particular difficulty over the admission of patients to hospital, but when all members of the team acknowledge that the social worker, in making an assessment of a disturbed psychiatric patient, is obliged by statute to select the least restrictive setting to provide care, there has been much greater agreement when such assessments are made.

Difficulties commonly encountered with drug treatment in community mental health teams

The case vignettes described above are selective and somewhat biased; they illustrate collaboration working well and smoothly. This is by no means the full story of multidisciplinary team working. One could argue that illustrating cases that showed differences of opinion between the members of the multidisciplinary team and the need for resolution of conflict would be more instructive, but as they would take much longer to describe they have been omitted here. Nevertheless, it is important to discuss differences of opinion because they are bound to occur. In a good community team, these differences promote better working and help to build up skills and the information base of all members. In a poorly functioning team they lead to fractious argument, the establishment of different cliques within the team, and battles between individuals instead of on behalf of patients.

With respect to drug treatment, we have identified five important areas of dissent that often cause problems. These are the five A's: absence of knowledge, attribution of benefit, ambivalence about the place of drug treatment, anger (mainly directed at medical staff) and antipsychiatry, a movement that still retains its devotees, even though it has conclusively been shown to have no scientific basis.

Absence of knowledge

The main purpose of writing this book is to correct the surprising degree of ignorance about drug treatment shown by many mental health professionals. Among the major areas of ignorance are the following beliefs:

- Drugs in various ways 'control' patients in the same negative way that a straitjacket does.
- Drugs invariably lead to dependence if they are given for long periods.
- Once you start taking drugs it is impossible to stop them.
- Drugs prevent other treatments from being successful.

These statements are countered in many other parts of this book. This does not mean that we are complacent about our knowledge of drug effects. Our ignorance still greatly exceeds our knowledge – in particular, the optimum length of treatment with any particular drugs is still a subject that can be debated extensively, and it is often only after a full multidisciplinary discussion that a reasonable decision can be made.

Attribution of effects

This problem is illustrated in case vignette 4.4. It is a well-known fact in psychology that when a stimulus is followed by a quick response it is more likely to be given special value by the subject. Psychological treatments tend to be delayed in their effects; drug treatment is more rapid.

As drug treatment involves the patient being a passive participant, if improvement is noted it is likely to be attributed to the drug therapy; similarly, if adverse effects are noted these too could be blamed more readily on drug therapy than on psychological treatment, whether or not they are true adverse reactions to the drug in question.

There is also sometimes difficulty in attributing improvement when several treatments are given to a patient. A nurse who has spent 10 hours counselling a depressed patient after a sudden death in the family will not take kindly to a doctor maintaining that the improvement the patient has shown after 2 months is almost entirely due to antidepressant therapy and that the bereavement counselling has been of secondary importance, or worse, unnecessary.

Although in short-term treatment those who praise the effect of drugs at the expense of psychological treatments may be correct, in the longer term the value of psychological treatment in preventing relapse is now well documented. Both behavioural therapy and cognitive therapy have been shown in several studies to have long-lasting value that buttresses the patient against relapse. This is illustrated in Figure 4.2; the benefits of drug treatment initially are more than countered in the long term by the protective effects of psychological treatment (providing the appropriate treatment has been chosen). This argues for collaboration and combination of different treatments, rather than a competitive league table in which sterile arguments are made in favour of one treatment or another being top of the pile.

Ambivalence

Unlike physical conditions such as pneumonia caused by a bacterial infection where there is no satisfactory non-drug alternative to an

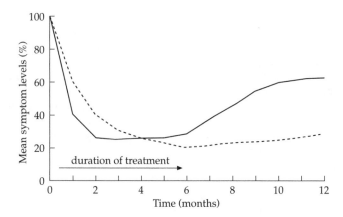

Figure 4.2 *Usual pattern of improvement and relapse after starting and stopping drug therapy (solid line) and psychological treatment (dotted line)*

antibiotic for treating the infection, in mental health disorders there is no comparable 'absolute indication' for drug treatment. There are some conditions in which drug treatment is almost essential, for example in mania and acute schizophrenia, but even then the adverse effects of treatment may make some try to avoid drugs wherever possible. In other conditions in psychiatry the arguments for using drugs become less and less convincing. This means that drug treatment has to jockey for position with other types of treatment and the choice of one mode of therapy over another may sometimes seem a random one. However, if a multi-disciplinary team is working well there are few difficulties in reconciling these opposing pressures. Thus, for example, it may be agreed to treat a person with a moderate degree of depression with, say, cognitive therapy in the first instance, and to consider drug treatment later if there are problems in treatment or symptoms persist. Alternatively, drug treatment may be chosen at the beginning with the intention of stopping it after 3 months, by which time it is expected that the cognitive therapy, begun at the same time as drug treatment, will have established a sound basis for continued health.

There is nothing wrong with being ambivalent about giving drugs; it goes with the territory. It is only when certain practitioners consider that drug treatment should *never* be given for certain conditions that conflicts can arise, even in the most harmonious of teams.

Anger

Anger may seem an odd subject to cover here, but drug treatment often does arouse a large number of emotions, especially anger, among health professionals and carers. The anger covers a wide range of subjects. We have noticed anger with the drug companies for seeming to have unlimited resources but apparently only being interested in courting doctors and getting them to prescribe their products. There is also anger with doctors for appearing to do so little (the prescription of a drug is an exercise lasting 2 minutes) and yet often achieving such powerful results; anger with other practitioners, patients or relatives for refusing a drug treatment when the prescriber considers it to be not only effective but essential; and anger with the patient for not getting better on psychological treatment so they have to be subjected to the perceived indignity of drug therapy.

It is important for all practitioners to be honest with themselves about their attitudes towards drug treatment. It is often useful to ask yourself whether you would be happy for a close relative to receive a psychotropic drug, and then to transfer that question to the situation in which drug treatment is being considered. If the answer to the question is a positive one, then any annoyance with the decision must be based on other considerations. You will need to ask yourself whether it is the way in which the decision has been made, the person who is making it, and how it affects your own role in treatment that may be responsible for the anger and annoyance you feel.

Antipsychiatry

The antipsychiatry movement, characteristically associated with the names of Laing and Esterson (1970) and referred to in Chapter 1, still has some adherents. Put simply, it can be argued that much major mental illness is not illness at all, but an understandable reaction of essentially sane individuals to the pressures of an insane society. If everyone around you behaves illogically and inappropriately then, so the argument goes, the only way to 'escape' from the pressures is to become mad oneself. Although the movement was backed initially by some slight evidence that the parents of schizophrenic patients behaved in a 'schizophrenogenic' way towards their offspring, subsequent research did not confirm these finding.

We were therefore faced with an attractive hypothesis that had been disproved. However, as so often happens with attractive hypotheses, many people were unable to let go of it and continued to argue its merits without any evidence. There are therefore still organizations in several countries where patients with major mental illness are managed without any form of drug treatment because their psychotic experiences are considered to be a liberating experience that will eventually lead to a 'breakthrough to health'. It is important to be humble in psychiatry and not to discount the possibility that for some patients this may indeed be the case, but our own experience suggests that the decision to avoid using drugs in the treatment of patients with severe mental illness should only be made rarely and after a great deal of consideration. It may sometimes be the best option, but only when desired by the patient after being given all the relevant evidence that they have been able to understand.

Further reading

Onyett, S. (1992). *Case Management in Mental Health*. London: Chapman & Hall.

5

Drug treatment of organic disorders

In psychiatry it is traditional to divide mental illnesses into two categories – organic and functional. This distinction is based on the likely aetiologies or causes of the disorders. For many disorders it is often difficult to make this distinction without a great deal of investigation and study, but it is important to do so, because once the cause of a disorder is known, it can radically affect the treatment given.

Organic disorders are those in which there is demonstrable structural damage to the brain, or brain dysfunction due to disease somewhere else in the body (often referred to as systemic disease). Examples of organic disorders arising within the brain include cerebral tumours, infections such as meningitis and encephalitis, and dementias. Systemic diseases include thyroid disorder and infections such as those affecting the chest and urinary tract.

Functional disorders are those in which no obvious brain damage has been identified. Examples of functional disorders include schizophrenia and depression. However, with the development of investigative techniques that can show brain structures and function without the need to penetrate the cranial cavity (collectively called neuroimaging), we know that many functional disorders may have an organic component. Computerized axial tomography (CT) and magnetic resonance imaging (MRI) have revolutionized investigation of organic disease in the brain, and there are now suggestions that a wide range of psychiatric disorders have underlying organic pathology (Lishman, 1993).

Organic disorders require treatment of the cause. This may be the surgical removal of a brain tumour, or the use of antibacterial medication in meningitis. In contrast, if a patient has a functional illness there is no obvious anatomical or pathological abnormality which can be treated. Antibiotics and surgery have no immediate therapeutic value and the clinician's efforts are concentrated on the treatment of the patient's symptoms. Depending on the diagnosis, this may involve antipsychotic medication, antidepressants, or psychological approaches including analytic psychotherapy and cognitive and behavioural methods.

Traditionally medical students and doctors in training are taught to consider their patients' diagnoses in a hierarchical manner, with organic disease at the top, followed by functional disorders and lastly the personality disorders. One of the reasons for this is to avoid missing an eminently treatable organic condition. For example, it may seem appropriate to treat a patient with a brain tumour who has predominantly depressive symptoms with antidepressant medication; however, when the correct diagnosis of organic disease is made it becomes clear that a surgical operation may be a far more effective (and possibly life-saving) method of intervention. This is not to suggest that the patient would not benefit from both treatments, but serves to remind the clinician that the primary diagnosis must not be missed.

Although at first this distinction between organic and functional illness seems clear, the concept may begin to falter when examined more closely. By convention organic psychiatric disorder does not include mental retardation, in which there is no obvious pathological cause. The paradox is continued with the inclusion of both epilepsy and the sleep disorders in which there is often *no* demonstrable structural pathology. Similar difficulties in the concept arise because with the passage of time and advances in our understanding of mental illness it has become apparent that disorders classified as functional *do* have demonstrable structural brain damage after all. For example, some brain scan studies of patients with schizophrenia have shown that the ventricular chambers within the brain are often enlarged and the brain tissue withered or atrophied (see Chapter 6). However, it is still generally accepted that the abnormalities in these functional disorders are at the microscopic or biochemical level and are only possible to detect when specialized diagnostic tests such as lumbar puncture and brain scanning are undertaken.

This chapter examines the various drug treatments available for managing patients with organic psychiatric disorders with particular emphasis on relevant aspects for community mental health workers. Throughout this and succeeding chapters, the general categories of the International Classification of Diseases (ICD) are followed (World Health Organization, 1992). This is a categorical system of disease classification developed since the beginning of this century under the auspices of the World Health Organization (see Chapter 4). It can be a very efficient form of communication. The diagnosis of Alzheimer's disease, the most common form of dementia, conveys a great deal of information in just two words. A diagnosis is a form of shorthand; if a picture is worth a thousand words a good diagnosis is worth quite a few hundred, but it needs to be used wisely and well to achieve this efficiency.

Delirium

The term 'delirium' refers to short-lived episodes of brain malfunction which are often called acute brain syndromes. Characteristic features include the sudden onset of confusion, reduced alertness, loss of memory, short-lived delusions (often of a paranoid nature) and dramatic loss of functioning. Acute states of delirium are not often encountered in community psychiatric practice but the characteristic sudden onset is a clue to correct diagnosis. In many instances there will be an underlying physical disorder or illness that accounts for the delirium and this will need to be investigated subsequently and treated.

Management of delirium

The patient in an acute attack of delirium is confused, often very frightened, and unpredictable in behaviour. If there is no support available in the home setting it will often be necessary for the patient to be admitted to hospital, but it is important to realize that this may make the confusion and acute symptoms worse, because the patient is being removed from a familiar environment. Neuroleptics (antipsychotic drugs or major tranquillizers) are the mainstay of drug treatment (see Chapter 6). Drugs such as chlorpromazine, thioridazine and droperidol are used both for their sedative properties and also their antipsychotic effects. It may sometimes be necessary to give these drugs intramuscularly or in liquid form to induce more rapid effects. Droperidol in relatively low doses (e.g. 5–20 mg) may be particularly useful in this respect because it is absorbed quickly and lasts for a short time. Judicious use of drugs of this nature may also help to keep the patient in a more familiar environment and reduce the need for hospital admission.

Case vignette 5.1

A community psychiatric team was called to visit Abimbola urgently as he was thought to be suffering from 'acute schizophrenia'. He was staying in a homeless person's hostel after being evicted from a refugee hostel because of disturbed behaviour. The staff at the homeless hostel said that he had been perfectly well on admission 3 days previously but in the last 7 hours had become extremely disturbed, maintaining that he had been bewitched by a woman who had cursed him in his home country, Nigeria, and was sending snakes through the walls and windows to harm him. On examination he was extremely distressed and in terror of being attacked by snakes. However, he also had a very high fever with a temperature of 40°C (104°F) and had marked shortness of breath and sweating. He also was unaware of the date, time and place, believing that he was in his home village 250 km away from Lagos in Nigeria. He was given droperidol 20 mg in the form of an elixir every 4 hours together with aspirin to reduce his fever. Fortunately both these drugs were available in the homeless hostel as other patients had previously received droperidol for schizophrenia. The next day he was completely well again and could not remember his experiences of the previous day. A fuller history taken when he was more lucid suggested strongly that he was having attacks of malaria. Abimbola had previously had malaria in Nigeria which had only been partially treated before he came to England. Subsequent investigations at the tropical medicine department confirmed that he did indeed have malaria and he was treated appropriately. He had no further episodes of delirium and the diagnosis of an acute toxic confusional state was made.

This example illustrates the importance of further enquiry and investigation after the episode of delirium has been treated. Although the community mental health worker cannot be expected to reach a diagnosis such as that of malaria unaided there are three questions that need to be asked whenever delirium is suspected.

Is there an underlying physical cause?

Simple examination of the patient should help to answer this question. Dehydration can be recognized by dryness of the mouth and a lax, loose skin; fever by a rapid pulse and breathing; jaundice by yellowing of the whites of the eyes; and anaemia by a sallow skin and paleness of the conjunctivae (the part of the skin in direct contact with the eyes). However, there are many other causes of delirium that are not easily recognized, including infections of the brain, electrolyte disturbance (particularly common after surgical operations) and some metabolic diseases (e.g. due to kidney failure). Because these conditions can often hinder the excretion and metabolism of drugs it is wise always to use low doses in the first instance.

Has the patient been exposed to any experience that could be the cause of delirium?

This question can only be answered satisfactorily if there is someone else who can talk about the problem other than the patient. Often there may be a clear relationship between the cause of delirium and its presentation; the most obvious is the acute delirium that sometimes follows alcohol intoxication, and delirium tremens, the most severe form of alcohol withdrawal syndrome.

Is there clear evidence of sudden onset of symptoms?

This is again dependent on an adequate history of the condition. Although chronic delirium can sometimes occur, it is not often observed in community psychiatric practice. Exposure to toxic substances such as arsenic can lead to chronic delirium but even then there should be clear evidence of a sudden change in behaviour. Other organic conditions, particularly the dementias discussed below, can show many of the features of delirium (although visual hallucinations are generally less common) and it is only their persistence that changes the diagnosis. It is also important to realize that delirium can be superimposed on a dementia or another organic illness at time of particular physical stress (e.g. after consumption of a moderate amount of alcohol or after a surgical operation).

The answers to these questions will help to decide whether an individual in a state of delirium ought to be admitted to hospital as an emergency or whether initial care can take place at home. A great deal depends on the circumstances in which the person is being seen. A nursing home staffed by qualified nursing personnel and visited regularly by medical staff will probably be able to cope with most cases of delirium without the need for admission to hospital, whereas a delirious person in a bed and breakfast hotel will almost invariably have to be admitted to a hospital bed.

Special problems in the drug treatment of delirium

It has already been mentioned that low doses of antipsychotic drugs can be useful in the initial treatment of delirious patients. There also needs to be awareness of the neuroleptic malignant syndrome, and the movement disorders created by neuroleptic drugs (discussed in Chapter 6). Although the symptoms of parkinsonism can be mistaken for delirium this is unlikely if an adequate assessment has been made. Treatment with antipsychotic drugs may often lower the blood pressure, a problem which is particularly common with chlorpromazine, and this may aggravate delirium by reducing the blood supply to the brain. This is another point in favour of using a drug with a rapid onset of action and short duration of effect, such as droperidol.

The dementias

Dementia literally means 'loss of mind'. It is a term used to refer to patients with chronic, degenerative, usually irreversible brain impairment which characteristically affects a wide range of brain functions. Some of the better-known types of dementia include Alzheimer's disease, and more recently, bovine spongiform encephalopathy (BSE) or 'mad cow' disease. Broadly speaking the dementias can be divided into three groups: Alzheimer's dementias; vascular dementias; and other types, the latter category containing a wide variety of uncommon dementias. These include Pick's disease, progressive supranuclear palsy, Creutzfeldt–Jakob disease, Wilson's disease, acquired immune deficiency syndrome (AIDS) dementia, BSE and Huntington's disease. Each of these groups is briefly discussed, although they are likely to appear in similar ways to the community mental health worker.

Alzheimer's dementia

Alzheimer's dementia is common. It affects at least 5% of people over 65 years old and probably 20% of those over 80 years old. Women are affected more commonly than men. The disease can conveniently be divided into two forms – type 2 (presenile) with an early age of onset before the age of 65 years, and type 1 (senile) with onset of symptoms after the age of 65 years.

The underlying cause has not yet been fully determined and although a variety of environmental agents have been identified over the years, none has been shown to have a clear causal relationship to Alzheimer's dementia. Examples include the suggestion that aluminium in drinking water may be a cause of the disease. What has become increasingly clear is the influence of genetic factors. These are implicated most conclusively in Alzheimer's disease type 2. This form of presenile dementia tends to run in families and some studies have shown a 50% chance of close relatives being affected. Evidence for genetic aetiology in type 1 or late-onset Alzheimer's suggests a looser association, with certain individuals inheriting more of a predisposition to the disease than others. This may have implications for the community mental health worker of the future, if and when techniques for genetic testing and determination of risk become more widely available. Obviously there are complex issues relating to the ethics of informing an individual that they are at high risk of developing dementia in later life, and there are implications not just for the patient but the whole family.

The onset of dementia in Alzheimer's disease is usually gradual, and involves a steady decline in intellectual function. Characteristically, patients do not present to health care workers early on in the course of the disorder. They may slowly deteriorate over several years before presenting for help, usually to their general practitioners. Indeed, studies have shown that general practitioners were only aware of approximately 80% of the severely demented and 30% of the mildly demented in their practice population. This relatively low rate of identification of sufferers is compounded by the fact that this group tend to lose insight (i.e. are unaware they are ill) early in the disease process. Consequently patients tend not to present themselves to medical services, and it is often frustrated and weary carers who finally persuade a dementing relative to agree to assessment.

Patients show progressive memory impairment, at first affecting recent memory but eventually extending to all parts of memory function. Sufferers become increasingly forgetful until in the later stages of the disease they are disoriented in time, place and person, with little ability to register either new memories or recall more distant ones. Typically the most remote memories remain accessible, although in time they too are lost. Other functions necessary for normal life become impaired, including the ability to manipulate objects (apraxia). For example, some patients are unable to carry out simple tasks such as dressing (dressing apraxia) or more complex actions which involve co-ordination of both hands. This is illustrated in many hospital wards for elderly psychiatric patients where the door separating the ward from the rest of the hospital has two handles which have to be operated simultaneously to open the door. A non-demented patient has no difficulty in opening the door; but a demented person is repeatedly frustrated by the inability to co-ordinate the actions of both hands.

Apraxia can cause major difficulties in carrying out simple tasks of daily living. Similarly, patients may have difficulties with the production of language which are very disabling. The earliest language skills to be lost are often those of language production, and affected people develop what is called *nominal aphasia* where they are unable to name things. Initially the individual will be unable to name less commonly used words (often known as low-frequency words). An example would be a watch-strap buckle or minute hand on the watch face. This progresses to a loss of commonly used (high-frequency) words such that the patient may be no longer able to name the watch itself. One serious implication of these neurological deficits is that it becomes increasingly difficult for carers to communicate with the patient, who develops combined loss of both comprehension and expression.

Other difficulties include epilepsy, urinary incontinence and both depressive and psychotic symptoms, such as hallucinations and delusions. Patients often have labile moods, rapidly switching from euphoria, with laughter and smiles, to tearfulness or anger. Behavioural disturbance ranges from aimless wandering, restlessness and aggressive outbursts to complete inertia. In the latter stages movement becomes slower with muscular rigidity and difficulty with walking, often with an unsteady gait.

All this has an impact on the person's life and general functioning and there is often a marked decline in social and interpersonal skills. Patients may be neither aware of their surroundings nor able to recognize and know who they are with. Prosopagnosia, the inability to recognize faces, and an inability to remember faces can be most distressing for relatives. Community mental health workers will often be a vital point of contact for such carers and their provision of support for carers is of paramount importance.

Vascular dementia

Vascular dementia is also common in the elderly. The underlying pathological finding, regardless of cause, is that of narrowing of the arterial blood vessels. 'Wear and tear' on arteries is associated with narrowing and 'hardening' as the vessel wall loses its elasticity. Consequently the vessel is unable to dilate and supply an adequate volume of blood to the tissues. This leads to vascular insufficiency, by which it is meant that the tissues receive neither an adequate blood supply nor a sufficient oxygen supply. Without oxygen, which the tissues need for vital metabolic processes, cell death occurs. In the brain such cellular death can cause dementia, as brain cells, once dead, cannot regrow. It is more common in men than women, which may have more to do with social factors such as smoking rather than the more obvious biological factors which have been implicated, such as the protective effects of oestrogens. The term 'vascular dementia' covers a range of disorders which are the result of vascular disease, whether this be due to a single stroke (blood clot or haemorrhage in the brain), or repeated 'ministrokes' – sometimes referred to as multi-infarct dementia. Important aetiological factors include those generally known to cause vascular disease, for example smoking, hypertension, diabetes and hypercholesterolaemia (raised cholesterol levels in the blood).

The main differences between Alzheimer's disease and vascular dementias are that the latter often have a sudden onset and progress in a stepwise fashion as a consequence of further abrupt episodes. This is in contrast to the steady deterioration seen in Alzheimer's dementia. In addition, it is said that insight remains preserved until a later stage of the disease in patients with vascular dementia. However, this is an oversimplification since the two conditions often occur at the same time.

Case vignette 5.2
Brian, a 74-year-old retired coal merchant, was brought to see his
general practitioner by his daughter who had cared for him since his
wife's death 2 years previously. Despite having chronic obstructive
airways disease he had remained relatively active both physically and
mentally until 3 months prior to consultation. Although he was
unable to walk far before becoming breathless his daughter would
drive him to the British Legion Club twice a week where he would
chat with other ex-servicemen and enjoy a game of cards and a pipe
of tobacco. Brian had noticed that over the last few months he had
become increasingly forgetful and his companions at the British
Legion had remarked that he was winning at cards less often than
previously. Brian's daughter had also expressed some concern about
her father and gave a history that his difficulties dated from an
episode 3 months previously when he had complained of dizzy spells.
At that time he had also collapsed at home and had been taken to
hospital in an ambulance. After a brief admission he was discharged
and it was felt that he had suffered a mild stroke.

His confusion worsened, particularly at night, although he did have
lucid moments during the day. Since then he had developed a mild
left-sided weakness but was still able to care for himself with a little
help from his daughter. However, over the following weeks he would
often appear perplexed and confused and his daughter noted that this
was usually worse at night. A cognitive assessment showed mild
impairment and it was felt that the most likely cause was a vascular
dementia. He was started on aspirin 75 mg once a day and advised to
stop smoking.

He continued to deteriorate and his daughter found it increasingly
difficult to care for him at home, particularly when he started to
wander at night. The community mental health worker and the
general practitioner were able to provide support and advice. The
community nurse arranged to visit regularly to monitor his mental
state and to give his daughter an opportunity to vent some of her
frustrations. In addition the district nurse was able to visit twice a
week to help Brian have a bath.

Over the following months his condition worsened in a stepwise
fashion and he became incontinent of urine. It was decided that his
daughter needed extra help and arrangements were made for a home
help to visit three times a week and a laundry service provided.
Despite this Brian became increasingly difficult to manage, would
wander, particularly at night, and on occasions he would lash out
aggressively at his carers. It was decided that further pharma-
cological treatment was appropriate and a low-dose neuroleptic was
prescribed (thioridazine 25 mg three times daily). This helped to
reduce his agitation and night wandering, cutting down the risk of
self-harm as well as making it easier for his carers to manage.

Brian's condition later deteriorated and one month after being started on thioridazine it was necessary to increase the night-time dose to 50 mg. This intervention helped ensure relatively restful nights for both Brian and his daughter, although with advancing disease, periods of residential respite care had to be arranged. He died at home 30 months after his dementia was first diagnosed.

Drug treatment of dementias

Drug treatments of dementias fall into two broad categories:

- those aimed at treatment of the underlying cause with the aim of arresting or reversing the changes in brain structure or function
- those aimed at symptom relief, and moderation of behavioural difficulties.

The first category will be influenced by the nature and cause of the dementia. Some important treatments are briefly outlined below.

In the early 1980s studies were published which suggested that the progression of Alzheimer's disease could be slowed by administering a combination of a drug called tacrine (or tetrahydroaminoacridine) and lecithin (Eagger *et al.*, 1992). This and subsequent studies showed that not only was deterioration halted, but in some cases an actual improvement could occur in the cognitive functioning of Alzheimer patients taking this drug combination. Unfortunately, not all subsequent replication studies have succeeded in showing this therapeutic benefit, although they have confirmed some of the significant adverse effects such as hepatitis. Ultimately this has led to a situation where the routine use of tacrine in clinical practice is prevented by the fact that it has not been granted a licence, although more recently a similar drug, donepezil, has been licensed for use in mild to moderate Alzheimer's disease. The theory behind these particular treatments rests on the cholinergic theory of memory impairment. Acetylcholine (ACh) is an important neurotransmitter or brain messenger (see Chapter 2) and experimental evidence has shown the following:

- The concentration of ACh is reduced in the brains of patients with dementia, who also have reduced concentration of enzymes involved in the production of ACh.
- Some drugs used in the treatment of patients with movement disorders specifically block or oppose the action of ACh and these drugs have been found to cause memory impairment in those who use them.

So the evidence points to ACh as having a central role in the biochemistry of memory impairment. Tacrine and donepezil act by inhibiting the enzymes that break down ACh and consequently tend to increase the overall levels of ACh in the brain. Lecithin is a precursor of ACh and maximizes its production. These two drugs therefore have complementary actions and increase the total amount of ACh available.

Case vignette 5.3
Chloe, a 68-year-old woman with Alzheimer's disease, lived with her husband in a bungalow. She had been experiencing increasing difficulty with her memory over the preceding year. Initially she was slightly absent-minded but her forgetfulness gradually worsened such that she was not able to remember what she had just done or what had just been said to her. Communication with her husband was necessarily impaired. In addition she developed problems dressing and found that she was unable to continue with the household tasks that had been a part of her daily routine for so many years. As Chloe's husband was himself unwell with angina he found it increasingly difficult to cope with the change in his wife. The couple were referred by their general practitioner to the local hospital which was a teaching hospital. In the Academic Department of Psychiatry for the Elderly a study was in progress comparing patients on standard treatments with patients treated with tacrine. Chloe was entered into the study with her husband's consent and randomly allocated to one of the treatment groups. In fact she was allocated to the group receiving tacrine plus lecithin. The medication was given three times a day, and the size of each dose was gradually increased from 25 mg to 150 mg.

Initially Chloe experienced mild nausea and headache but this seemed to resolve gradually after the first week. In view of the risk of liver toxicity associated with tacrine the psychiatrist in charge of her care ensured that a blood test was undertaken regularly every 2 weeks to monitor Chloe's hepatic function. Fortunately Chloe's community mental health worker was able to collect the blood sample since he made regular calls to monitor her progress, as well as being able to perform venepuncture. After 3 months on tacrine, cognitive testing undertaken in the local hospital by neuropsychologists showed a mild but significant improvement in Chloe's mental functioning. Perhaps what was more important was the apparent halt in the progression of the dementia rather than the actual improvement, since the improvement was only detected by using sophisticated cognitive tests. The benefit was also obvious to the community nurse and to Chloe's husband, who had noticed that there had been a slowing down of the rate of deterioration particularly with regard to problems with small everyday tasks and communication. Unfortunately after 4 months on the treatment Chloe's liver function started to deteriorate, although she herself remained asymptomatic. Initially this was monitored more closely with no alteration to the dose, but with evidence of increasingly abnormal liver function, it was decided to stop the tacrine before she developed significant and potentially irreversible hepatic damage. Follow-up showed that withdrawal of tacrine led to a gradual return of her liver function to normal. Sadly, her dementia continued to progress and her mental condition deteriorated.

In the case of *multi-infarct dementia* (MID), any drug that prevents the progression of advancing vascular disease deserves attention. The main drug treatment is aspirin, given on a once daily basis at a dose of 75 mg (a lower dose than that used routinely for pain relief). Aspirin is a thrombolytic agent (i.e. it reduces the clotting of blood platelets) and thereby reduces the incidence of adverse vascular events in an individual, for example by reducing the number of 'ministrokes'. Similarly, any drug that is effective in the treatment of hypertension (high blood pressure) is also valuable in the treatment of MID. Antihypertensives are drugs that lower blood pressure. There are many of these, ranging from drugs such as frusemide, which also acts as a diuretic, through to propranolol and nifedipine. It is beyond the scope of this book to examine these drugs in detail, but it is relevant to point out that some antihypertensives, of which reserpine is the best-known example but which now is seldom used, are clearly established as causing depression. The newer drugs are less likely to do this, although propranolol has also been implicated when given in large doses.

Multi-infarct dementia is also common in patients with diabetes who are at risk of developing blood vessel disease and damage to capillaries. This damage, referred to as microangiopathy, can be limited by good diabetic control, and for this reason, successful diabetic regimens from the outset of the illness pay dividends for the future by reducing the incidence of dementing conditions in later life. Other non-drug treatments are also helpful in the treatment of patients with MID, including help in stopping smoking, and advice about healthier diet. The earlier these regimens can be instigated the better, both with regard to treatment of MID and its prevention.

Drug treatment of behavioural problems

All the dementias, regardless of the underlying cause and differences in specific symptomatology, have certain features in common. Consequently there are general approaches to management which can be useful in most people who are affected. The following problems are amenable to drug treatments:

- Behavioural abnormalities – agitation, wandering, restlessness, irritability and aggressive outbursts, insomnia.
- Depressive symptoms – low mood, labile mood, disturbed sleep pattern, anorexia.
- Psychotic symptoms – delusions, hallucinations.

Patients with dementia often develop behavioural problems. Major tranquillizers are expedient and remain the mainstay of medical treatment but, in general, psychological approaches are preferred and should probably be the first line of treatment. However, when there is no response to behavioural or cognitive methods the clinicians and carers may have to resort to drug treatments. Agitation and restlessness in those with chronic brain syndromes is common and low-dose neuroleptics can be an appropriate and effective choice of treatment. Although these drugs are 'antipsychotic' they are often effective as sedatives in doses lower than those for the treatment of psychosis (see also Chapters 6 and 8). The following vignettes illustrate how these drugs can be successfully used in patients with dementia, but also illustrate some of the drawbacks.

Case vignette 5.4

Dennis was a 71-year-old man with vascular dementia. He was living with and being cared for by his daughter and her family. When he sustained yet another stroke there was a marked deterioration in his behaviour. Rather than the placid, withdrawn man that he had been before, Dennis became intensely restless, wandered around the house, and often seemed unable to sit still. His daughter was increasingly worried that he would wander off and either get lost or be run over, and she put extra locks on the inside of the doors within the house. She began to feel that she could never turn her back for a moment lest her father got into trouble and injured himself. Dennis's grandchildren also began to find his behaviour distressing and the youngest, only 9 years old, found his agitated pacing and mumbling frightening.

At times Dennis's restlessness seemed to peak, and at these times – usually in the evening or at night – he would become irritable and on occasions physically violent. His daughter was becoming worn down by the struggles that developed whenever she tried to wash or feed him, and the grandchildren showed fearfulness and tended to stay in their bedrooms to avoid him. The district nurse provided psychological support to Dennis's daughter as well as practical assistance with bathing. However, things continued to worsen. The community mental health worker assessed his mental state and decided to inform Dennis's general practitioner about his recent deterioration and suggest that it would now be appropriate to begin some form of tranquillizer medication.

The general practitioner agreed and Dennis was given a prescription of promazine 25 mg three times daily. Unfortunately this made no difference and the restlessness persisted. The dose was therefore increased to 50 mg three times daily, but again with little demonstrable benefit. Since promazine has only modest calming or sedative effects (as opposed to its marked ability to cause drowsiness) it was decided to change the medication to droperidol 5 mg three times daily. This was extremely effective at reducing Dennis's agitation but unfortunately because of its parkinsonian effects, the drug caused him to become stiff and wooden in his posture and movements. To combat this a compromise was reached by reducing the dose of droperidol to 5 mg twice daily and adding the antiparkinsonian drug procyclidine 5 mg twice daily. This was both enough to remove the parkinsonian symptoms and reduce his restlessness. It was possible to achieve this balance because of the ability of the community mental health worker (a nurse) to visit regularly and monitor both beneficial and adverse effects of the drug.

Wilson's disease

Wilson's disease is a rare inherited disorder of copper metabolism. It leads to increased and damaging levels of copper in the blood stream and consequently in a number of important organs including the brain. If untreated it is fatal. Clinical features range from depression to dementia. The most common presentation is with symptoms of behavioural disturbance, personality dysfunction, depression or intellectual impairment. Not surprisingly in view of this wide range of presenting symptoms it is a difficult disease to diagnose and research suggests that as many as 20% of patients are initially seen by a psychiatrist before the correct diagnosis is made. Once the disorder has been contemplated, a simple blood test which measures the level of copper in the blood stream can verify the diagnosis (caeruloplasmin level).

Management of these patients involves not only treating the cause but also symptomatic relief. Primary treatment is aimed at reducing the level of circulating copper by dietary restriction and the use of chelating agents such as D-penicillamine. A chelating agent is a drug that is able to 'mop up' excess amounts of metallic ions such as copper with its own molecular structure acting as a 'sponge'. The drug concerned can then be eliminated from the body instead of causing damage in the liver and kidneys.

Parkinson's disease

Parkinson's disease is a common neurological disease which affects 1 in every 200 people over the age of 70 years. It is in essence a disturbance of movement and is characterized by a triad of symptoms – tremor, rigidity of the limbs and slowing of voluntary movements (bradykinesia). Most mental health workers are probably familiar with the typical clinical symptoms of a patient with Parkinson's disease, because these symptoms are simulated almost exactly by the parkinsonian side-effects of anti-psychotic drugs. However, the latter condition is often described as 'pseudoparkinsonism' because there are some differences, including the symptom of motor restlessness (akathisia) which is rare in parkinsonism but very common in the drug-induced type (see Chapter 6).

Almost all patients with parkinsonism, however caused, walk with a stuttering, shuffling gait, tend not to swing their arms fully, and are prone to falls. Their faces are usually mask-like and expressionless, and their speech slurred and monotonous. Fine movements are difficult and handwriting often becomes small and difficult to read (micrographia). This slowness and paucity of movement and expression contrast starkly with a coarse tremor which typically affects the hands (pill-rolling tremor) and head (titubation). The tremor is most noticeable when the limbs and body are at rest, is improved by voluntary movement and is made worse by anxiety.

The drug treatment of Parkinson's disease was revolutionized in 1967 with the discovery of levodopa (L-dopa). The excitement surrounding this discovery included the administration of L-dopa to patients with a postencephalitic form of Parkinson's disease (encephalitis lethargica), and interested readers are referred to a fuller account by Oliver Sachs (1990), and the film based on it (*Awakenings*).

The discovery of the therapeutic effects of L-dopa helped to unravel some of the mysteries of the underlying disease process in Parkinson's disease, namely those of the biochemical abnormalities. The most likely explanation is that there is a deficiency of dopamine nerve cells in a specific part of the brain called the substantia nigra. This part, which derives its name from its black pigmentation, is found in the midbrain, the area connecting the cerebral hemispheres with the brain stem and spinal cord; in other words it is a central part of the brain not only anatomically but also functionally, since it is an area connecting nerve pathways together rather like a telephone exchange. Dopamine is an important transmitter substance, enabling messages to be passed from one nerve to another (see Chapter 2). It is widely distributed throughout the nervous system but its function within the substantia nigra is related to the control of movement. This area of the brain is concerned with the general co-ordination of movement and allows muscles to operate in a smooth and controlled fashion. Reduced function, as in Parkinson's disease, interferes with this procedure and all complex movements become clumsy and badly co-ordinated.

Levodopa is a precursor of dopamine. Following its absorption into the body it passes into the central nervous system where it is converted to dopamine. (Dopamine itself is not an effective drug since, owing to its biochemical nature, it is poorly absorbed from the gut and only passes into the brain in tiny quantities.) Levodopa itself has similar problems and the total amount that passes into the brain is small in comparison with the total dose. Most of the drug remains in the general circulation (outside the brain) where it has no therapeutic effect, but where it can cause troublesome adverse effects mainly through conversion to dopamine. Consequently L-dopa usually needs to be administered together with another drug (e.g. carbidopa, benserazide) which prevents conversion of L-dopa to dopamine outside the brain. It is also important for each mental health worker to realize that L-dopa can produce psychotic symptoms in some patients and that it is generally avoided in psychiatric patients because of this tendency.

AIDS and HIV infection

Acquired immune deficiency syndrome (AIDS) results from infection with the human immunodeficiency virus (HIV), also called the human lymphotrophic virus type III (HLTV-III). The syndrome has been widely reported in both the popular and the scientific press. Although the first case in the USA was reported by the Centers for Disease Control (CDC) in Atlanta in 1981, it is likely that the disease was present much earlier but not identified. The infectious agent is a lentivirus or slow virus and is transmitted from person to person via the transfer of bodily fluids. The main reported methods of transmission include sexual intercourse (whether between male homosexual or heterosexual partners) and via the reception of infected blood or blood products. The latter route has been most important in injecting drug abusers using non-sterile, shared, 'dirty' needles and patients with haemophilia receiving factor VIII (before the advent of HIV screening). Although the virus has been isolated in blood, vaginal secretions, semen, saliva, tears and breast milk, there have to date been no recorded cases linked to infection via tears or saliva. Transmission from mother to baby (vertical transmission) can occur in utero or as a result of birth trauma.

Infection may be asymptomatic or associated with a mild flu-like illness. The development of antibodies (or seroconversion) occurs over the following weeks or months. The virus multiplies by incorporating viral genetic material, also known as ribonucleic acid or RNA, into the patient's cells. The patient's cells are known as the 'host cells' since they provide a home for the viral material. This viral material alters the structure and composition of the host cell genetic material (deoxyribonucleic acid, DNA) and the genetic template of the cell becomes changed. Since it is the genetic template that tells our cells what to do and what proteins to make, this has a profound effect on the functioning of the host cell. Cells start producing abnormal proteins and a variety of cell processes are upset. One of the consequences is that the immune system malfunctions and this is characterized by a reduced population of T cells (white cells involved in fighting infection). The ability of the infected person to resist infection (and cancer) is consequently impaired.

Clinical symptoms of illness may not occur for years since the virus has a long latent period. When they do occur, clinical manifestations include tumours such as the much-reported (and previously rare) Kaposi's sarcoma and opportunistic infections such as pneumonia caused by less common organisms such as fungi. These infections are called 'opportunistic' since the infecting organism multiplies because it has the opportunity to become established, whereas normally it would be seen off by the body's immune defences. Death when it occurs is often the result of infection in an individual with a severely impaired immune system.

The psychological manifestations of infection with HIV are many and varied. What has become clear is that the virus is 'neurotropic', in other words it specifically infects nervous tissue such as the brain. Virus particles have been isolated from the cerebrospinal fluid and from brain tissue itself. It is now apparent that some of the psychiatric manifestations of HIV infection can be directly attributed to infection of brain tissue rather than to immunosuppressant effects. Psychiatric complications include:

- Functional illnesses such as 'AIDS panic' (common after initial diagnosis), adjustment disorders, depressive disorders with both somatic and psychotic features, and obsessional disorder.
- Organic illnesses including encephalitis, meningitis, tumours within the nervous system, vascular problems, specific nerve dysfunction and dementia (King, 1993).

There are few drug treatments specific to AIDS and their efficacy is questionable. Zidovudine (azidothymidine, AZT) (Retrovir) has been used extensively to try to halt the disease process. Although it is of limited value alone, it has now been shown to delay the progress of the disease when used initially with other drugs (the DELTA trial) (Delta Coordination Committee, 1996).

Huntington's chorea

Huntington's chorea is an inherited disorder. After a normal childhood and early adult life patients develop the characteristic symptoms when they are 40–60 years old. Clinical symptoms include the following:

- Memory loss, disorientation and general intellectual deterioration are characteristic.
- Progressive abnormality of movement develops, including jerking (choreiform) and writhing (athetoid) involuntary movements.
- Anxiety and depression are common.
- Psychotic symptoms (delusions and hallucinations) occur frequently.
- Gradual damage to muscles leads to problems with swallowing and feeding, and incontinence.

We now have a much greater understanding of the nature of the underlying genetic abnormality in Huntington's disease. However, there are as yet no specific drug treatments for this condition. Some success has been reported with tetrabenazine. This drug was initially introduced as an antipsychotic but has since been shown to have more useful functions treating movement disorders such as tardive dyskinesia (associated with use of antipsychotic medication) (see Chapter 6) and the writhing and jerking movements of Huntington's disease. Tetrabenazine reduces the amount of amine neurotransmitter substance in some nerve endings and this is thought to be its mode of action in the treatment of movement disorder. Benzodiazepines may also reduce the abnormal movements to some extent.

Multiple sclerosis

Multiple or disseminated sclerosis (MS) is a progressive disease affecting the nervous system. Some nerve cells are surrounded by a protective casing of fatty material called myelin. This myelin is wrapped around the nerve cells to form a sheath which helps to speed up the transmission of nerve impulses. Consequently myelinated fibres conduct nerve impulses quickly and unmyelinated fibres (without the sheath of myelin) conduct impulses slowly. In MS myelin is destroyed and the nerve cells are stripped down to the basic fibres. It is not clear why this occurs, and a number of theories of aetiology have been put forward with suggestions ranging from a reaction to acute viral infections, to genetic causation. The nervous system can be 'hit' at any spot but commonly the optic nerve and the cerebellum (the brain's balance centre) are affected early. It is also common for the patient to have multiple sites of demyelination and for these sites to vary over time. Patients often present with painful eyes and impaired vision, with a variety of neurological disturbances depending on the areas affected. These include weakness, sensory loss, unsteady gait, tremor and slurred speech.

Drug therapy in patients with MS is based on treatment with steroids. There are a number of deleterious effects of steroids including weight gain and osteoporosis as well as psychiatric disturbance such as psychosis. Psychiatric complications are common and include mood disturbance, personality change and cognitive impairment. The most common psychiatric complication is the development of a depressive illness and it is likely that these episodes of depression represent an integral part of the disease process and not only the psychological response of the patient to chronic illness and disability. There may be euphoria in more advanced cases which appears quite inappropriate to the affected person's severe disability.

In depressed patients with MS, conventional antidepressants can be very useful. People with MS are an extremely important group in whom depression may go undetected. It is vital that those involved in the care of such patients do not forget to look out for the signs and symptoms of depression.

Syphilis

Although much less common now than in the nineteenth century, syphilis does still occur and indeed since the advent of AIDS has been increasing in frequency in some groups. Syphilis follows infection with *Treponema pallidum*, a micro-organism called a spirochaete, usually transmitted through sexual contact (although it can be transferred to the fetus through the placenta). Traditionally the stages of the disease have been described as primary, secondary and tertiary. Primary syphilis refers to the time shortly after infection, which may be subclinical or characterized by genital chancres or ulcers. Secondary syphilis refers to the development of a skin rash approximately 2–3 months after infection. This rash is often associated with fever, general malaise and sometimes blood anaemia (reduced number of red blood cells). Tertiary syphilis refers to the long-term complications that arise years after inadequately treated infection. Such complications may affect the cardiovascular system and the central and peripheral nervous system. In the latter cases four syndromes may occur:

- Meningovascular syphilis – syphilitic involvement of the meninges or membranes lining the brain. The main features include paralysis, muscle wasting and pain due to nerve entrapment.
- Tabes dorsalis – this is due to infestation of the spinal cord with spirochaetes. The parts of the spinal cord associated with locomotion tend to be preferentially affected and the clinical symptoms and signs include an unsteady gait. Associated features include loss of sensation, particularly on the trunk.
- Localized gummata – these are lesions that may afflict any number of anatomical sites from the skin and mouth to the liver, brain and bones.
- 'General paralysis of the insane' – this is uncommon and due to widespread lesions throughout the nervous system. Clinically patients may have any number and variety of symptoms ranging from loss of

Table 5.1 *Medical conditions that can present with mental symptoms*

Organic disorder	Common presentations to mental health services	Clues to presence of organic disorder
Alcohol-induced dementia (Korsakov's psychosis, Wernicke's encephalopathy)	Mood disturbance (both mania and depression), fantastic stories that are not corroborated by others, delirium	History of long-term heavy alcohol use
Glandular fever and similar acute viral infections	Depression, fatigue (also see chronic fatigue syndrome in Chapter 9)	Recent history of flu-like illness (also including toxoplasmosis)
Post-concussional syndrome and other results of head injury (e.g. post-traumatic dementia)	Depression and anxiety	Clear onset of symptoms after single or repeated head injury (e.g. boxing)
Brain tumours	Memory loss, persistent headaches (sometimes misdiagnosed as anxiety), epileptic seizures, depression	Gradual onset of symptoms, personality change
Multiple sclerosis	Mood symptoms (both depression and mania (euphoria), excessive fatigue, confusion)	Clear evidence of loss of function (both in feeling and movement) in different parts of the body at different times
Cancer (particularly of stomach, bowel and lung)	As for brain tumour with secondaries, depression	Marked loss of weight (beyond that expected in depression), persistent physical symptoms
Autoimmune diseases, e.g. systemic lupus erythematosus (SLE)	Mood disturbance (both elevated and depressed mood and anxiety), psychotic symptoms (often as a consequence of therapy particularly linked with steroids), confusion	Not easy for the community practitioner; these diseases can affect all systems of the body, the patient generally looks unwell and can present different mental and physical features at different times
Endocrine disorders (e.g. hypothyroidism)	Mood disturbance, (depression, anxiety)	Change in appearance, intolerance of cold

See Trimble (1988) for fuller information.

Table 5.2 *Drug and physical treatments that can cause mental symptoms*

Drug or physical treatment	Common presentation of symptoms	Explanation
Repeated ECT administration	Persistent memory loss, cognitive impairment, apathy	Loss of brain cells following trauma during administration of treatment (not yet convincingly demonstrated)
Some hypotensive drugs (to reduce blood pressure) such as reserpine, debrisoquine, bethanidine, propranolol (in high dosage), atenolol	Depression, fatigue, suicidal ideation (usually indistinguishable from other depressive syndromes)	Reduction in amine levels in the central nervous system (see Chapter 8)
Benzodiazepines and other sedative drugs (e.g. alcohol, chlormethiazole)	Depression, panic, delirium, epileptic seizures	Occurs after sudden withdrawal of drug in people who are dependent on it (thought to be due to deficiency of gamma-aminobutyric acid, GABA)
Tricyclic antidepressants	Panic, anxiety	Much less common than with benzodiazepine withdrawal, but can occur when high doses of drug are stopped suddenly. Can be avoided by gradual reduction
Digoxin, barbiturates, levodopa, aspirin, benzodiazepines, lithium and many others	Delirium, confusion, disorientation, oversedation, cognitive impairment	Usually follows deliberate or accidental overdose of drug, and symptoms are those demonstrated when the drug reaches toxic levels in the brain

Table 5.2 (*continued*)

Antipsychotic drugs	Depression and 'pseudodepression' due to misinterpretation of symptoms	Depression may be consequence of dopamine blockade; pseudodepression more common when the limited movement and facial features of parkinsonian symptoms are misinterpreted
Caffeine (in coffee, tea and cola), antiasthmatic drugs such as salbutamol (tablets or inhaler), terbutaline, decongestants (e.g. ephedrine, pseudoephedrine, phenylephrine)	Panic, headache, tension, tremor, generalized anxiety, insomnia, mood variability	These drugs are stimulants and can therefore create anxiety symptoms. Their involvement is often recognized by detecting the relationship between giving the drug and the development of symptoms shortly afterwards

sensation and power to psychiatric symptoms such as psychosis and depression.

Prevention of the primary infection is the optimum intervention, but if infection does occur, patients should receive a full 14-day course of procaine penicillin. Should complications arise suggesting that the primary infection was inadequately treated a further course of antibiotics is necessary, and should be given for a longer period of 3 weeks.

Promoting awareness of organic mental disorders

It is in the field of organic disorders that community mental health workers can often feel at a disadvantage because of limitations in their training. However, although it is clearly inappropriate for workers who have no training in general medicine to attempt to encompass all the conditions that can present in psychiatric form and therefore be encountered by the community mental health worker, it is very helpful to be aware of medical conditions that may cause mental symptoms. Tables 5.1 and 5.2 list the most important conditions that can present with, or are complicated by, psychiatric symptoms. These are separated into conditions that are intrinsic to the disease concerned and those that are consequences of the treatment for that condition, mainly by drugs ('iatrogenic' or literally doctor-made, as they would not have occurred without the treatment).

The community mental health worker can be aware of these possibilities by taking a full medical and drug history. It is particularly important to write down the names of any drugs taken by the patients, preferably by checking the names and dosage of each drug from supplies held in the patient's possession. Even if these do not at first appear to be helpful, further discussion of the problems in the multidisciplinary team should help to establish whether there is a medical condition that could be at least partly responsible for the mental symptoms presenting for treatment.

A large part of successful clinical practice is knowing when and where to turn for help outside one's immediate clinical sphere of reference. It is in the field of organic mental disorders that this skill is often exercised most importantly. We hope this chapter has helped to set a few ground rules for this.

Further reading

King, M. B. (1993). *AIDS, HIV and Mental Health*. Cambridge University Press.
Lishman, W. A. (1987). *Organic Psychiatry*, 2nd edn. Oxford: Blackwell.
Sacks, O. (1985). *Awakenings*. London: Picador.
Trimble, M. R. (1988). *Biological Psychiatry*. Chichester: John Wiley.

6

Drugs and community treatment of schizophrenia

What is schizophrenia?

Schizophrenia is the name given to a group of serious mental disorders which may affect as many as 1% of the population at some time in their lives. More than most types of mental disorder, schizophrenia can disrupt every aspect of a person's life. There are many theories about what causes schizophrenia, but although much can be done to help, so far none of the theories has led to ways of preventing or curing the condition.

Schizophrenia is characterized by:

- particular disturbances of perception and experience (*positive* or *first rank symptoms*)
- disorganized thinking, feeling and behaviour
- reduced emotional and verbal expression and communication (*negative* or *defect symptoms*)
- a tendency for the condition to endure for years, often for life, albeit with relapses and remissions.

The major effect that schizophrenia has on the way people think, feel and behave undermines their ability to make and keep relationships, and to function effectively in a competitive society. Not surprisingly, schizophrenia can cause untold misery, not only for the people directly affected by the disorder, but for their friends and families as well. The fear and mistrust shown by society towards people with serious mental disorders such as schizophrenia can add stigma and material hardship to the self-neglect and emotional impoverishment which are often part of the illness.

Is schizophrenia a myth?

There are many puzzling aspects of schizophrenia, and because the condition can have devastating and potentially stigmatizing effects, some people have wished to deny that it exists at all. Following the writings of radical psychiatrists like Thomas Szasz and R. D. Laing, at one time it was fashionable to view the person labelled as schizophrenic as being a victim of society in general, and of families and doctors in particular. The notion that they might be suffering from a mental illness was vigorously refuted.

It was believed that physical or psychological abuse or persecution might render a sensitive person 'schizophrenic'. Following from this, it was sometimes claimed that people with schizophrenia were somehow suffering on behalf of other people, or undergoing psychological experiences which amounted to spiritual 'voyages of discovery' from which the rest of society could benefit. This quasi-mystical view of schizophrenia was connected with the use of psychotomimetic drugs such as LSD and mescaline which grew in the 1950s and 1960s like the 'magic mushrooms' which were being ingested in large quantities. This interest followed much older religious rituals and practices of peoples like the indigenous Mexicans as described by influential authors such as Aldous Huxley, and later Timothy Leary. The 'antipsychiatry movement' strongly opposed the idea that medical treatments such as psychotropic medication might help a condition like schizophrenia. Antipsychotic drugs were condemned as instruments of repression and control ('chemical straitjackets') at the same time as the benefits of psychotomimetic drugs were being extolled.

It is understandable that those who have had personal experience of such an unpleasant condition as schizophrenia should wish to abolish it. However, many of the antischizophrenia polemicists were – and still are – 'armchair clinicians' who can afford to keep a safe distance from the harsh realities of mental illness. Whilst critical examination of the limitations of the concept of schizophrenia is useful as a stimulus to improve knowledge and treatment, to argue that schizophrenia is not a respectable subject for a scientific or clinical endeavour could mean that millions of affected people would suffer from neglect, just as they used to in the past.

Integral to the *illness concept* of schizophrenia is the need to help through tried and tested treatments such as medication and particular types of psychotherapy. Also, where applicable, the concept of mental illness in general and of schizophrenia in particular excuses people from total responsibility for inappropriate or criminal behaviour committed under the influence of symptoms such as hallucinations and delusions.

Illness and psychosis

Schizophrenia is regarded as a mental illness by psychiatrists (and, we hope, by all community mental health workers) because it causes suffering and disability, and puts the affected person at a clear social and biological disadvantage or handicap. The term 'illness' does not necessarily imply the presence of physical disease, although ever since the condition was first described at the beginning of the nineteenth century, it has been believed that there is something wrong with the brain in schizophrenia. For many years, extensive investigations found nothing to substantiate this belief, but evidence has gradually accumulated confirming that schizophrenia is indeed likely to be due to subtle abnormalities of brain structure and function (Bebbington and McGuffin, 1988; Crow, 1991).

Schizophrenia is classified as a psychosis, by which is meant a serious mental disorder characterized by wide-ranging and sometimes dramatic disturbances in people's perceptions, thoughts, feelings and behaviour. In addition, and more enigmatically, psychosis always seems to involve some impairment in a person's ability to make judgements about external reality. Associated with this, there is often a serious interference with a person's sense of themselves and their relationships to other people, and their self-care and sense of self-preservation are also often undermined. Most strikingly, a person with a psychosis is likely to experience false perceptions (hallucinations) and develop false beliefs (delusions) which are often bizarre and terrifying, and in which they maintain unshakeable conviction despite all the evidence to the contrary. Hallucinations are perceptions of sensory stimulation, e.g. hearing voices when no stimulation is actually occurring. There may be little or no understanding on the part of the affected person that there is something wrong with them, rather than with the outside world, and this loss of contact with reality or insight is a striking and necessary feature of psychosis (Table 6.1). We all can experience hallucinations and false beliefs at various times of our lives, but provided we have an awareness of the unusualness of these experiences, we cannot be said to suffer from a psychosis.

Table 6.1   *Defining psychoses*

Psychoses are serious mental illnesses involving abnormalities of:

- perception (e.g. hallucinations)
- thought content and form (e.g. delusions, incoherence of speech)
- mood (e.g. depression, elation, blunting)
- behaviour (e.g. extreme over- or underactivity, and repetitive, bizarre or violent actions).

Additional features:

- loss of insight and contact with reality
- impaired interpersonal relationships and social adjustment
- impaired self-care and self-preservation.

There are four main types of psychosis, which all tend to overlap and may be difficult to tell apart (Figure 6.1). Some types of psychosis are associated with obvious disorders of the brain such as occurs after head injury or with the development of a tumour, or in various types of epilepsy (Table 6.2). It is this common association between known brain disorders and psychotic phenomena that suggests to us that even when there is no obvious brain disorder or disease, psychotic symptoms are probably reflecting underlying brain dysfunction. It must be stressed, however, that the mere existence of hallucinations and strange beliefs is insufficient to qualify for a description of psychosis, and these phenomena can certainly exist without anything being obviously wrong with the brain.

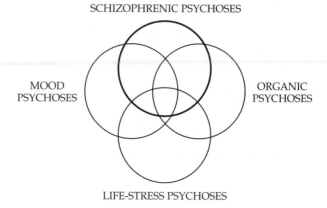

Figure 6.1   *The four main types of psychosis overlap in terms of clinical features and possible underlying causes*

Table 6.2   *Organic psychoses*

Organic psychoses are strongly associated with:

- physical or chemical damage to brain cells
- abnormal brain development or functioning
- degeneration of brain cells
- impairment of 'cognitive functions' such as attention, memory and intellect, sometimes resulting in disorientation and confusion and clouding of consciousness when alertness is reduced
- presence of drugs or toxins

Non-organic or 'functional' psychoses, which include schizophrenia, are mainly distinguished from organic conditions by exclusion, that is, they are *not* associated with obvious brain damage or disease, or with drugs or toxins, although if any of these are involved later, they may make the original condition worse.

Although it now seems likely that, even in functional psychosis, there are subtle but important changes in brain structure and function, these are not obvious or necessary for making a diagnosis. This depends entirely on what people do and say, and how the disorder progresses or recovers. Unlike the situation with organic psychosis, cognitive functions such as attention and memory are often, on superficial examination, apparently normal, and the level of arousal and consciousness is rarely impaired in the functional psychoses except in unusual states such as catatonic stupor (a state of complete non-responsiveness in which the person is fully conscious and awake). Where there are noticeable disturbances in attention and memory, this can often be explained by the presence of distressing psychological symptoms, or by a lack of motivation to take part in psychological testing. However, an important clinical advance in recent years has been the recognition that subtle cognitive impairments may be crucial in functional psychoses such as schizophrenia.

Misunderstandings of other people's feelings, motives or intentions, and both over- and underestimation of dangers and risks may, for example, explain paranoid feelings, social withdrawal and poor social skills, as well as apparently irrational attacks of anxiety and depression, aggression or self-harming behaviour. Some theorists believe that the difficulties in appreciating the mental states of others which often occur in people with schizophrenia is linked to abnormal functioning of particular parts of the brain (Frith and Done, 1989; Liddle, 1993). This may lead not only to problems with interpersonal relationships and communication, but also to important abnormalities in feeling, perception and thinking. Thus being abnormally unaware of one's own wishes, intensions and decisions to act, may result in some of the false perceptions and beliefs that underlie schizophrenia. The same lack of awareness of one's own mental state may lead to an apparent lack of feeling and expression.

Other theorists have argued that the cognitive abnormalities which may be central to the state of schizophrenia result in 'irrelevant features of ordinary things appearing more important than the whole object or situation' (World Health Organization, 1992), or in other words, not being able to 'see the forest for the trees'. If the immediate environment has much more impact on the person with schizophrenia than awareness of their own mental state, reductions in stimulation (boredom) or over-stimulation (stress) will be difficult to cope with. This was exactly what was observed many years ago when researchers realized the impact of the hospital environment on people with schizophrenia living in mental hospital wards (Goffman, 1961).

The symptoms and syndromes of schizophrenia

Although schizophrenia is certainly not a myth, there are arguments against it being a distinct mental illness. Despite the accumulating evidence that known brain disorders can cause a condition like schizophrenia, and that in some cases of 'ordinary' schizophrenia disordered brain structure and function can now be demonstrated, in the main it is still only possible to make the diagnosis on the basis of what people say and do. Not surprisingly in the absence of an 'acid test' for diagnosis, there may be a considerable uncertainty and lack of agreement about what actually constitutes schizophrenia in an individual case.

The term 'schizophrenia' used to be applied in a very vague and general way to any situation where a person was acting strangely, hearing voices, or professing strange and eccentric beliefs. Put simply, people whose behaviour and thinking could not be understood by 'normal' people were regarded as 'crazy' or schizophrenic. This 'dustbin' attribution theory is obviously false. Many people we cannot understand are quite rational, or, if irrational, have an understandable explanation for their odd beliefs that has nothing to do with schizophrenia. Not surprisingly perhaps, the condition defined in this way appeared to be extremely common but variable in its presentation, and from a scientific point of view, a fairly meaningless concept because of its heterogeneity. It is only when attempts are made to define the condition precisely and in a narrow, restricted sense, that it can be shown to represent a valid and reliably recognizable disorder. A 'narrow' definition of schizophrenia includes the presence of particular types of auditory hallucinations and abnormal experiences (*first rank symptoms*), all of which suggest that the person is having difficulties in identifying their thoughts, feelings and intentions as their own. Instead, some of their experiences appear to be imposed upon them from outside, and their own thoughts may appear as voices arguing or discussing their actions. Alternatively, thoughts may seem to be withdrawn or broadcast from their mind, or 'alien' thoughts may occur to them as though inserted into their brain. Their actions may also seem to be initiated or controlled by other people or outside forces rather than by their own will (passivity experiences).

In addition to these particular and extremely puzzling experiences, a person with schizophrenia may show abnormal patterns of mood, rather than any particular type of strong feeling. For example, anxiety and depression, or feelings of elation, may come and go quite suddenly with little or no apparent connection with outside circumstances. This disconnectedness or discontinuity of emotional expression is often associated with disconnected thoughts and speech, so the person may switch from one topic to another apparently without connecting links. When this disconnection of thinking becomes particularly severe, speech may be so jumbled as to be barely intelligible ('*word salad*').

At the same time, general inertia and impoverishment of thought and behaviour may insidiously develop, making the person with schizophrenia seem 'burnt out' or like a zombie, a pale shadow of their former self. This *negative syndrome* or *defect state* is the most socially disabling feature of schizophrenia, and is the aspect of the disorder that clearly distinguishes it from other kinds of mental illness. Unfortunately, it is also the aspect of schizophrenia that is least well understood and least easily helped. Although various types of drug treatment can effectively damp down false perceptions and delusional beliefs during the acute stages of the illness, and perhaps to a lesser extent help improve disorganized behaviour and incoherence of speech, negative symptoms benefit much less from drug treatment. Psychosocial treatments are most valuable here, and it is essential to adopt a holistic approach which considers the impact of the mental disorder on a person's inner life and personality, as well as on their relationships with others, and their role in society.

In the late 1970s a British psychiatrist, Tim Crow, proposed that *positive symptoms* of schizophrenia such as delusions and hallucinations were due to overactivity of systems in the brain that use dopamine as a chemical neurotransmitter. Dopamine was known to be released by drugs such as amphetamines ('speed') which could cause a type of schizophrenia after prolonged use by addicts, and blocking the effects of dopamine was apparently the main action shared by all antipsychotic drugs available at that time. In contrast, Crow suggested that the negative syndrome consisting of poverty of speech and flattening of affect was due to damage or structural change to the brain, as revealed by the recently invented CT brain scan (Crow, 1980).

Subsequent research has shown that it is unlikely that dopamine systems are actually abnormal in the brains of people with schizophrenia. It seems that the dopamine blocking effects of antipsychotic drugs are palliative rather than curative, and are affecting mechanisms in the brain which indirectly bring about an improvement in psychotic symptoms. In a similar way, the effectiveness of an aspirin for helping a headache does not mean that headaches are due to a lack of aspirin. The hypothesis that negative symptoms are always accompanied by signs of brain damage has also been refuted to some extent, but there is no doubt that Tim Crow and his theories triggered off a new wave of enthusiasm for brain research in schizophrenia.

Later clinical research in this field showed that in addition to the positive and negative syndromes of schizophrenia (now renamed *reality distortion syndrome* and *psychomotor poverty syndrome* respectively), a third *disorganization syndrome* has emerged (Liddle, 1987). The disorganization syndrome comprises thought disorder and the incongruous or disconnected emotional behaviour that occurs in schizophrenia, although less commonly than the symptoms making up the reality distortion and psychomotor poverty syndromes. All three syndromes can occur within the same individual at the same time, although the poverty syndrome tends to make a relatively late appearance, and indicates a more severe form of illness. The disorganization syndrome is next in terms of onset and severity of illness, but the reality distortion syndrome mainly dominates the clinical picture in the earlier stages of the illness. Although often severe in its immediate impact, the reality distortion syndrome is still compatible with a reasonable chance of short-term recovery and long-term remission of illness.

The boundaries of schizophrenia with normality and other mental illnesses

When narrowly defined, schizophrenia is a severe, long-term mental disorder which can be reliably identified in people from all over the world (Jablensky et al., 1992), regardless of culture, colour or creed. It is fairly distinct for example from psychoses caused by extreme stress, which are usually of sudden onset, brief in duration, and may occur in otherwise normal people, with a strong influence from cultural and social factors. The incidence of 'narrow, severe' (*nuclear*) schizophrenia is fairly constant throughout the world and therefore appears to be little influenced by differences in the physical and social environment. This would be an unusual finding for any disease or illness with environmental causes (e.g. infections), since cultural and geographical factors usually play a major role in these disorders. Rather, nuclear schizophrenia appears to be mainly genetically determined and fundamentally connected with the human condition, and presumably with the make-up of the brain.

In contrast, 'broad, mild' schizophrenia blurs into less severe forms of mental illness or personality disorders, or even into extremes of normal behaviour and experience. As a rule, 'broad, mild' schizophrenia cannot be defined so precisely or as reliably as nuclear schizophrenia. Not surprisingly, 'broad, mild' schizophrenia is more common than 'narrow, severe' schizophrenia, and the incidence probably varies by a factor of three or four across countries and cultures. The incidence, course and outcome of 'broad, mild' schizophrenia are more likely to be affected by the physical and social environment than by genetic factors. However, the dividing line between nuclear schizophrenia and milder forms of schizophrenia can also be blurred and there appears to be a hierarchy or continuum, with 'narrow, severe' schizophrenia at the top, spreading down via 'broad, mild' schizophrenia, to personality disorders and neurotic problems at the bottom. This explains a common observation that in nuclear schizophrenia the features of other conditions further down in the hierarchy are present at various times during the course of the illness (Figure 6.2).

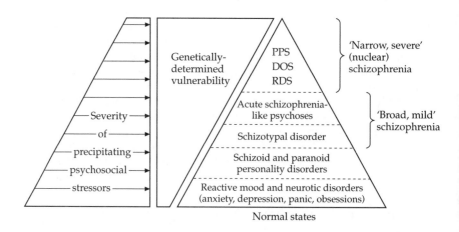

Figure 6.2   *The 'narrow, severe' – 'broad, mild' continuum concept of schizophrenia, the hierarchy of syndromes, and the relative roles of genetic and environmental (e.g. psychosocial) trigger factors. Syndromes nearer the apex of the clinical syndrome triangle are clinically more severe, but blend in with milder syndromes nearer the base of the triangle. Each syndrome in the hierarchy has some clinical features which are not shared by syndromes lower down in the hierarchy, but which are common to the more severe syndromes higher up. Genetic factors strongly determine vulnerability to the more severe syndromes, with less contribution to the more mild syndromes. In contrast, psychosocial stressors strongly influence the milder states, but are less relevant to the more severe forms of illness (DOS, disorganization syndrome; PPS, psychomotor poverty syndrome; RDS, reality distortion syndrome)*

When the condition of schizophrenia was first subjected to intensive study at the end of the nineteenth century, it was stressed that the condition usually starts early in life and often persists thereafter, albeit with fluctuations in severity over time. This is in contrast to other forms of functional psychosis, which after first flaring up, will then disappear completely, although with a tendency to recur later in life. These other types of psychotic disorder are typically associated with marked disturbances of mood such as depression or euphoria, and were dubbed *manic-depressive insanity* by Kraepelin (see Chapter 7).

Whilst this latter type of mood psychosis is often associated with hallucinations, false beliefs or delusions, and abnormal thought processes, all of these tend to be compatible or *congruent* with the disturbance in mood. For example, severely depressed people may hear voices telling them that they are sinners who deserve to die. Similarly, a person with mania, who feels expansive in mood and hyperenergetic, may develop the false belief of having superhuman powers. In contrast, although depression, elation and anxiety may all occur at various stages in schizophrenia, the false beliefs and perceptions are often out of keeping with or unrelated to the prevailing state of mood or feeling. Later in the course of schizophrenia, a person's mood may show the puzzling and characteristic 'shallowness' or 'blunting' which gives the impression that the person is no longer capable of experiencing the normal range and intensity of feeling that they had shown before becoming ill.

Although schizophrenia can be distinguished from other kinds of mental illness such as mood psychoses, there appears to be considerable overlap. Just as 'normal' people can be more or less prone to psychotic experiences and thought processes, with a continuum between what is normal at one extreme and what represents severe schizophrenia at the other (Figure 6.2), so the dividing line between schizophrenia and other kinds of psychosis can be similarly blurred. This has led to the idea of a *continuum of psychosis*, with schizophrenia representing one end of the spectrum and manic-depressive psychosis the other (Crow, 1986). In between there appears to be a range of conditions that have features of both types of disorder, but which are distinct in various other ways. This concept has gained considerable support, and one of the implications is that rather than talking about a person fitting into the category of schizophrenia, instead one should say how much schizophrenia their condition represents. This implies that it is impossible to be dogmatic about the label of schizophrenia, which would help reduce some of the stigma associated with the term.

Course and outcome of schizophrenia

Although severe forms of schizophrenia occur with about the same frequency in all societies (about 10–15% of all cases diagnosed), the long-term outcome in slightly less severe types of the illness appears to be quite variable in different parts of the world. In developing countries, many more people have a very good outcome than in highly developed western countries (50% versus 5%) (World Health Organization, 1979).

The reasons for this are probably complicated, but one of the most likely explanations is that in developed countries there is less tolerance of serious mental illness, and affected people can cope less well with a demanding and competitive society. Lack of tolerance of people with schizophrenia is likely to lead to additional adverse circumstances and stress, which appear to increase the likelihood of relapses of illness and reduce the extent to which recovery can occur. It seems ironic that in cultures where mental health services are most developed and sophisticated, the outcome of schizophrenia is least encouraging. The highly evolved mental health services that advanced countries can offer therefore appear barely able to keep up with the extra pressures that society imposes on people with mental illnesses like schizophrenia.

It used to be claimed that the outcome of schizophrenia was invariably poor, with little or no chance of complete recovery. This bleak outlook probably arose because the condition was studied in people who were already selected for poor outcome by the fact that they were in large mental institutions. Nowadays it is known that even with a narrow definition of schizophrenia, albeit one that allows the diagnosis to be made after a brief period of illness, a quarter or more of people who develop the condition can show a marked and substantial recovery. Unfortunately about 10–15% of people with schizophrenia remain very severely affected indeed, with either no recovery or even an exacerbation of symptoms over time. However, there is usually a tendency for the acute active symptoms of illness to become less noticeable over the years at the expense of the accumulation of disabling negative features. For the remainder of the people with schizophrenia, recurring episodes or relapses of acute disturbance can be expected to occur against a background of long-term mental disability and personality impairment.

No treatments have so far been found that will alter this pattern of outcome, although the frequency and severity of relapses, and the severity of overall impairments, disabilities and handicaps can be greatly reduced by medication and by psychosocial treatments. Cutting down the frequency and severity of relapses not only reduces distress and the socially damaging short-term effects of acute mental breakdowns, it is also likely to reduce the impact of the illness on people's long-term social functioning (relationships, employment), as well as possible detrimental effects on brain functioning. However, even taking an optimistic view, half of the people who develop schizophrenia will continue to need a great deal of help and support for years to come (Table 6.3).

Causes of schizophrenia

Schizophrenia-like disorders may result from damage to – or abnormal development and functioning of – certain parts of the brain. When these changes are obvious and their causes known, the conditions are called 'organic' (see above), and are not normally referred to as schizophrenia at all. Examples include the mental disturbances caused by:

- prolonged use of certain drugs (e.g. amphetamines)

Table 6.3 *Outcome in schizophrenia, 5–10 years from onset*

Aspect of disorder	Percentage of patients	Outcome
Symptoms	15	Complete recovery
	60	Partial recovery, relapsing
	15	Chronic 'negative' (defect)
	10	Chronic 'positive' (florid)
Social	50	Self-supporting
	40	Sheltered housing
	10	Long-term 24 hour care
Global	25	Much better
	50	Better but affected
	15	No better
	10	Worse

- brain damage due to trauma, infection or disease
- certain types of epilepsy mainly affecting the temporal lobes of the brain.

For schizophrenia as a whole, multiple causes are likely, either acting alone or in combination, but none is known for certain. For 'narrow, severe' or nuclear schizophrenia, it now seems probable that subtle but important abnormalities of brain structure and function resulting from a disorder of brain development are involved. These abnormalities appear to be influenced by environmental factors before or shortly after birth, and also by the person's genetic inheritance (Murray *et al.*, 1985).

The three syndromes of schizophrenia referred to previously have now been investigated using special brain scans (positron emission tomography, PET). The syndromes have been shown to be linked to altered physiological activity in particular sites in the brain. In the normal brain, these same brain areas appear to be involved in particular tasks which can help to explain what is going wrong in the brain of schizophrenic patients. Thus a task involving the monitoring of one's own mental activity appears to rely on nerve-cell function in the parahippocampal gyrus of the temporal lobe, mainly on the left side of the brain. This is the same brain area that tends to be abnormally inactive in people with schizophrenia who are experiencing the reality distortion syndrome of hallucination and delusions. This finding confirms the idea put forward by the British neuropsychologist Chris Frith, that the positive symptoms of schizophrenia result from problems in monitoring one's own mental activity (Frith and Done, 1989). This may cause people to experience their own thoughts and actions as being imposed from outside, or to hear their own thoughts as other people's 'voices'. Contrary to Tim Crow's original hypothesis, more recent research by him and others has shown that the positive symptoms of schizophrenia are associated with subtle changes in brain structure in the temporal lobe including the parahippocampal gyrus, especially on the left side, just where the PET studies have shown up abnormalities in the living brain (Liddle *et al.*, 1992). Even more strikingly, there is evidence that these structural abnormalities arise during development of the brain before or shortly after birth, that is, many years before the onset of the schizophrenic illness (Crow, 1991).

In normal people PET scans have shown that a task of verbal fluency involving 'spontaneous mental activity' increases nerve cell function in the left dorsolateral prefrontal cortex, the brain area that is underactive in schizophrenic patients with the negative or psychomotor poverty syndrome. This suggests that the negative syndrome reflects a reduction in frontal lobe function and in the spontaneous generation of thoughts, feelings and actions, which is certainly compatible with how people with this syndrome appear.

Similar correlations between particular mental tasks and the parts of the brain (the right anterior cingulate gyrus and thalamus) affected in the disorganization syndrome, suggest that eventually it will be possible to understand all the symptoms and syndromes of schizophrenia in terms of disturbances in the normal function of particular areas of the brain. Functional and structural brain anomalies in schizophrenia tend to be either mainly on the left or right side of the brain or (less commonly) equally on both sides. During the growth and development of the brain before and shortly after birth, there is normally an increasing asymmetry between left and right sides of the brain which appears to bestow upon human beings their particular ability to use language. This 'laterality' of cortical function is reduced in schizophrenia, and the two sides of the brain appear less dissimilar in size, although with subtle but important abnormalities in brain cell structure in particular areas (Crow, 1991).

Factors likely to contribute to the abnormal brain development that leads to schizophrenia can broadly be divided into genetic and environmental causes.

Genetic factors in schizophrenia

It has long been known that schizophrenia tends to run in families because of an inherited (genetic) susceptibility to the condition. Thus although the risk of schizophrenia to the general population is about 1%, it is about ten times this figure if a close relative also has the condition. Despite a great deal of research in the field of medical genetics, no particular genes have been reliably associated with schizophrenia. In view of the fact that 'organic' schizophrenia-like conditions can be produced by a diverse range of effects on brain mechanisms (e.g. drugs, infections and epilepsy, see Chapter 5), it is likely that there are numerous genes involved in the inheritance of schizophrenia. In this sense there may be several or many different types of schizophrenia, which despite superficial similarities in clinical features, may have diverse causes and genetics.

Genetic factors in schizophrenia appear strong, as indicated by adoption studies in which children of affected parents have been found to show the same ten-fold increased risk of developing schizophrenia, despite the fact that they were separated from their biological parents and lived with normal adopted parents from early infancy. However, genetic factors are unlikely to explain all cases of schizophrenia, because many affected people have no family history of the condition. Even more tellingly, in identical (monozygotic) twins who have an identical genetic make-up, one twin may develop schizophrenia but the other will not in more than 50% of cases (Kringlen, 1987). Interestingly, the brain structure of the affected twin as revealed by brain scanning techniques appears to be less 'normal' than that of the affected twin, even though not necessarily obviously abnormal compared with the general population. This suggests that brain mechanisms are probably always altered in 'narrow, severe' schizophrenia, but whether this is cause or effect cannot be determined at this time.

The genetic factors that determine cerebral laterality and the human capacity for language and communication may also be involved in the cause of schizophrenia.

Schizophrenia and the physical environment

Non-genetic causes for the brain abnormalities observed in schizophrenia are being hotly debated, and mostly focus on infections occurring while the baby is developing in the womb. Physical trauma to the brain at birth or in infancy is another possibility. It seems likely that these early environmental factors may act alone or increase the expression of a genetically-determined predisposition to schizophrenia. For example, a genetically-determined abnormal immune reaction to a particular viral infection may cause disturbance of brain growth or brain damage which eventually leads to schizophrenia when the child grows up. Presumably the stronger the genetic predisposition, the greater the likelihood of developing schizophrenia with only mild or no adverse physical circumstances (Figure 6.2).

It is well established that schizophrenia is more common in areas of social deprivation such as inner cities. This used to be thought to be entirely due to people with schizophrenia 'drifting' or moving into poor areas where they were more likely to remain and blend in with the general neglect and deprivation. Although this 'drift hypothesis' is still probably true to some extent, it is now believed that long-term exposure to poverty and adverse social circumstances may actually 'breed' and increase the risk of developing schizophrenia (Lewis et al., 1992).

Psychosocial causes of schizophrenia

The link between schizophrenia, city life and poverty suggests that adverse factors which are more common in the city dwellers' physical environment, such as pollution, drugs, poor nutrition, head injuries and infections, may be involved in the development of the condition. However, it is just as likely that psychosocial factors particularly associated with poor city life such as long-term stress, loneliness, alienation and racial harassment may be important too. Although these putative psychosocial causes of schizophrenia seem inherently more likely to apply to the 'broad, mild' type of schizophrenic disorder, what evidence there is suggests that they may also apply to 'narrow, severe' schizophrenia. Although we are a long way from being able to demonstrate the adverse psychosocial factors that cause schizophrenia, these factors are certainly of importance in determining the severity of the disorder as measured by the number of relapses or flare-ups of acute mental disorder, once the condition has become established.

Thus it seems that genetic, physical and psychosocial factors act in concert to predispose to and precipitate schizophrenic illnesses and to affect their outcome. The vulnerability model of schizophrenia helps to synthesize and illustrate these ideas (Figure 6.3).

Treatment and management of schizophrenia

Drug treatment of schizophrenia is aimed primarily at the symptoms and signs resulting from the characteristic impairments in cognitive, perceptual and motor functions. However, as schizophrenia is (in the

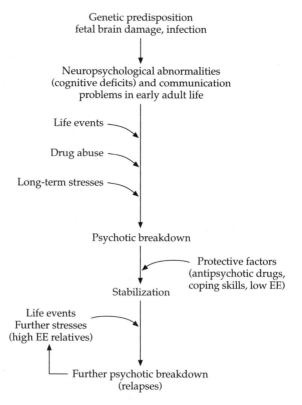

Figure 6.3   *Vulnerability model of schizophrenia*

present state of our knowledge) incurable, drug treatment can never be more than partially successful in helping people with schizophrenia. Inevitably the affected person will have to cope with a range of problems, disabilities and potential handicaps for which other kinds of help will be needed (Table 6.4), although without reasonably effective drug treatment, practical help and psychosocial therapy will have much less impact.

Table 6.4 *Problems and needs in schizophrenia*

Health and Safety
Acute relapses of psychosis
Long-term cognitive, perceptual, emotional and behavioural
impairments
Protection from self-neglect, self-harm and violence to others
Physical health problems
Inadequate diet

Disabilities in daily living
Poor hygiene and appearance
Poor care of personal environment
Problems in interpersonal skills and relationships
Overdependence on others
Loneliness and isolation
Poor household skills and budgeting

Social handicaps
Ignorance, misunderstanding and non-acceptance of illness
Lack of social support
Criticism and hostility from family, friends and neighbours
Stigmatization by others
Vulnerability to exploitation by others
Unemployment and lack of leisure opportunities
Poor housing
Lack of transport and telephone
Poverty

Psychosocial management of problems in schizophrenia will need to be closely integrated and co-ordinated with drug therapy if both types of approach are to be really effective. The role of the key worker is vital, since a close personal relationship is probably the single most important factor in motivating a person with schizophrenia to continue to accept help over a long period.

Key workers are also well placed to monitor the effects of drug treatment and to assess the benefits and drawbacks of medication through their knowledge of the clients and their circumstances. If problems such as side-effects are picked up by the observant and well-informed key worker, the worker will need to have the experience and confidence to give appropriate help and obtain further expert advice if needed. The key worker who is knowledgeable about medication issues will also be in a good position to help the client understand and accept the importance of drug therapy. Since the key worker is also likely to be providing care and services which are perceived by the client as having immediate relevance and value, the key worker's advice on drug treatment is likely to be heeded, and their advocacy of medication will have a good chance of overcoming any negative feelings that the client may have about it.

Table 6.5   *Suggestions for how to work with people with schizophrenia*

General aims
To give reassurance, advice and education
To provide practical guidance and to set examples of reasonable behaviour
To help with reality testing
To bolster self-esteem and confidence

General awareness
People with schizophrenia often feel powerless, threatened and afraid, despite having the ability to make others feel the same; similarly they may feel mixed up, uncertain or despairing despite appearing unrealistically confident, dogmatic or unconcerned
Contact with other people may be both desired and feared, and may produce overdependence on, or suspiciousness or hostile rejection of those who try to help

Specific tips
Listen carefully to what the person says and what this conveys about their feelings and experiences
Try not to be put off by bizarre ideas or incoherence of speech, but consider what feelings are involved
Avoid being overfamiliar or too formal
Probe carefully with questions, but do not cross-examine, criticize or argue
Do not pretend to agree with the person's odd or delusional ideas or beliefs, but acknowledge that their feelings and experiences are real to them
Avoid laughing at what the person does or says unless they are clearly trying to be humorous
Respond to anger and hostility calmly and with reassurances that you wish to help
Be frank and down to earth, and if a person goes off on a tangent, or becomes vague or irrelevant, bring the conversation back to everyday matters that are causing difficulties or concern
Do not talk too much
Do not prolong the contact if the person is obviously finding it difficult

Suggestions for ways of working with people with schizophrenia are outlined in Table 6.5. In order to avoid disappointment and disillusionment on the part of both client and carer, it is important that the expectations of improvement are kept to a reasonable level, whilst avoiding a sense of pessimism or 'therapeutic nihilism'. It may take a long time to see any changes in a person's problems or disabilities, although even small changes in certain areas may have a big impact on the individual, and result in a significant improvement in their quality of life as they perceive it.

The management of schizophrenia is considered here as six topics:

- antipsychotic drugs
- acute episodes of psychosis
- relapse prevention
- persistent symptoms and disturbed behaviour
- compliance with medication
- other practical management problems.

In a book about drug treatment, it is not possible to deal comprehensively with all aspects of the management of schizophrenia. In each section the focus is on drug treatment, but with consideration of psychosocial interventions and the interplay between the two types of approach.

The properties of antipsychotic drugs: what do they do and how do they work?

Before 1950 there were no important specific drug treatments for schizophrenia or other psychoses. Rauwolfia alkaloids, long used in Indian medicine, were rediscovered by the psychiatric profession in the 1930s but had too many side-effects for routine use. Acutely disturbed psychotic patients were often managed by physical restraint and given powerful sedative drugs such as paraldehyde or barbiturates in order to quell episodes of acute overarousal and excitement. Despite the fact that people were rendered drowsy or even unconscious by these drugs, their underlying psychotic disturbance usually remained unaffected. Furthermore, these powerful sedative drugs were dangerous because slightly exceeding the required dose would result in potentially fatal suppression of respiration. This was less likely to happen with paraldehyde, because being a highly irritant liquid, it was difficult to administer even in adequate amounts.

There were a few other physical treatments available for severely disturbed psychotic patients including electroconvulsive therapy (ECT) and insulin coma therapy. Despite its reputation to the contrary, ECT is safe, and it is still occasionally used for the treatment of unusually acute forms of schizophrenia, since it can produce a remission of psychotic symptoms when other treatments have failed. Nowadays the use of ECT is mainly restricted to psychotic patients in a state of extreme withdrawal (catatonic stupor) who are in a life-threatening situation through self-neglect. This can happen in schizophrenia but is more common in mood

Table 6.6 Clinical properties of different classes of antipsychotic drugs given orally. The drugs are usually given in divided doses, although a single dose at night may suffice

Class of drug	Typical daily dose[1] (mg/day)	High daily dose[2] (mg/day)	Neuroleptic actions			Other actions	
			Antipsychotic[3]	Sedative– anxiolytic	Extrapyramidal	Anticholinergic effects	Postural hypotension
Phenothiazines with aliphatic side-chain e.g. chlorpromazine (Largactil)	500	1000	++	+++	++	++	++
with piperidine side-chain e.g. thioridazine (Melleril)	400	800	++	+++	+	+++	+++
with piperazine side-chain e.g. trifluoperazine (Stelazine)	15	60	++	++	+++	+	+
Butyrophenones e.g. haloperidol (Serenace)	10	40	++	++	+++	+	+
Diphenylbutylpiperidines e.g. pimozide (Orap)	8	20	++	+	++	+/0	+/0
Benzamides e.g. sulpiride (Dolmatil)	1000	2400	++	+	+	0	+/0

Table 6.6 (*continued*)

Dibenzodiazepines e.g. clozapine (Clozaril)	350	900	+++	+++	0	++	++
Benzisoxazoles e.g. risperidone (Risperdal)	6	12	++	+	+	+	+++

Key: 0, no effect; +/0, uncertain effect; +, mild; ++, moderate; +++, marked.

[1]These doses are approximately equivalent therapeutic doses.
[2]At or below the advisory maximum dose in the *British National Formulary*, where given.
[3]Response to equivalent therapeutic doses.

psychoses, and in the latter it may be the treatment of choice in manic patients or in severely depressed, deluded people who are actively suicidal. Despite being complicated and hazardous, insulin coma therapy enjoyed a vogue for a number of years and was widely believed to be effective for treating psychotic symptoms. However, controlled evaluation eventually showed it to be no more effective than the 'tender loving care' that patients received during its administration (Ackner *et al.*, 1962).

Although in the early 1950s there was still an emphasis on institutional treatment for people with major mental illnesses such as schizophrenia, there was a strong desire on the part of mental health professionals to shorten patients' stay in hospital, and to move towards community-oriented care. The philosophy of community care received an enormous boost after 1952 with the introduction of chlorpromazine, the first truly specific antipsychotic drug. The introduction of chlorpromazine made an enormous impact on the management of psychiatric patients, even those who did not benefit directly from its tranquillizing and antipsychotic effects. Chlorpromazine inspired a new optimism in mental health care and led to an enlightened change in attitudes which enabled many more patients to leave hospital. When chlorpromazine was first introduced into medicine, it was used in anaesthesia to increase the analgesic and sedative effects of other agents. Patients who received it showed a remarkable indifference to stressful circumstances, even though they were still reasonably alert. This prompted psychiatrists to try its effect in a number of patients with mental illness. One or two doses of chlorpromazine did indeed produce a remarkable calming or tranquillizing effect on previously distressed and hyperactive patients, so that they appeared both emotionally and physically unreactive to their surroundings without being heavily sedated. As the drug was used over several days, characteristic movement disorders very like those occurring in Parkinson's disease began to emerge. These included slow resting tremor of the extremities, stiffness of the arms and legs, slow, shuffling gait, etc., and there was usually also a drop in blood pressure and an increase in pulse rate, especially when patients stood up (postural hypotension). Most remarkable of all, as psychiatrists continued with the treatment, to their surprise patients began to show a reduction in their characteristic delusions and hallucinatory experiences, and in those patients with thought disorder, an improvement in their ability to express their ideas coherently. As treatment was maintained, patients showed further improvements in their general behaviour, social interaction and self-care.

Over the next twenty years, many other drugs with similar properties to chlorpromazine were introduced into psychiatry. In this chapter the term 'antipsychotic drugs' is used to describe these substances, but the terms 'neuroleptics' and 'major tranquillizers' are also commonly used to describe the same drugs. To begin with, drugs with a similar chemical structure to chlorpromazine were produced. These belong to the chemical class called *phenothiazines*, and they differ from each other in the extent to which they produce various side-effects, and also in their clinical potency; the more potent the drug, the less is needed to produce a particular therapeutic effect. In the late 1950s and 1960s, drugs were

Table 6.7 *Long-acting antipsychotic drugs (intramuscular depot injections).[1,2] All these drugs have very similar clinical properties despite minor differences in their side-effects*

Class of drug	Example	Trade name	Typical dose[3]	High dose[4]
Phenothiazines	Fluphenazine decanoate	Modecate	25 mg every 2 weeks	100 mg every 2 weeks
	Pipothiazine palmitate	Piportil	50 mg every 4 weeks	200 mg every 4 weeks
Butyrophenones	Haloperidol decanoate	Haldol Decanoate	50 mg every 4 weeks	300 mg every 4 weeks
Thioxanthenes	Flupenthixol decanoate	Depixol	40 mg every 2 weeks	160 mg every week
	Zuclopenthixol decanoate	Clopixol	250 mg every 2 weeks	500 mg every week
	Zuclopenthixol acetate[5]	Clopixol Acuphase	100 mg single dose	400 mg over 4–8 days

[1] To simplify dose equivalence calculations, doses can be expressed as mg per week, although weekly injections are not usually recommended. The rate at which active drug passes from the injection site into the blood stream depends on the surface area rather than the volume of the depot drug injected. With this qualification, and assuming steady state conditions and normal liver functions, a dose (mg) of depot drug injected weekly is approximately equivalent to twice the dose injected fortnightly, or four times the dose injected monthly.

[2] These drugs are dissolved in vegetable oil and only become active gradually as they are released from the oil into the blood stream.

[3] The doses given are approximately equivalent to 125 mg chlorpromazine by mouth per day (350 mg chlorpromazine for this dose of Clopixol Acuphase).

[4] At or below the advisory maximum dose in the *British National Formulary*.

[5] This is not strictly a depot preparation.

produced with chemical structures different from the phenothiazines, but with similar clinical properties. However, some of these alternative drugs are up to a hundred times more potent, or in other words can be used in a hundredth of the dose to produce the same antipsychotic effect as chlorpromazine (Tables 6.6 and 6.7). Interestingly, nearly all these drugs were first identified as being potentially useful in schizophrenia and other psychoses by the fact that when given to animals they produce a lowering of activity, and a characteristic trance-like state called catalepsy, which is similar to the catatonic stupor sometimes seen in psychotic patients, and which the drugs help to resolve.

By the middle of the 1960s the effectiveness of these drugs in the acute treatment of schizophrenia had been demonstrated by double-blind placebo-controlled trials (Table 6.8). Approximately 75% of acutely psychotic patients showed a marked improvement on drugs such as chlorpromazine, compared to only 25% on inactive placebo. Controlled trials confirmed that merely sedating patients with barbiturates produced no benefit over a placebo treatment. Intriguingly, a sedative drug called promazine was more effective than placebo but less effective than chlorpromazine. Later it was shown that promazine had many of the pharmacological properties of chlorpromazine and other phenothiazines but to a lesser degree (Figure 6.4) (Casey et al., 1960).

Table 6.8   *Global change in acute schizophrenia after 6 weeks treatment with phenothiazines (e.g. chlorpromazine) or placebo*

Treatment	Improvement		No change or worse %
	Marked (%)	*Slight (%)*	
Placebo	25	25	50
Phenothiazines	75	15	10

Data from NIMH (1964).

By the late 1970s several dozen antipsychotic drugs had been introduced, all with different clinical potencies. At this point it was discovered that the single property that correlated with differences in clinical potency was the ability of the drugs to block the effects of dopamine at particular receptor sites in the brain. Dopamine is a naturally occurring amine, known to be a chemical neurotransmitter in the brain, involved in the control of mood and motor activity. The most potent drugs, for example haloperidol and pimozide, are also the most selective for dopamine (D_2) receptor blockade, with relatively few other pharmacological effects. In contrast, low-potency drugs such as chlorpromazine

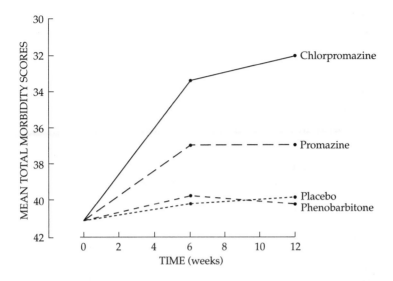

Figure 6.4 *Reductions in symptom (morbidity) scores in acute schizophrenic patients treated with chlorpromazine compared with placebo or phenobarbitone (a barbiturate). Only chlorpromazine had a significant therapeutic effect (adapted from Casey et al., 1960)*

have a wide range of effects on other neurotransmitter systems in the brain, and also effects elsewhere in the body such as the eyes and skin. The wide-ranging actions of chlorpromazine had already been recognized, hence its first trade name 'Largactil'.

The wide spectrum of pharmacological effects of low-potency antipsychotic agents means that when these drugs are given to schizophrenic patients there are many side-effects owing to their pharmacological actions on other systems. Prominent amongst the side-effects are drowsiness and sedation, changes in blood pressure and pulse, a lowering of the seizure threshold with a tendency to produce epileptic fits, dry mouth, blurred vision, constipation and difficulty in passing urine (Table 6.9). In contrast, the more 'pure', high-potency drugs produce only one major type of side-effect in the short term, i.e. parkinsonian movement disorders. It was soon realized that these parkinsonian effects are also due to dopamine receptor blockade in the brain, although at sites in the brain (the extrapyramidal system) different from those presumably involved in the antipsychotic action (cerebral cortex and limbic system). Low-potency antipsychotic drugs also have a potential to produce parkinsonian effects, but some of their other pharmacological actions (anticholinergic effects, Table 6.9) act as built-in antidotes to the parkinsonian-inducing properties of the drugs.

Table 6.9 *Adverse effects of antipsychotic drugs*

Effects on the nervous system
Drowsiness, lethargy, muzziness

Epileptic fits in susceptible patients (1 in 1000); more common with clozapine (3 in 100)

Parkinsonian symptoms (resting tremor, shuffling gait, slowness, difficulty initiating movement, rigidity)

Other 'extrapyramidal' movement disorders including muscle spasms, involuntary movements and restlessness; tardive dyskinesia

Neuropleptic malignant syndrome: rare, cause unknown, associated with confusion, stupor, fever, sweating, rigidity; may be fatal if left untreated

Effects on other systems
Dry mouth, blurred vision, constipation, urinary retention (anticholinergic effects)

Sexual problems (reduced libido, impotence)

Weight gain, enlarged breasts, menstrual irregularities, infertility (uncommon)

Palpitations, hypotension, dizziness

Jaundice and liver problems (rare)

Blood disorders due to bone-marrow depression (e.g. agranulocytosis), quite rare with most drugs but occurs in 1–2% of people on clozapine

Allergic skin rashes and sensitivity to light (especially chlorpromazine)

Limitations of antipsychotic drugs – side-effects and treatment resistance

As the wave of enthusiasm for chlorpromazine and related drugs began to recede, it became apparent that there were two major limitations with these drugs. Firstly, the drugs produce many unpleasant side-effects, some of which are hard to recognize, or take months or years to show themselves (Table 6.10). It was soon appreciated that these adverse affects are an important reason for patients not wanting to take their medication. In addition, a sizeable minority of patients with schizophrenia (25% or more) show little or no benefit from medication with these drugs, whatever dose or duration of treatment is tried.

It is only relatively recently that advances in drug therapy have been made which partly overcome some of these difficulties. In the late 1980s,

Table 6.10 *Movement disorder side-effects caused by antipsychotic drugs*

Side-effect	Treatment
Acute spasms (dystonias) Especially involving eye muscles, face and neck; usually occurs early in treatment and may affect men more than women; chronic spasms may also occur	Reduce dose of antipsychotic medication, give anticholinergic drug such as procyclidine (Kemedrin) or orphenadrine (Disipal)
Drug-induced parkinsonism Rigidity of limbs, tremor at rest, reduced arm swing, shuffling gait and slowness, mask-like expression Occurs in mild form in over 50% of treated patients at some time, severe symptoms in 15–20%	As for acute spasms
Subjective inner restlessness (akathisia) Urge to fidget and pace up and down on the spot; may occur in over 50% of treated patients; can be very distressing, but easily missed or mistaken for anxiety or agitation (which it can provoke)	Dose reduction is best strategy; anticholinergic drugs may not be helpful, but beta-blockers (propranolol) often are
Late-onset involuntary movements (tardive dyskinesia) Especially chewing, sucking and grimacing; occurs in 20–40% of long-term patients, especially elderly women; may reflect aging process, exacerbated by presence of psychosis and exposure to antipsychotic drugs	Difficult; movements will be suppressed temporarily by increase in dose of antipsychotic drug, only to get worse again in the longer term; therefore reduce dose of antipsychotic medication if possible; clozapine may make better with no long-term 'breakthrough' of movement disorder, and improved treatment of psychosis

a drug which had been in use since 1965, but had been withdrawn in many countries because of severe toxic side-effects, was recognized as having superior efficacy in schizophrenic patients. This drug is clozapine. It has been shown to be particularly helpful in up to half of the patients who have previously failed to respond to other more conventional antipsychotic drugs. Clozapine is also more effective in treating the schizophrenic 'defect state' which other drugs hardly help or may even make worse. Although clozapine has a few, very serious adverse effects, it is notable for being relatively free of extrapyramidal or parkinsonian actions, and can even be used to treat patients in whom movement disorders such as tardive dyskinesia (Table 6.10) have been induced by previous antipsychotic drug therapy. Furthermore, many people find that clozapine is relatively free of the unpleasant subjective effects produced by more conventional antipsychotic drugs. The most serious adverse effect of clozapine is the tendency to cause reduced immunity owing to depression of the bone marrow, with a serious reduction in white blood cell count (agranulocytosis) in a small proportion of people (1–2%) (Table 6.11). Clinical signs of infection (e.g. sore throat, fever) in patients taking clozapine must therefore be investigated by measuring the white blood cell count. 'Ordinary' causes of infections such as colds or influenza will usually be associated with a rise in white cell count, whereas in infection due to suppressed immunity the white cell count will be abnormally low. The second problem with clozapine is a tendency to lower the seizure threshold and cause epileptic fits, especially if the dose is increased too quickly. Sometimes people taking clozapine have also to be maintained on anticonvulsant medication, although the anticonvulsant drug carbamazepine (Tegretol) should be avoided as this also has a tendency to reduce the white cell count.

Despite these rather alarming difficulties, clozapine was reintroduced into clinical practice in the UK in 1990, and it is now widely used for selected patients who have severe symptoms that have not responded well to other drug treatments (*British Journal of Psychiatry*, 1992). Its use is very closely monitored, and patients have to undergo once-monthly blood tests for as long as they are taking the drug, which can only be prescribed by a specialist. The use of clozapine appears to be justified because, despite its high cost and potential hazards, it gives hope of a significant improvement in the psychiatric condition of people who may be otherwise regarded as unsuitable for living in the community because of the severity of their psychotic symptoms and behavioural disturbance. Unfortunately, because of the risk of serious side-effects, clozapine cannot be given as a long-acting injection, so one has either to rely on the patient's accurate self-administration or resort to close supervision by care workers.

So far, it is not clear how clozapine acts to produce its superior antipsychotic actions, nor its serious side-effects, although there are many clues and hypotheses. Not surprisingly, the hunt is on for a drug that shares clozapine's useful features but is much safer. Risperidone is a possible candidate (see Table 6.6). This drug is already widely used, although whether it is as effective as clozapine seems doubtful. The same applies to two recently introduced drugs, sertindole and olanzapine. However, like clozapine, all three drugs are 'atypical' in producing few extrapyramidal (movement disorder) side-effects.

Table 6.11 *Clozapine and blood disorders causing low immunity. Blood (haematology) results and physical well-being of all people taking clozapine (Clozaril) must be monitored regularly. Weekly blood samples are taken during the first 18 weeks of treatment, with samples every 2 weeks thereafter for the first year of treatment. For long-term maintenance treatment, blood samples every 4 weeks are sufficient*

White blood cell count (WBC) status	Action
'Green' WBC $> 3.5 \times 10^9/l$ and neutrophils $> 2.0 \times 10^9/l$	Continue clozapine, repeat blood sample for WBC in 1, 2, or 4 weeks as appropriate
'Amber' WBC > 3.0–$3.5 \times 10^9/l$ and/or neutrophils > 1.5–$2.0 \times 10^9/l$	If patient clinically well, continue clozapine, but repeat blood sample *twice weekly* If patient has any clinical signs of low WBC (fever, sore throat, etc.), STOP clozapine. Only start prescribing again when symptoms go and status is 'green'
'Red' WBC $< 3.0 \times 10^9/l$ and or neutrophils $< 1.5 \times 10^9/l$ and/or platelets $< 100 \times 10^9/l$	STOP clozapine Arrange emergency blood sample (telephone the Clozaril Patient Monitoring Service) Refer patient for urgent medical review

If patient develops fever, sore throat, etc. at any time, consider (a) twice-weekly blood tests, and, depending on level of clinical suspicion of neutropenia or agranulocytosis, (b) emergency blood test and stop drug. Restart drug only when symptoms clear *and* WBC status 'green'. Build up dose slowly if clozapine restarted after an interruption of more than 2 days.

Drug treatment in the acute phase of psychosis

People who are going through an acute psychotic breakdown are often confused, terrified and behaviourally disturbed. The major tranquillizing effect of antipsychotic drugs such as chlorpromazine or haloperidol can produce an immediate benefit by reducing anxiety and agitation and promoting settled behaviour. Provided doses are carefully adjusted to the individual, this improvement can usually be achieved without making the person excessively drowsy. In extremely disturbed people, or those who are violently aggressive, it may be safest to administer the medication by intramuscular injection because this works more quickly and more reliably. This may sometimes have to be done against the person's wishes, in the interests of their own and other people's well-being and safety. In an emergency this can be done under common law in the UK, but if this procedure needs to be repeated, the patient should be assessed for treatment under the Mental Health Act.

In the past it was believed that major tranquillizing drugs were perfectly safe when given in the short term, even if administered in high doses by injection. For this reason, when a person failed to settle quickly after being given a major tranquillizer in usual dosage, it was common practice to rapidly increase the dose. When the patient's mental disturbance and behaviour did eventually settle down, it was usually concluded that this was a result of the high doses of medication. We now know that this is often a mistake. Most patients will settle readily enough on low to medium doses of these drugs, if given the chance, and people who do not respond to initial medication will probably not show much additional benefit if the dose is increased further. It has become more widely appreciated that, given in very high doses, these drugs are not as safe as once thought. There have been a number of well-publicized tragedies where disturbed and overaroused patients suffered heart attacks after being given high doses of these drugs. Although sudden death can occur in any traumatic situation, or even without any apparent cause whatsoever, it does seem reasonable to use high doses of these drugs as sparingly as possible.

If an acutely disturbed person who is believed to be suffering from psychosis does not become calm on a moderate dose of an antipsychotic drug, rather than using higher and higher doses, a different type of tranquillizing drug such as diazepam (Valium) is usually added (Pilowsky et al., 1992). In a crisis every effort should be made to calm and reassure the patient by personal contact and 'talking them down', only using emergency drug treatment when it is apparent that a dangerous situation is developing which cannot be easily contained by calm words and firm handling alone. Regular, low to moderate doses of a major tranquillizer will usually bring about a calmer state of mind in psychotic patients and help prevent a crisis of disturbed behaviour arising in the first place.

Once the behavioural overarousal and anxiety have reduced, the acutely psychotic patient still requires help to settle their distressing symptoms. These symptoms usually take the form of various kinds of hallucinations, experiences of having thoughts or actions interfered with from outside themselves, and terrifying beliefs of being persecuted, threatened or harmed. Sometimes these beliefs are bizarre, e.g. patients believe that they are being attacked by aliens from outer space, or that they themselves have been transformed into an insect. Not surprisingly people in these situations often feel desperate, and are sometimes driven to make suicide attempts or to become violent. For these reasons, during periods of severe acute disturbance, people with schizophrenia may need a place of safety or refuge where they can receive 24-hour help and care by skilled staff. This is still usually achieved by arranging an admission to the local psychiatric inpatient unit, which is often attached to a district general hospital. When a person is refusing admission and treatment, and is thought to be putting the health and safety of themselves or others at risk, it may be necessary to admit them under a compulsory order (or Section) of the Mental Health Act. This usually requires the recommendation of two doctors and an application by a specially trained approved social worker. The patient's next of kin may also be involved and in any case the family will be consulted.

Once drug treatment has commenced, the patient will need support and encouragement to continue with it, as at this stage many psychotic people are not convinced that the treatment they are receiving is necessary or even helpful. In people who are particularly reluctant to take treatment, medication may be prescribed by injections, preferably using a drug with an effect lasting over several days (e.g. zuclopenthixol acetate injection, Clopixol Acuphase, see Table 6.7). Because an antipsychotic effect is likely to take days or weeks to develop, the care staff must be patient, and do all they can to reassure and support the person going through the psychotic experiences.

It is usual to start with low doses of whichever antipsychotic drug is selected. The choice of drug is usually arbitrary, although if the person has responded well to a particular medication in the past, it makes good sense to use this for the current episode. If the person has broken down and suffered a psychotic relapse despite continuing on their usual medication, it may be justifiable to increase the dose of this if there are grounds to suspect that inadequate amounts are reaching the brain. This can occur as a result of changes in the amount of drug absorbed from the gut (e.g. due to drinking excessive tea or coffee), or more usually because of erratic consumption of tablets. Even so, the aim is to use doses of medication that produce little drowsiness and no (or only slight) movement side-effects, such as stiffness, tremor or slowness. If the person is sensitive to these drug-induced movement disorders, but becomes more disturbed when the dose of antipsychotic is lowered again, it is usually best to maintain the dose but administer an anticholinergic drug which reduces the severity of most movement disorders (see Table 6.10).

Patients who feel reasonably comfortable on medication and show an early improvement in their psychotic symptoms are, not surprisingly, likely to do well in the longer term. In contrast, people who quickly experience unpleasant subjective effects, feel little or no initial benefit with respect to their psychotic symptoms, or show marked sensitivity to the parkinsonian movement disorder effects of the drug, are likely to do less well on the medication in the longer term. Under these circumstances, it may be better to switch to another drug (e.g. one of the new atypical neuroleptics) at an early stage, rather than trying to persuade the patient to persist with medication to which they are clearly not reacting well. For reasons that often remain unclear, some people only respond to one particular drug, and this can only be discovered by painstaking trial and error. Whatever drug is chosen, the aim is to keep the dose to a minimum whilst ensuring reasonable effectiveness, always remembering that the drug may take several weeks or even months to work fully, and that the process probably cannot be speeded up by using higher, less well tolerated doses (Kinon *et al.*, 1993). Once again, supplementing antipsychotic medication with a benzodiazepine such as diazepam will often help to settle persisting anxiety and behavioural disturbance, with little risk of producing dependence or addiction.

This whole process is essentially empirical, and benefits from a high degree of clinical experience on the part of the people who are assessing the patient's mental and physical state and adjusting the medication accordingly. The assessment will be much more meaningful if carried out by people who are familiar with the patient and with the environment in which they usually live and work. For example, side-effects of medication or psychotic symptoms that seem minor in the clinic or hospital ward may be highly incapacitating or stigmatizing in the context of the person's daily life. Conversely, when their problems are assessed by a stranger in the rather intimidating setting of a hospital or clinic, a psychotic patient may appear much more disturbed and disabled than when seen in familiar surroundings.

It was established early on that most, if not all, symptoms and problem behaviours shown by acutely psychotic patients can be improved by antipsychotic medication, in comparison with a placebo or inactive treatment (Figure 6.5). Even symptoms or behaviour that can be described as 'negative' by virtue of the fact that they represent the absence of normal feelings or behaviour, e.g. lack of self-care or social withdrawal, tend to respond well to drug treatments in people who will respond at all. These types of negative symptoms are probably consequences of active features of psychosis such as paranoid fears, auditory hallucinations, etc. At this stage it is uncommon for more serious, treatment-resistant negative symptoms to be apparent. The latter include marked apathy, poverty of speech and reduced emotional range and reactivity (flattening and blunting of affect). On the whole these 'primary' true negative or defect symptoms tend to show little improvement with conventional antipsychotic drugs. However, clozapine appears to be helpful in up to a half of those people who are severely disabled by negative symptoms, although it may take a year or more for clozapine to have its full beneficial effect. If there are coexisting positive symptoms, as is usually the case, these will be helped as well by clozapine.

In most cases symptoms and problems will have resolved sufficiently after a few weeks or months to consider discharging patients back to their homes if they have been admitted to hospital, or alternatively, if they have been managed in the community, to consider reducing the high level of support that may have been needed to help them stay out of hospital. Unfortunately, however, a significant proportion of people with acute schizophrenia (e.g. 20%) fail to show much early improvement, and 6 months after the flare-up of their mental illness may still be too ill to leave hospital and live more independently. It is difficult to predict this state of affairs in the early stages of the illness, although people who have shown a poor response to treatment in the past will continue to show a slow and incomplete resolution of acute episodes, and will tend to respond poorly in the future.

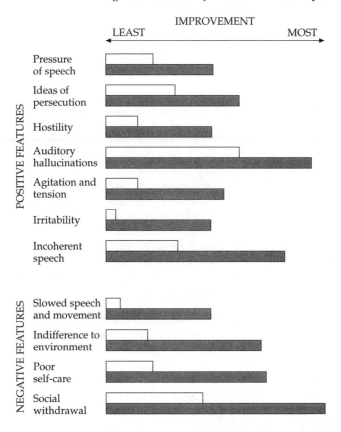

Figure 6.5 *Relative improvement in individual symptoms of acute schizophrenia on antipsychotic drug (shaded bars) or placebo treatment (white bars). Positive features are defined empirically as representing the presence of abnormal mental states or behaviour, and negative features as representing the absence of normal features (adapted from NIMH, 1964)*

Throughout the period of an acute psychotic relapse, people need a high level of reassurance and containment that can best come from contact with skilled care staff whom they know or get to know well. Consistency and continuity of care is important to help the patient get over the worse effects of their acute mental illness. If the person has friends or relatives who can provide this level of containment and support without becoming unduly stressed themselves, this may be a positive factor in helping people recover. However, often friends and relatives are so overinvolved and upset themselves that their attempts to help may only make matters worse (Kuipers *et al.*, 1992). Under these circumstances the person may well be better off in hospital or in a residential setting where they can receive skilled support from mental health professionals in the community. The emphasis in treatment is to try to bring the person back into contact with reality, without aggressively challenging or devaluing their psychotic experiences or beliefs. Concentrating on normal everyday things that a person feels comfortable with is often a useful strategy, and intrusive probing into the 'meaning' of their abnormal experiences (or the lack of it) is not usually helpful at this stage.

Particular problems arise when the affected person feels persecuted and paranoid, and develops extreme fear or mistrust of the people around them who are trying to help. The need to give drug treatment under duress (i.e. under a Section of the Mental Health Act) for a protracted period bodes badly for the future, for it is uncommon for treatment to restore a person's 'insight' sufficiently for them to look back with acceptance on their compulsory treatment, or to continue with it in the future when they are no longer under compulsion to do so. At an early stage, it is essential to try to correct any misunderstandings that the person with schizophrenia or their friends or family may have about the effects and purposes of drug treatment. For example, many people feel that drug treatment represents a form of 'chemical straitjacket' or punishment. Although the major tranquillizing, behavioural-controlling effect of these drugs may be important in the acutely disturbed phases of a mental breakdown, this is usually not needed or intended later on. It has to be communicated to all concerned that the eventual aim of drug treatment in schizophrenia is to help a person feel better and return to a *more normal* routine.

Unfortunately, even when adverse side-effects are largely avoided, it is common for acutely psychotic patients not to be aware of any subjective benefit at all from drug treatment, even though objectively the symptoms and disturbed behaviour show an obvious improvement. Under these circumstances, people usually ascribe their improvement to other factors, e.g. support from their relatives or a change in diet, which although not necessarily insignificant or unimportant, are usually – in the experience of the mental health professionals involved – of secondary importance or relatively incidental. Even when people can accept that they have been 'ill' or have been suffering from a 'nervous breakdown', they often do not agree that they feel better as a result of drug treatment. This disagreement is a strong predictor of poor compliance with medication later on.

Sometimes a person with an established schizophrenic illness experiences a flare-up or relapse of active psychotic symptoms, despite the fact that they are reliably taking antipsychotic medication in what appears to be an adequate dose. In the past it was probably not sufficiently recognized that relapses can occur due to recent life events, or even 'spontaneously', despite people being on full doses of antipsychotic medication. Although a temporary increase in medication may be worth considering in these circumstances, it is just as likely that the full benefits of the drug have already been reached, and that there are no advantages in adding more of the drug, even temporarily. Instead it may be better to use other strategies to help a person recover from their upset, e.g. short-term extra support at home or a brief admission to hospital. If further drug treatment is considered necessary, the additional short-term use of a drug from a different class altogether (e.g. an anxiolytic drug such as diazepam) may be effective.

A person with schizophrenia can become depressed just like anybody else, although the risk of depression and other mood disorders is probably higher in people with schizophrenia. If a depressive episode occurs while they are taking low doses of antipsychotic medication, or no medication at all, it is usually worth restarting or increasing the dose of antipsychotic medication, rather than trying an antidepressant drug. This is because the depression is often 'part and parcel' of the schizophrenic illness, which needs more active treatment with an antipsychotic drug. However, in situations where people with schizophrenia show clear-cut signs of a depressive illness, or if their depression is clearly reactive to other events, e.g. the realization as insight returns of how ill they have been, then an antidepressant drug may well be helpful as an additional treatment. Unfortunately, the delayed effect of antidepressant drugs makes it difficult to evaluate this strategy quickly, and side-effects of some antidepressants have the potential to make antipsychotic symptoms worse, even when combined with antipsychotic drugs.

Another situation that may cause difficulties is where patients have suffered a psychotic breakdown as part of an ongoing schizophrenic disorder, but against expectation, their psychotic disturbance settles spontaneously without the need for any antipsychotic medication. Particularly if this is a person's first experience of mental illness, it tends to confirm in their minds that they are not really ill at all, but that their condition was 'just stress' and therefore nothing to be seriously concerned about. What evidence there is, suggests that a spontaneous resolution of a first episode of a schizophrenic illness does not necessarily predict a good future outcome, and drug treatment is often advisable eventually.

Optimizing treatment with antipsychotic drugs – adjusting doses

Compared with other drugs used in medicine and psychiatry, antipsychotic drugs are relatively safe and rarely cause serious or lethal complications, even in overdose. Selective reporting in the media of sudden medication-related deaths can give misleading impressions about their safety. However, it is undeniable that many patients experience unpleasant and distressing side-effects, which in some cases may be intolerable. Fortunately, adverse effects are related to dose and can usually be reduced or minimized by keeping doses as low as possible. Individuals differ considerably in the doses that they require for an adequate antipsychotic effect, and this has to be arrived at by a careful process of trial and error.

In recent years there has been a greater effort to use the minimal effective doses of these drugs in order to reduce side-effects and to maximize the benefits of treatment. It has been found that for many drugs, doses lower than those used in the past are effective and well tolerated in the average patient. For people who are unlucky not to respond adequately to conventional doses of antipsychotic drugs, a further increase in dose will not usually be helpful (Beckman and Laux, 1990; Kinon et al., 1993). However, a small minority of patients definitely do require and tolerate doses of antipsychotic medication that are above average. This is probably because of problems, usually unidentified, resulting in lower than usual drug levels in the blood and body fluids. In contrast, some people seem to need lower than average doses to achieve optimal therapeutic effect and may actually be made worse by doses above this, even when side-effects are not particularly obvious. In these cases, sometimes remarkable improvement in mental symptoms can result from dose reduction.

Reasons sometimes given for using a high dose of an antipsychotic drug are, firstly, that the patient only improves when the dose is increased, and secondly, attempts to reduce the dose result in relapse of psychosis. These reasons can be misleading because insufficient time may have been allowed for the patient to respond to lower doses, and relapse on dose reduction may have been the result of giving high doses. In order to understand this, it has to be appreciated that high doses of antipsychotic drugs taken over long periods may cause compensatory supersensitivity or 'upregulation' of dopamine systems in the brain, resulting in rebound overactivity of dopamine when the dose of medication is eventually reduced (see Chapter 2). This will cause a relapse of psychosis in the same way as sometimes happens when a person with schizophrenia takes a large dose of amphetamine ('speed').

Where there are doubts about the appropriate dose of antipsychotic medication, or problems with side-effects, it may be worthwhile measuring the level of the drug in the blood if this can be arranged. For some commonly used drugs, e.g. haloperidol, it is now reasonably well established that for the great majority of people, an antipsychotic response occurs at blood levels below a certain limit (for haloperidol, 20 ng/ml of plasma). Interestingly, now that the effects of the drugs can be observed in the living brain using special techniques (e.g. PET scans), it has been shown that the full effects of antipsychotic drugs on dopamine receptors is also usually achieved at blood levels below this limit. Furthermore, the amount of drug binding to dopamine receptors in the brains of people who show a good clinical response to medication is similar to that occurring in people who have not responded. The implication of this is that, despite having apparently similar illnesses, different people with schizophrenia have different disorders of brain function which respond differently to drug treatment. This further implies that there is unlikely to be a universally effective drug treatment for schizophrenia. Instead, a range of drugs with different biological modes of action are likely to be needed to help deal with the different underlying disturbances in brain functions.

Optimizing treatment by dealing with adverse effects

Adverse affects of antipsychotic drugs can be divided into those affecting the nervous system and those affecting other systems of the body (see Tables 6.9 and 6.10). It is important to be able to recognize and identify adverse side-effects because appropriate action and treatment is usually required, both to relieve distress and possible exacerbation of psychosis, and also to avoid jeopardizing future compliance with medication. In the case of the blood disorder (agranulocytosis) produced by clozapine, the patient may first present with an apparently trivial fever and sore throat. A failure to recognize and respond promptly to this complication could be dangerous (Table 6.11).

The most effective and conservative response for dealing with side-effects is dose reduction, although this may risk a relapse of active mental illness. Fortunately, in most instances, the dose of antipsychotic medication needed to provide optimal therapeutic effectiveness is lower than that causing adverse effects such as parkinsonian movement disorders (McEvoy *et al.*, 1991). Sometimes there is a paradoxical increase in parkinsonian side-effects when reducing high doses of some antipsychotic drugs. This is probably because anticholinergic effects of the drugs, which counteract parkinsonian side-effects, are only prominent at high doses, and decrease more rapidly than dopamine blocking effects as doses go down. This may leave dopamine blockade relatively unopposed by anticholinergic actions, and so parkinsonian side-effects reappear (see Figure 2.3).

Where parkinsonian movement disorders are produced by antipsychotic drugs, additional anticholinergic drugs such as orphenadrine or procyclidine are often used to boost the antipsychotic drug's 'built-in' anticholinergic properties, and so oppose the effects of dopamine blockade in the extrapyramidal system. In cases of acute muscular spasm or dystonia, which can be very distressing and alarming especially if it affects the eyes, mouth or throat, an injection of an anticholinergic drug such as procyclidine can produce rapid relief. However, these drugs should only be used when they are really necessary as they may tend to counteract the beneficial antipsychotic actions of medication (Johnstone *et al.*, 1983) and can lead to abuse for their euphoriant effects.

An antipsychotic drug-induced compulsive desire to fidget and move (akathisia) can be very distressing indeed. If the problem has been present for a long time, people may be observed to 'jog on the spot' but deny that it is causing them any discomfort or distress. Dose reduction is usually the best strategy for akathisia, particularly in the acute phase, although an alternative strategy is to give benzodiazepines such as diazepam, or beta-blockers such as propranolol. It is important to ensure that the drugs used to beat side-effects do not cause adverse effects of their own. Whenever several drugs are prescribed together (*polypharmacy*), the problems arising owing to adverse interactions between the drugs can be a bigger problem than the original side-effects of the antipsychotic medication (see Chapter 3).

Associated with akathisia, although possibly distinct from it, is an unpleasant subjective state (*dysphoria*) which people find difficult to describe but which is highly objectionable. This may occur in up to a third of people taking antipsychotic drugs, and usually reveals itself early on in treatment. If it does occur, it tends to predict a poor response to drug treatment, possibly because of poor compliance with medication later on. Interestingly, there is some evidence that clozapine is relatively free of this mysterious problem.

Maintenance medication to help prevent relapses

For most people affected by it, schizophrenia is a long-term, even life-long, disorder. After substantial recovery from the first episode of schizophrenia, between 40% and 60% of people may show a further episode of active mental illness in the following year (Gaebel and Pietzcker, 1985). This figure will have almost certainly risen to about 70–80% by the second year, depending on the severity of the person's inherent biological vulnerability to psychosis, and on their exposure to stress, both in the short term and long term. The 'biological' factors that predict vulnerability to sustained or further episodes of illness are diffi-cult to pin down; but being male, early onset of negative symptoms and a poor response of positive symptoms to antipsychotic medication are all features suggesting a high likelihood of relapse and 'chronicity'. Disorganized thinking as shown by incoherence of speech may also be a poor prognostic feature, although this is one of the less common features of acute schizophrenia. Apart from the absence of poor prognostic features, there are not really any factors that can reliably identify in advance the 15–20% of people with schizophrenia who will have a good outcome.

Psychosocial factors leading to increased stress and relapse vulnera-bility have been studied in recent years (see above). Probably the best psychosocial predictor of the likelihood of relapse is the presence of a critical or hostile attitude in the household to which the patient returns after recovery from the episode of psychosis. Even overprotectiveness can be stressful to the person with schizophrenia and increase their likeli-hood of relapse. This exposure to high 'expressed emotion' (EE) can double the risk of a person suffering a further relapse of illness in the first year (Vaughn and Leff, 1976), and this risk seems to increase with time as negative attitudes amongst friends and families appear to increase.

For people with established schizophrenia who go into remission and discontinue their medication, the chance of a further relapse of psychosis is high (Hirsch et al., 1973; Hogarty et al., 1974). After 2–3 years, on average about 85% of people in this situation will have relapsed at least once (Figure 6.6). Numerous studies have shown that maintenance antipsychotic medication can reduce the risk of relapses considerably, even though people may still have residual symptoms of mental illness, and will also have to put up with the problems of taking long-term medication. Reducing exposure to high EE and other stresses can also help a great deal. Research has shown that a reduction in the person's contact with high EE relatives or carers to less than 35 hours per week (e.g. by attending a day centre or working at a part-time job) can have as great an effect in reducing the risk of relapse over a 1-year period as staying on maintenance antipsychotic medication. Furthermore, the protective effect of both treatment strategies appears to be additive (Figure 6.7). Family therapy using a combination of behavioural and educational approaches can reduce high EE and increase the ability of family members to cope more effectively with problems that arise as a consequence of their relative's mental illness. Family therapy can also improve the individual's compliance with taking medication, and equips

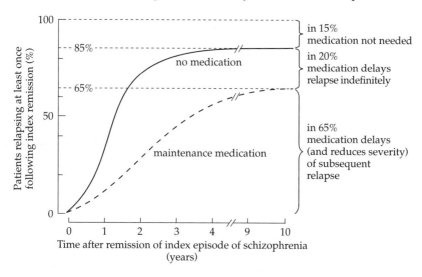

Figure 6.6 *The prophylactic effect of maintenance antipsychotic medication in preventing or delaying relapses of acute psychotic illness in schizophrenia (adapted from the work of Hirsch, Hogarty and others, see Bristow and Hirsch, 1993)*

family members to detect early signs of a relapse of illness and to arrange appropriate future help. Family interventions therefore are much more effective if they form part of a package of care which includes conventional mental health services. However, this kind of therapy and support is not acceptable to all families, and is irrelevant if the person with schizophrenia lives alone. Furthermore, the treatment is expensive and needs to be maintained over a long period (e.g. 2 years or more) if the benefits are to have a lasting impact (Kuipers *et al.*, 1992).

When should maintenance medication be phased out?

If a person's social circumstances are reasonably favourable, and assuming that their first episode of schizophrenia did not have any of the features indicating a poor prognosis (see above), it may be worth considering a gradual reduction and phasing out of antipsychotic medication after a year of relative or complete remission. Since between 15% and 20% of people who recover from a classic schizophrenic illness would, if given no further treatment or help, remain well for the foreseeable future, it is certainly worth considering this step. However, one has to be realistic about the chances of further problems arising, and if another relapse does occur, the usual advice is to continue with permanent maintenance medication, assuming that no other complications or contraindications arise later. For example if tardive dyskinesia develops, this might prompt a further attempt at withdrawal from medication, or a switch to an antipsychotic drug such as clozapine which will not usually make the tardive dyskinesia worse, and may even improve it.

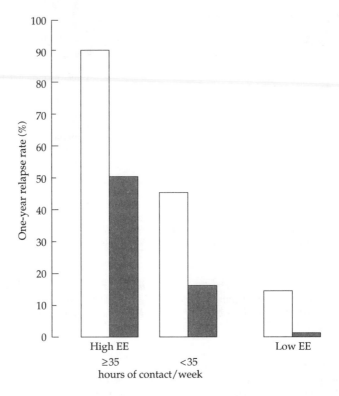

Figure 6.7   *The rate of relapse of acute illness in schizophrenia is increased by exposure to high expressed emotion (EE), and reduced by less or low EE and by maintenance antipsychotic medication (shaded bars; no medication, white bars). Adapted from Vaughn and Leff (1976)*

If a person is to remain on long-term medication indefinitely, the use of long-acting (depot) injections would seem to be an obvious choice because the patient will no longer need reminding to take tablets at least once or twice per day. However, many people are opposed to the idea of long-acting injections, and apart from the issue of compliance (see below) and the avoidance of irregular absorption of drugs taken by mouth, there are no other real advantages to this form of medication to justify insisting on it.

Establishing the minimum effective dosage for maintenance in a particular patient is a difficult issue. In practice it is usually a matter of trial and error, and possibly having to learn from the lesson of reducing the dose too far so that a relapse or partial relapse is the consequence. In recent years a considerable amount of research has looked into the question of maintenance dosages generally, and only now is a consensus emerging (Johnson, 1988). The dosage of antipsychotic medication for maintenance can usually be considerably lower than that needed to bring about a remission of the acute illness. For example, an average antipsychotic dose of chlorpromazine is about 500 mg per day, whereas for maintenance treatment, a dose of 125 mg a day may suffice. This dose of chlorpro-mazine is equivalent to approximately 25 mg of fluphenazine decanoate injected every 2 weeks (see Table 6.7), and this tends to be the standard treatment used in studies of maintenance drug treatment in schizo-phrenia. When considering groups of patients, further reductions in the dosage of maintenance drug appear to result in a significant increase in the risk of relapse. For example, a 50% reduction in maintenance dose may increase the average risk of relapse from 10% to 30% over the following year. However, lower doses are associated with a reduction in side-effects, although not to a very marked degree. Nonetheless, a low-dose strategy for maintenance is worth considering if the person on the receiving end makes freedom from side-effects a higher priority than protection from relapse.

Early warning of relapse and intermittent drug treatment

An alternative strategy in an attempt to reduce the overall amount of long-term medication is for the patient to come off regular medication but to receive special education in recognizing early signs of an imminent relapse. For any person, the type of symptoms that herald a relapse of psychosis tend to be consistent from one occasion to the next, and for this reason have been dubbed the person's *relapse signature* (Birchwood and Tarrier, 1994). Typical early warning symptoms include feeling depressed and on edge; having trouble sleeping, with disturbing dreams; feeling preoccupied and remote from family and friends; loss of interest and indecisiveness, etc. It is sometimes helpful for the person to write down their 'relapse signature' on a special *crisis card* so that at the earliest sign of trouble, they can be shown this card by family, friends or carers to remind them that their current problems and feelings are likely to be warning signs of a relapse. This is important because loss of appreciation of illness is a common problem as the psychosis develops.

The idea is that having previously identified and accepted the risk of an impending relapse, the person agrees to take some medication and adopt other coping strategies to help prevent the relapse getting out of control. Unfortunately, when this approach is tried in practice the relapse rate is double that of patients on continuous treatment. Furthermore, there is little difference in the overall intake of medication and the ensuing problems with side-effects. Despite these disappointing results, many people like the idea of an intermittent dosing strategy and may agree to a compromise arrangement whereby they take low-dose (suboptimal) maintenance treatment, but supplement this with higher doses when early warning signs of relapse are noted.

Managing persistent symptoms and behavioural disturbances

Many people with schizophrenia continue to experience psychotic symptoms and show long-term behavioural disturbances despite continuing to take antipsychotic medication. Before deciding what to do, it is important to assess accurately how troubling and disabling these persistent difficulties are. For this, there is no substitute for knowing as much as possible about the affected person and their way of life. Only then can reasonable management plans be made – which may include the option of doing nothing at all.

Hallucinations and delusions

If it is obvious that persistent symptoms such as hallucinations and delusions are significantly interfering with a person's peace of mind and quality of life, the first step should probably be to optimize the effects of antipsychotic medication. If no side-effects are apparent or complained about, it is usually worth gradually increasing the dosage until side-effects can just be detected. The dose of medication can then be reduced by one step, and adequate time given for the change to have an effect. Conversely, if side-effects are already present, a dose reduction may be a more effective strategy. Side-effects such as sedation and muzziness can sometimes make positive psychotic symptoms worse, so this strategy is always worth considering. However, the suggestion of a dosage reduction in a person who is still troubled by active symptoms is sometimes not well received by the person's friends and family or other carers, and sometimes the patient also objects. However, if the dosage is reduced gradually, a slight deterioration in mental state indicating that it was the wrong strategy after all will easily be correctible, and no harm will be done.

If dosage alterations or a change to another antipsychotic drug fail to make any helpful difference, usually the next strategy is to add other drug treatments to see if these can have an augmenting effect on the original medication. Drugs found to be useful in this situation are carbamazepine, sodium valproate, lithium and propranolol, amongst others. Finding a helpful augmentation treatment is nearly always a matter of trial and error, but it should probably be left to a specialist psychiatrist rather than to a general practitioner who may lack the necessary knowledge and experience, especially if problems arise. Certainly the potential for adverse reactions always increases when combinations of drugs are used in this way, which is one reason why it should not be embarked upon lightly.

This certainly applies to the use of clozapine. This drug has been shown to have a helpful therapeutic effect against a range of positive and negative symptoms of schizophrenia, even in people who have not responded well to other drugs, either because symptoms did not improve, or because side-effects were intolerable. Clozapine can help up to a half of such patients, although it may take 6–12 months for treatment to show its full benefit. As mentioned in the previous section, clozapine can have major hazards and can only be prescribed by a consultant psychiatrist after treatment has been started in hospital. For the first 18 weeks, weekly blood tests are necessary, followed by twice-monthly and then monthly blood tests for as long as the person takes the drug. Because of its potential hazards clozapine cannot be given by long-acting injection, which in addition to the necessity for frequent blood tests, means that there are often problems with compliance, and this is a common reason for treatment failure with clozapine. However, the high level of care and attention that people receive while taking clozapine may have additional therapeutic benefits. Apart from the occasional use of anticholinergic drugs to help control excessive salivation (a common side-effect of clozapine), all other psychotropic drugs are best avoided. Prescribing other antipsychotic drugs at the same time as clozapine may counteract some of its benefits, and in view of the already high level of concern about its adverse affects, it seems imprudent to raise these anxieties further by adding opportunities for adverse drug interactions.

While attempts are made to optimize drug treatment for persistent positive psychotic symptoms, other more general measures should be taken to help the person cope should the drug treatment strategy fail. These general measures include reducing the person's isolation, while avoiding stress and overarousal and other factors that could trigger an exacerbation of psychotic symptoms. For example, people who are distressed by hearing voices or who believe that they are being persecuted and harmed in some way, are likely to remain disturbed if they react by withdrawing into themselves. On the other hand, if their circumstances bring them into constant conflict with others, this could inflame their psychotic experiences and beliefs. The aim is usually to encourage patients to increase their social contacts in small, easily manageable steps, with opportunities to withdraw for periods of 'time out' when situations become too stressful. Relaxation exercises and other anxiety management techniques will enhance the effectiveness of this time-out strategy.

The next phase is to try specific cognitive behavioural techniques to help the person control and cope with their persistent psychotic symptoms. In attempting this, it is important to win the person's trust by adopting an open-minded attitude towards their psychotic experiences and beliefs. The aim is to neither contradict nor collude with their beliefs and experiences, but to create an atmosphere and opportunity to constructively re-examine what they are going through. The therapist attempts to understand and validate what the patient believes and is experiencing, while at the same time pointing out that other people experience reality differently.

In dealing with hallucinations, it is usually best to proceed in three stages (Birchwood and Tarrier, 1994). The first stage involves distraction techniques, which although of limited and short-term benefit, can give the person confidence that their distressing symptoms can be brought under control. These techniques involve encouraging the patient to concentrate on some other activity when they are experiencing auditory hallucinations. Talking to others or to themselves under their breath, listening to music and taking part in physical activity are all sometimes helpful. Some patients find wearing earplugs, even in one ear, to be a helpful technique, although how or why this should help remains obscure.

The second stage involves focusing on the auditory hallucinations so that the patient can gain a greater sense of mastery and control over them. Initially the therapist aims not to challenge the patient's belief that the voices are coming from some outside source. Instead the patient can be advised to react to the voices as though they were the speech of a real but unwelcome intruder. Initially this may be alarming and threatening to the patient, so focusing on voices should be done when the patient is otherwise feeling relaxed and secure. Should the experience get too alarming, the patient should be instructed in relaxation techniques to help them keep control. In focusing on the voices and considering their content, it may help to question them and write down what the voices say. The patient can then be encouraged to doubt the credibility of the voices or even to tell them to 'shut up' or 'mind their own business'. In this way the patient may be able to learn to evoke and reduce the voices at will, and so feel more in control.

The third stage in this process is to encourage the patient to attribute the voices to their own mental processes. It may be acceptable to the patient to believe that the voices are a reflection of their 'unconscious mind', and this will help them come to terms with the fact that the hallucinatory voices are often very unpleasant and derogatory.

Persistent delusional ideas can be dealt with in a similar way, although it is always best to start with less firmly held beliefs and only to move on to more fixed delusional convictions once some success has been achieved. In the early stages, the implications and ramifications of the delusional ideas can be explored, followed by a review of alternative possibilities or explanations. The patient is encouraged to test out the relative merits and reality of their delusional beliefs and the alternative explanations that are arrived at through discussions with the therapist.

Negative symptoms and socially disruptive behaviour

If these problems persist for any time, it is difficult to devise changes in medication that will make any useful difference. Clozapine can usually help negative symptoms when conventional drugs have failed, and the new drugs risperidone, sertindole and olanzapine may also have a useful effect. However, with all these drugs, it is the negative symptoms which arise secondarily to positive symptoms rather than true primary negative symptoms which are most likely to improve. Impulsive irritability and aggressive behaviour can sometimes be helped by adding carbamazepine or lithium to antipsychotic drug regimens, but the success rate is not high. It is important to exclude adverse effects of antipsychotic medication which may be making these problems worse. For example, drug-induced parkinsonism may mimic or exacerbate negative symptoms, and akathisia or impaired concentration or confusion due to excessive medication might be factors in explaining socially inappropriate or aggressive behaviour.

In devising psychosocial strategies for management, it is important to set goals for progress at an appropriate level. If the goals are too ambitious, patients will rapidly become discouraged, whereas if they are too easy, they will provide no incentive and lower self-esteem further. It is often a good idea to start with physical fitness issues as these have obvious relevance to most people and can be tackled easily compared with more complicated tasks involving skilled behaviour or social inter-action. As with positive psychotic symptoms, optimizing the environ-ment is very important to give negative symptoms and socially disruptive behaviour the best chance of improvement. Reducing both isolation and boredom on the one hand and overarousal and stress on the other can have a helpful impact.

Negative symptoms and socially inappropriate behaviour or poor hygiene can be a heavy burden for carers and family and friends. In helping the affected person, it is nearly always important to try to help carers as well. Family members often have a sense of grief as a reaction to their relative's long-term mental illness, since a person with schizo-phrenia is often a pale shadow of what they were and might have been. Relatives often feel guilty, sometimes believing that it was their fault the schizophrenic illness occurred in the first place. The sense of guilt can be exacerbated by understandable feelings of anger towards the person with schizophrenia who may appear to reject or take for granted their rela-tive's concern. In supporting carers and family members, an attempt is made to help them avoid excessive hostility towards their relative, and while acknowledging the possible validity of their anger, to help prevent blame of the affected person. Similarly, families can be encouraged to stop treating their affected relative like a helpless child. Overprotec-tiveness should be discouraged and carers should be supported in their attempts to foster as much autonomy and independence as possible in their affected relative, even when in the short term this may involve taking a few risks and weathering a great deal of anxiety. Family members can often get a great deal of help and support by attending carers' groups. In addition to providing a forum for learning and education about schizophrenia, these can contribute a sense of hope and purpose to what otherwise may seem a meaningless and hopeless problem.

Social withdrawal and poor self-care are problems that cause particular worry and distress to carers, if not to the person with schizophrenia. Both these problems can reflect either 'primary' negative symptoms, or be secondary to active psychotic symptoms such as delusions and hallucina-tions. It is important to decide which is the case, because even persistent positive symptoms are usually easier to manage than primary negative symptoms. Social withdrawal, if not secondary to active psychotic symp-toms, often reflects anxiety about social interactions or a general apathy about doing anything. In the first case, social withdrawal may be an attempt to avoid anxiety-provoking situations, but if so, this will set up a vicious cycle, since avoidance will only further increase the fear of social contacts. In the case of apathy, there may be a general lack of reinforce-ment or pleasure from social situations, but the problem will only get worse if social contacts are minimized. The management therefore is to encourage the person to make small steps to increase their social contacts, anticipating and dealing with the anxiety that may be produced in the process, and providing personal encouragement and support through the key worker role. If it is thought that the person with schizophrenia is experiencing persistent lack of pleasure (*anhedonia*) owing to a depressive condition, antidepressive medication added to their antipsychotic drugs can sometimes help.

In the case of poor self-care, in addition to being secondary to positive symptoms of psychosis, the other two main associated factors are lack of motivation and lack of skills, often combined with high levels of social anxiety. As with social withdrawal, lack of motivation is helped by encouraging small steps of improvement using praise and powerful personal reinforcement from the key worker. In dealing with absent or lost skills, social skills training involves breaking down tasks into small steps that can be approached in a hierarchy of difficulty. A general principle here is that skills acquired in one setting are often only partially generalized to other situations. For this reason most people with schizophrenia who show long-term social skills deficits need to have help in this area maintained over an indefinite period, and particularly when there is a change in the setting in which they carry out their daily routines.

Poor concentration is a problem that is often encountered in people who have had schizophrenia for some time. This too may be caused by the distracting effects of hallucinatory experiences, or may reflect the effects of overmedication with sedative drugs. In many cases, however, it appears to reflect a cognitive deficit associated with long-term mental illness. Whatever the cause, it will almost certainly add to problems such as apathy and social withdrawal. In helping to deal with poor concentration, tasks that present difficulty are broken down into small steps which can be dealt with over brief periods with the aid of frequent prompts and as much reinforcement as possible. While doing this, distractions and extraneous stimuli should be kept to a minimum. If improvement in poor concentration has resulted in a task being successfully completed, this will not necessarily encourage the person to try again, so the coping skills used will have to be continually reinforced.

Depression and low self-esteem are common in people with long-term schizophrenia and are often the consequence of the many losses and problems that this condition is associated with. Material impoverishment, unemployment, social isolation and loneliness are all factors leading to depression in schizophrenia. Periods of improved insight may increase people's awareness of their losses and disabilities, and so contribute to their depression and despair (*postpsychotic depression*). Antidepressants may be helpful in these situations, but probably more important is supportive psychotherapy from a trusted and consistent therapist, who, while not denying the losses and sense of waste that the person has experienced as a result of the illness, can also improve the person's sense of self-worth, and perhaps inject a small dose of realistic hope and optimism through the expression of their concern.

Poor compliance with prescribed treatment

Having already made the point that maintenance antipsychotic medication is far from ideal, but better than nothing for the majority of people with schizophrenia, it becomes a major goal to ensure that people do take the medication that they are prescribed. This can be a problem, since the people who are probably most in need of their medication are the ones most likely not to take it reliably, if at all. On average between a third and a half of people prescribed medication by mouth for long-term mainte-nance treatment of schizophrenia do not take their drugs, and with another third of patients, compliance with medication is probably irreg-ular and erratic.

There are many reasons why people with schizophrenia may not take the drugs that they are prescribed. Probably the most common reason is the experience of unpleasant side-effects, which often convinces patients that the treatment is worse than the condition for which they are taking medication. Linked to the off-putting influence of side-effects, is the fact that people with schizophrenia may deny that treatment had been of any benefit, or that if it was of help, the need for it has passed now that they feel better. It is common for people with schizophrenia not to appreciate the need for long-term medication in order to prevent relapses of illness, and even careful and sympathetic explanation may fail to convince them. Rejection of the need for treatment is often regarded as an indicator of poor insight, so there is a risk of circularity if a lack of insight is claimed to be a cause of low compliance with medication. Although the aspect of insight that reflects people's acceptance or denial of illness does appear to correlate with compliance with medication, interestingly it is not neces-sary for people to agree with their doctors about exactly what is wrong with them in order to agree to take their medication. For example, a person may agree to take antipsychotic medication on the grounds that it helps them sleep or cope with feelings of anxiety, even though this may not be the main reason that the medication has been prescribed.

People who have a hostile or mistrustful attitude towards people trying to help them are very unlikely to take medication prescribed by the same people. Unfortunately mistrust and hostility can sometimes be made worse by having to enforce treatment, e.g. under a Section of the Mental Health Act. When this is done in the interest of people's health and safety, it is always hoped that treatment will eventually restore insight and banish hostility and mistrust, despite the fact that the treat-ment had to be started with coercion.

Unfortunately it often turns out that a person who is forced to have treatment never entirely forgives those who treat them in this way, and can never be fully convinced that it was done in good faith, and in order to help them. If treatment is only partially successful in dealing with paranoid beliefs specifically centred on medication, e.g. that drugs are a form of poison, then this will militate against compliance with medica-tion.

It is a common experience that many people with schizophrenia attribute symptoms of their illness to side-effects of medication. Even more commonly, friends and relatives often believe that the apathy and blunted emotional expression (affect) characteristic of schizophrenia are adverse effects of medication. Sometimes they are right to believe this, as drug-induced parkinsonism can often be mistaken for negative symp-toms, even by experienced staff. This is especially likely if they do not know the patient well, and make the unwarranted assumption that the person has been in an apathetic, withdrawn state for a long time when this is not the case. Perhaps the side-effect that most commonly leads to patients not complying with their medication is akathisia, because this complaint is sometimes not taken seriously enough by the staff who are responsible for prescribing and monitoring the medication. In contrast, abnormal involuntary movements especially tardive dyskinesia often cause more worry to staff than to the person affected, and are not usually directly linked to non-compliance with medication. The apathy and inactivity associated with negative symptoms can, however, make an important contribution to poor compliance with medication, simply because the person may not be bothered to attend for treatment or to pick up their prescription. Poor concentration and forgetfulness, which can be negative symptoms of schizophrenia, can also lead to poor compliance.

Finally, an important reason for people refusing to take medication is that they object on principle to being given medication to deal with what they view as a personal or spiritual problem. They may believe that drug treatment devalues their experience of illness, and represents a humiliating and stigmatizing imposition. In this they are often supported by friends and family, and even by carers and professionals working with them. These negative attitudes towards medication are often fostered by misunderstanding and misinformation about drug treatment, although the fact that some prescribers are very insensitive to people's feelings on this matter does not help.

A number of ways of helping people comply better with their medication can be suggested. Probably the single most important strategy is a full and frank explanation about the reasons medication is being prescribed and the risks and benefits associated with it. A willingness to compromise and go along with the patient's wishes about medication will help inspire confidence in a frightened and mistrustful patient, and help compliance even if the medication regimen selected may not be optimal in other ways. Although the process of negotiation and compromise may take a long time, it is usually worth it. Specific practical strategies may include giving patients only enough oral medication for a short period (e.g. 2–4 days) so that they are less likely to mislay their tablets or hoard them. Administering medication at a day centre and linking this with an enjoyable experience of a meal or social event can also help make the medication more palatable. When the medication is administered or supervised by a person whom the patient likes and respects, it is much more likely that they will take the medication that is prescribed.

Giving antipsychotic drugs in the form of depot injections can certainly help compliance, as administration of the injection can be linked with rewarding experiences such as personal counselling, attendance at a therapy group or a social event. Depot injections are also more reliable in that erratic absorption of drugs by mouth is avoided. However, many people are extremely put off by the idea of a regular intramuscular injection in the buttocks, especially if they have grave misgivings about the need for medication anyway. If this is the case, it is usually best not to press the issue of depot medication too far for fear that it will alienate the patient and damage any trust that has been established. However, if all else fails, and the person appears to be showing deterioration in their mental state as a result of non-compliance with medication, it may be necessary to consider admission to hospital under a Section of the Mental Health Act so that treatment can be re-established in hospital.

Other practical management problems in schizophrenia

When a patient doesn't want to be seen

A common problem in trying to help people with schizophrenia is their total rejection of the idea that they need any help at all. This is not usually conveyed by any detailed argument on their part, but rather they tend to 'vote with their feet' and avoid contact with health workers whenever possible. The people who do come into contact with the affected person – relatives, friends and neighbours – are often only too convinced that the person is ill and in need of treatment. Although it sometimes has to be accepted that there is little to be done to help someone who is actively rejecting help, persistence and compromise usually do pay off. This is sometimes called *assertive outreach*. In reality it is no more and no less than not giving up easily in trying to help somebody, and in the process trying to establish some degree of trust and co-operation. It is often possible to get a 'foot in the door' by providing at least something that the person acknowledges they want and need. If this can be offered as part of an overall treatment package including medication, then some progress can be made. Sometimes it has to be accepted that no active treatment will be tolerated by the patient, but at least they will trust the mental health worker enough to stay in contact. This is often extremely valuable, since the health worker can monitor whether the patient's condition has deteriorated sufficiently to warrant admission to hospital under a compulsory order of the Mental Health Act. At the very least, the mental health worker may be able to obtain information from friends, relatives or neighbours who do see the person on a regular basis, and to agree with them on a management plan should matters deteriorate unacceptably.

To treat or not to treat?

Sometimes there is disagreement within a multidisciplinary team about the potential value of drug treatment for a particular person's problems. Health workers may be echoing their client's own negative attitudes about drug treatment, or polarizing the issue into an either/or argument in deciding the relative merits of several management approaches including drug treatment. Since in most situations, and particularly in schizophrenia, drug treatments are helpful adjuncts to other kinds of help and therapy, this polarized attitude may occasionally reflect prejudice or ignorance. On the other hand, doctors in particular have a tendency to overestimate the value of medication, and should be careful not to press their case for medication at the expense of other approaches which may be just as valid or more helpful. As a generalization, if there are disabling symptoms, drug treatment is likely to be of some benefit, assuming that side-effects and other problems can be kept to a minimum. Where the person's difficulties are mainly interpersonal or social in nature and origin, at best drug treatment will only complement and enhance other approaches. However, in cases of established schizo-phrenia, the arguments for some form of prophylactic drug treatment are very strong. Low-dose regimens or intermittent treatment in response to early signs of psychotic relapse appear to be second-best compromises which may have to be adopted in order to engage the person in other forms of more acceptable treatment.

Starting treatment

Because people are often apprehensive about starting medication, this process has to be handled sensitively and with due awareness of the frightening nature of some drug side-effects. It is known that a sizeable minority of people when first given antipsychotic drugs experience unpleasant subjective sensations which may put them off taking medica-tion for good. Explanation beforehand can be helpful in preventing rejec-tion of treatment for this reason, but the better strategy is to carefully supervise the effects of a 'test dose' of medication, giving the patient lots of explanation and reassurance in the process. Although this carries the risk of alarming the patient, in practice this rarely seems to happen, and the message that comes across is one of concern and expertise on the part of the person prescribing the medication.

Distinguishing side-effects of medication from untreated or untreatable effects of illness

Although psychotic drugs have a major tranquillizing action which will appear after one or two doses, the antipsychotic effect takes weeks or even months to reach its peak. In the meantime side-effects may have emerged which confuse the clinical picture. There is no substitute for careful and sustained clinical observation of the patient's responses, with frequent reassurance to the patient that things are going well. Although skill and experience are needed in this monitoring process, just as impor-tant is in-depth knowledge of the patient, and familiarity with the settings and routines of their daily life which may be affected by the administration of medication.

Negative symptoms of schizophrenia versus extrapyramidal side-effects or oversedation

As the acute symptoms and disturbance of a schizophrenic relapse begin to settle, negative symptoms of schizophrenia often become more notice-able. This is partly because the active positive symptoms tend to mask negative symptoms. Also, following recovery from an acute florid illness, there is sometimes an increase in the severity of negative symptoms compared with the patient's mental state before the relapse. A similar consideration applies to depressive symptoms which are often 'revealed' as more active psychotic symptoms begin to settle, particularly if the patient's returning insight leads them to feel despondent or despairing about their situation. However, it is also the case that during an acute relapse, antipsychotic medication is often administered in higher dosages than is used for maintenance treatment. For this reason, as the acute symptoms recede, oversedation and extrapyramidal side-effects of high-dose antipsychotic medication should be anticipated. Clinically, negative symptoms of schizophrenia are easily confused with depression or with sedation and parkinsonian features due to medication. The patient may appear unspontaneous and lacking in emotional expression in all these conditions and show slowness of movement and lack of spontaneity in speech and action.

In schizophrenia there is often an impaired awareness of or ability to describe alterations in mood, so patients themselves may not complain of any problems. However, in terms of everyday activities, lack of facial expression, lack of reactivity and slowness can have damaging effects. There is a pressing need to improve the situation, but if it is inaccurately ascribed to 'untreatable' negative symptoms of schizophrenia, nothing may be done. In contrast, drug-induced extrapyramidal side-effects or parkinsonism can be readily treated, and depression may be amenable to antidepressant drugs or supportive psychotherapy.

The way out of these difficulties is firstly to exclude parkinsonian features by carefully examining the patient to check for other signs of parkinsonism such as a resting tremor of the extremities, characteristic rigidity of the limbs, and dribbling and drooling due to overproduction of saliva. A shuffling gait and reduced arm swing are also characteristic. Once there is a reasonable level of suspicion that extrapyramidal or parkinsonian symptoms are responsible for the patient's 'negative state', a trial of anticholinergic medication (e.g. procyclidine), preferably by injection, should settle the matter by producing some detectable (albeit short-term) relief of the problem. If this is confirmed, regular oral anti-cholinergic medication for a while, combined with reduction in the dose of antipsychotic medication, would be the obvious strategy. If after going through these procedures, it is concluded that the person is affected by negative symptoms or depression, these have to be distinguished from each other by careful consideration of what is on the person's mind. For example, although it may be difficult to get the person to speak about their feelings, their emphasis on pessimistic ideas and a lack of pleasure and enjoyment in accustomed activities may be a pointer to a depressive condition rather than negative symptoms.

Anxiety versus akathisia

People with schizophrenia are often prone to feelings of anxiety and tension, usually as part of a general pattern of mood instability and vulnerability to stress. Anxiety often produces feelings of tension and motor restlessness, and an unpleasant subjective feeling or *dysphoria*. These symptoms can closely resemble the drug-induced syndrome of akathisia, which is a highly unpleasant sensation associated with an irresistible desire to fidget (Table 6.10). When the problem has been present for a long time, the unpleasant subjective aspect of the problem seems to recede and the person can be observed to be fidgeting or pacing on the spot without any expressed discomfort. Distinguishing anxiety from akathisia can be a particular problem when the affected person finds it difficult to put their feelings into words. Anxiety may herald the imminent relapse of their psychosis, and may provoke the mental health worker to recommend more antipsychotic medication. In contrast, antipsychotic drug-induced akathisia is best handled by a reduction in medication if this can be achieved without causing a deterioration in the person's mental state.

Fortunately, drugs used for treating akathisia (beta-blockers and benzodiazepines) can also be helpful in treating anxiety states. The conditions are best distinguished by careful consideration of the history of the complaint and by keeping a high level of suspicion about akathisia, which is much more common than people used to believe. Reducing the dose of the antipsychotic medication should bring about some relief, and if so this will fairly reliably distinguish it from anxiety.

Drug-induced muscle spasms versus 'hysteria' or 'acting out' behaviour

The muscle spasms or dystonias which antipsychotic drugs can provoke often produce bizarre behaviour such as the eyes rolling up and the patients sticking out their tongue and being unable to speak properly. In addition spasm of the neck may restrict patients to holding their head in a fixed abnormal position. All these features can sometimes be attributed to 'hysteria', 'acting out' or simply faking. The injustice that this does to the patient's distress is extreme and it would be inexcusable to fail to recognize such an important side-effect of medication. It can even be a dangerous complication if the muscle spasms affect the throat or muscles of respiration. Fortunately there is a simple way of making the differential diagnosis, since acute dystonias will respond, at least in the short term, to an injection of an anticholinergic drug.

When the muscle spasms have been present for a long time, it may be more difficult to tell them apart from bizarre or 'manneristic' postures and behaviour due to the psychosis. Long-standing dystonias are less responsive to anticholinergic medication, and their persistence may lead the affected person to behave strangely as a secondary reaction to the way people treat them in response to their odd appearance (Barnes and Braude, 1985). Careful examination and a trial of anticholinergic medication over several days or weeks is the best way forward.

Drug-induced constipation and incontinence versus self-neglect

Antipsychotic drugs can produce a number of side-effects affecting the gastrointestinal system, especially constipation. If this becomes a long-term problem the bowel can become obstructed, and there can be an overflow of loose, watery stools causing faecal incontinence. Severe constipation can also provoke urinary incontinence. Furthermore, the anticholinergic side-effects of antipsychotic drugs tend to produce retention of urine, especially in the elderly, and this too can result in overflow incontinence of urine. A person who is showing faecal or urinary incontinence may also be exhibiting behavioural disturbance that is an integral part of their mental illness, although not obviously related to delusional ideas or hallucinations. Disorders of movement and arousal in schizophrenia are termed *catatonic* and incontinence may be a feature of this.

The management of catatonic states is more vigorous treatment of the underlying psychotic disorder, whereas if the problems are being produced as side-effects of medication, then a dose reduction or a switch to a different drug with fewer side-effects may be the answer. Once again it is important to make a careful evaluation of the history of the problem and to look for any other signs of anticholinergic side-effects, e.g. dry mouth, blurred vision and dilated pupils. If these are detected, it may also be important to reduce or stop any anticholinergic medication that is being concurrently prescribed for parkinsonian side-effects. If these 'side-effect' tablets were indeed found to be responsible for the constipation or urinary incontinence, this would be a good example of treatment for side-effects causing side-effects of their own and compounding the patients' problems.

Catatonic states versus neuroleptic malignant syndrome

In rare cases, catatonic states can be severe and result in extreme lack of responsiveness (stupor, rigidity of the limbs, fever and sweating, etc.). These signs can easily be confused with the rare but potentially dangerous neuroleptic malignant syndrome which is believed to be provoked by antipsychotic drugs in susceptible people. Treatment of the neuroleptic malignant syndrome involves stopping antipsychotic drugs, giving an intravenous infusion of saline if the patient is not drinking adequately, and administering muscle relaxants if the rigidity of the muscles increases and results in high fever and dangerous changes in blood chemistry. Treatment of severe catatonic stupor may require administration of electroconvulsive therapy, but in other respects the management is similar to that of the neuroleptic malignant syndrome, particularly in immediately stopping antipsychotic drugs and administering muscle relaxants such as benzodiazepines. In any case the management of these highly alarming and potentially dangerous states should be in hospital under specialist supervision.

Mental confusion secondary to psychosis or toxic effects of drugs

In people who are experiencing severe and terrifying psychotic symptoms, the clinical picture may often be of marked perplexity, disorientation and confusion. Adverse reactions to drugs can sometimes result in a toxic confusional state owing to an impairment of the level of consciousness and depression of the nervous system. Once again, when the problem is due to deterioration of illness an increase in medication is indicated, whereas in the case of drug-induced adverse reactions management involves reducing or stopping the medication. The main factor distinguishing psychologically-determined confusion from toxic or organic confusion is the level of consciousness or arousal. In toxic confusional states the person is usually slightly drowsy, although this may not be easy to detect if they are also frightened and disturbed. Once again this type of problem is sufficiently serious to warrant referring the person to hospital for further assessment and management.

Drug and alcohol abuse

People with schizophrenia are believed to be especially at risk from heavy usage of recreational or illicit drugs and alcohol, presumably because they take these substances in an attempt to relieve their disabling and distressing experiences of mental illness. Cannabis in particular appears to be used in an attempt to self-medicate negative symptoms of schizophrenia, and in this regard it may be partially successful, although at the risk of possibly aggravating active psychotic features. Stimulant drugs like cocaine ('crack') and amphetamines ('speed') can certainly worsen psychotic symptoms in a proportion of schizophrenic patients, although paradoxically there have been reports of amphetamines actually bringing about an improvement in others. Alcohol abuse often exacerbates psychotic symptoms in schizophrenia and adds to problems of self-neglect and poor compliance with medication, which may already have complicated the person's management.

Anticholinergic drugs may be abused by patients because they sometimes have a mood-lifting or 'high' effect which people value as a relief from their negative symptoms. Unfortunately these anticholinergic drugs can partially cancel out the antipsychotic actions of their other medication, and if taken in very high doses, anticholinergic drugs can produce a *toxic psychosis* in their own right. A disturbed patient who appears actively psychotic but is showing clinical features of anticholinergic drug poisoning (dilated pupils, dry mouth, fast pulse and high temperature, etc.) should be referred for immediate specialist assessment as the condition can be dangerous.

Summary and practical guide for dealing with problems in schizophrenia

As a summary of some of the practical issues discussed in this chapter, Table 6.12 outlines the psychosocial management and related medication issues in the principal problem areas encountered in the long-term treatment of schizophrenia. Table 6.13 summarizes 12 common problems or situations arising in the management of schizophrenic patients, with notes on how to understand what is going on and what to do about it. This should only be regarded as a crude guide, but at least it is reassuring that the management of such a complicated and sometimes bewildering condition as schizophrenia can be boiled down to just a few points, no matter how simplistic.

Table 6.12 *Psychosocial management and related medication issues in five related problem areas encountered in long-term treatment of schizophrenia*

Problems	Psychosocial management	Medication issues
1. Persistent symptoms and behavioural disturbance	Supportive counselling Cognitive behavioural therapy	Dose increases/decreases Exclude side-effects that may exacerbate mental symptoms Change antipsychotic drugs Try augmentation with added drugs Try new drug (clozapine, risperidone, etc.)
2. Problems of daily living: relationship problems loneliness poor hygiene and appearance poor housekeeping and budgeting	Problem solving, and practical and social skills training Use of day centres and drop-ins Behavioural family therapy	Drug and alcohol abuse Side-effects of medication (constipation, incontinence) exacerbating hygiene problems
3. Impaired social functioning: non-acceptance of illness ignorance and stigma poor housing unemployment and poverty	Social skills training Education Advocacy and legal advice Improved housing Work counselling and retraining	Social unacceptability of medication Non-compliance with medication
4. Increased stress reaction	Coping strategies Family stress management	Temporary increase in dose or change to another medication
5. Relapses of florid mental illness	Crisis intervention 'Crisis cards' and 'relapse signatures'	Temporary increase in dose or change to another medication Consider treatment in hospital under the Mental Health Act

Table 6.13 *Schizophrenia – problems to look for and what to do about them*

	Sign	Meaning	Action
1.	Patient talks to him/herself or shouts and waves as though at something or somebody	Possibly hearing *voices* or seeing *visions*, or more than usually troubled by these, indicating mental illness	If associated with recent stress, symptoms may settle spontaneously or with temporary increase in dose of usual maintenance antipsychotic medication. Otherwise may need short-term hospitalization. If health is at risk, or is danger to self or others and refusing help, may need to be hospitalized under the Mental Health Act
2.	Patient seems very suspicious or *paranoid*, or is preoccupied with and insistent about odd, unrealistic ideas	Patient may be suffering from *delusions*, which with *hallucinations* are key features of *psychosis*	As above
3.	Incoherent speech, jumbled meaning and words. May stop speaking mid-sentence	Patient's thoughts are disjointed and disorganized. May experience thoughts being withdrawn or inserted into mind	As above
4.	Patient is unusually dirty and dishevelled, wearing odd clothes or showing *bizarre behaviour*	May reflect delusional beliefs or disorganized thinking	As above
5.	Patient seems depressed and more than usually worried and tense without obvious explanation or reason	May represent the early stage of a relapse of acute mental illness, or the emergence of insight following loss of contact with reality during psychotic breakdown	Look into the possibility of correctible personal and social problems; arrange supportive counselling; advise small increase in antipsychotic medication (antidepressant drugs may be helpful); enquire about suicidal ideas or plans (suicidal acts are often unpredictable, but may be *driven* by voices or delusions)
6.	Patient seems very restless and fidgety, unable to keep still or pacing on the spot	May be same as (5), or more probably a side-effect of antipsychotic medication called *akathisia*	Reduce dose of antipsychotic medication if this not likely to make mental illness worse or cause relapse; try effect of *beta-blockers* (propranolol) or benzodiazepine (diazepam)

Table 6.13 (*continued*)

7.	Patient unexpectedly insists on stopping antipsychotic medication, but cannot or will not say why	May reflect delusional ideas about treatment, or may be suffering embarrassing side-effect (e.g. impotence) or symptoms difficult to describe (e.g. akathisia or *dysphoria*)	Be sensitive to patient's feelings and motives. Try to negotiate dose reduction rather than stopping completely. If patient still insists, do not reject patient because patient rejects medication
8.	Patient has slow tremor of hands and other parts of the body at rest	Parkinsonian side-effects of antipsychotic medication	Reduce dose of antipsychotic medication if possible, or try short-term (4–8 week) treatment with antiparkinsonian medication, e.g. procyclidine, orphenadrine etc. (use sparingly because may make psychosis worse and has potential for other adverse effects)
9.	Patient shows spasms of face, eyes, mouth, tongue, throat, etc., often just after starting antipsychotic medication	Acute muscle spasms (*dystonia*), a distressing, sometimes serious, but thankfully transient side-effect of antipsychotic drugs	Needs immediate treatment with antiparkinsonian drug, e.g. procyclidine, preferably by injection initially, followed by a short course of tablets
10.	Patient shows constant jerking or writhing movements of mouth, tongue, face, etc.	Movements may be *voluntary*, and part of patient's mental illness, or *involuntary*, representing a neurological disorder (e.g. *tardive dyskinesia*)	Refer for specialist assessment by consultant psychiatrist
11.	Patient seems emotionally *flat*, with mask-like expression and little spontaneous talk or movement; moves slowly and stiffly with little arm swing	May represent *negative features* of schizophrenia (defect state), and/or a parkinsonian-like condition produced by antipsychotic medication	Assess the effect of one or two doses of an anti-parkinsonian drug (e.g. procyclidine); consider reducing antipsychotic medication
12.	Patient is more or less mute and motionless; apparently unresponsive, although conscious and reasonably alert; may be adopting odd positions and postures for long periods	May be *catatonic stupor* due to worsening of mental illness and/or additional physical illness; if also stiff and pyrexial (>38°) may be rare but very serious complication of antipsychotic medication (neuroleptic malignant syndrome)	Refer for general medical and specialist psychiatric assessment in hospital

Further reading

Bebbington, P. and McGuffin, P. (eds) (1988). *Schizophrenia: The Major Issues.* London: Heinemann.

Birchwood, M. J. and Tarrier, N. (eds) (1994). *Psychological Management of Schizophrenia*. Chichester: John Wiley.

Kuipers, L, Leff, J. and Lam, D. (1992). *Family Work for Schizophrenia: A Practical Guide*. London: Gaskell.

Laing, R. D. (1959). *The Divided Self*. London: Tavistock.

7

Drug treatment of mood disorders

The mood disorders referred to in formal classifications are those of depression and mania. This is confusing in many ways, because there are far more moods than these two, including anxiety, anger, ecstasy, fear and irritability. However, both mania and depression are extremely important psychiatric syndromes and so have been given their own category in ICD-10. Unfortunately, although in their classical forms both mania and depression are easy to identify, the range of conditions covered under these headings are complex and have defied attempts at a clear-cut classification which brooks no argument. Because of this, there have been many classifications of mood disorders, and it may be useful to give a brief history of these classifications and the different terms that have been used over the years. This can usefully be divided into three phases.

Classification of mood disorders

Phase 1 (1890–1930)

Although mania and depression had been recognized as illnesses for many centuries, it is only since the 1890s that there has been an acceptable classification of these disorders. The father of psychiatric classification, Emil Kraepelin, a Swiss psychiatrist, initiated this by separating manic-depressive psychosis from schizophrenia. He observed that patients in the mental hospital of which he was superintendent had two types of mental illness. Both types began early in adult life but had different courses (natural histories). The first tended to come in episodes, in which elation and overactivity were present at some times, and depression and despair at others. The episodes could last for variable lengths of time but in between them the people returned to their normal selves. The second group usually became ill a little earlier in life and more slowly, and developed symptoms of social withdrawal, false beliefs (delusions), odd perceptual experiences such as hallucinations, and the feeling that their minds were being controlled. Sometimes there was overlap between the first and the second groups (i.e. both could have delusions at different times) but an important difference was that the second group did not improve, but rather tended to deteriorate over time.

Unlike patients in the first group, those in the second group never returned to how they were before they became ill (premorbid functioning). Kraepelin labelled the first group's disorder 'manic-depressive psychosis' because mood disturbance was the most prominent feature. As mania and depression seemed to occur at different times the condition seemed to be a single one and any patient who had an episode of mania was liable to get an episode of depression subsequently, and vice versa if the initial presentation was that of depression. The second group's disorder was labelled 'dementia praecox' (precocious dementia) because his view was that the patients in this group after many years were indistinguishable from those of older patients with dementia. As they reached this state at a much younger age the diagnosis of 'dementia praecox' was considered to be appropriate.

Subsequently, another Swiss psychiatrist, Eugen Bleuler, coined the word 'schizophrenia' (shattered mind) to describe the second group. This term has been generally adopted because evidence that schizophrenia is a form of early dementia has not been substantiated (although in some forms of schizophrenia there is cognitive impairment at a later stage of illness), and the main clinical feature is a disruption or dislocation of all mental processes such as thinking, feeling and perception (see Chapter 6).

This classification only covered the most severe forms of mood disorder and most of the people to whom it applied were patients in mental hospitals. Those with milder forms of depression were normally included under the heading of neurosis and neurasthenia and regarded as the province of the new discipline of psychoanalysis.

Phase 2 (1930–1980)

Although the category of manic-depressive psychosis remained almost unchanged, it was realized that other forms of depression were not adequately covered by this general title. It was also realized that 'neurosis' was too broad a term to cover all the milder mood disorders. A debate developed among psychiatrists as to whether there were two forms of depression, one which was a consequence of circumstances (e.g. loss of a loved person) and another which was biologically determined and independent of circumstances, or just one condition of which these were the two extremes (Kendall, 1976). Those who felt the distinction was an important one used the terms 'reactive depression' (or depressive neurosis) and 'endogenous depression' (sometimes termed 'depressive psychosis') to identify the two categories. However, the other group of psychiatrists involved in classification felt that this distinction was not a useful one and that all patients with depressive disorders could be included under one grouping. In the 50 years between 1930 and 1980 the 'separatists', if we can use this name, won the argument and the terms 'reactive' and 'endogenous' depression became widely used.

Phase 3 (1980 onwards)

A number of research studies cast doubt upon the separation of reactive and endogenous depression during the late 1970s (Sartorius et al., 1980). In particular, the notion of a disorder that was entirely endogenous (i.e.

determined from within) received heavy criticism. Almost all forms of depression were found to be associated with life events (usually involving loss); these may have been either close to the episode of depression or many years removed, but there was little evidence that people developed their episodes of mood disorder entirely independent of any external circumstances. Nevertheless, there continued to be confusion because manic-depressive psychoses, now more commonly called affective or mood disorders and separated into the bipolar type (i.e. episodes of both depression and mania) and the unipolar type (i.e. episodes of only depression or mania), were regarded as having some endogenous features. Furthermore, genetic studies suggested that these conditions are inherited to a significant degree. It was also difficult to know where depression as a range of disorders ended and the mood or affective psychoses began. The argument that neurotic depression had a different outcome from psychotic depression also was shown to be suspect (Lee and Murray, 1988).

In the last few years we have returned to a simpler classification. In this, manic episodes are separated into those of hypomania (mild mania) or severe mania (just called mania) involving psychotic symptoms. Depression is separated into mild, moderate and severe episodes. Some of the features that used to be regarded as essential in the endogenous type of depression – symptoms of anorexia, weight loss, waking in the early morning, loss of libido (sexual interest) and a diurnal mood swing (feeling worse in the morning) – are together grouped as the 'somatic syndrome' of depression and can also be included as a subgrouping of the classification. Whereas it used to be thought that the somatic syndrome could only occur in severe depression, it is now appreciated that it can occur in milder forms of depression and so its presence is not necessarily an indicator of the severity of depression. However, if psychotic symptoms are present they are always regarded as indicating severe depression.

The diagnosis of mood disorder is likely to continue to change, but the system followed here is that of ICD-10, the International Classification of Disease, 10th revision (World Health Organization, 1992). This not only separates mood disorders as they present at a point in time but also takes into account their course. Thus mood disorders are separated into:

- Episodes (e.g. manic episode or depressive episode), which describes the mental status at the time the diagnosis is made.
- Bipolar affective disorder (either the manic phase or the depressive phase of an established affective psychosis).
- Recurrent depressive disorder (i.e. there have been clear-cut past episodes of the same condition).
- Persistent less severe mood disorders (not covered in any of the above).

It would be beyond the scope of this book to discuss in detail the further subclassification of mood disorder, but two aspects deserve mention. Firstly, what used to be called 'cyclothymic personality disorder' is now felt to be a mild variant of manic-depressive disorder and is therefore included among the persistent mood disorders mentioned above. Secondly, schizoaffective disorders, which at various times have been regarded as mood disorders, are now grouped amongst the schizophrenias. It is also fair to add that depression is not completely removed from the neurotic disorders, an issue discussed in Chapter 8. All in all, although we have tried to put mood disorder in one place in the latest classification it is clear that it escapes from its cage quite easily and is attached to other disorders within the psychiatric classification.

Main clinical features

Most mental health workers reading this will be familiar with the clinical presentation of patients with mood disorders, but for the sake of completeness the main features of each are discussed.

It is helpful to think of mood disorders as occurring across a spectrum with mania at one end and severe depression at the other. In between there are intermediate stages which are represented in Figure 7.1. We all occupy a position along this spectrum at any one time and we may oscillate from one point on the spectrum to another. For example, someone who has been previously well may gradually become depressed, initially with mild depressive symptoms which then become more severe. The same individual may recover and have repeated episodes of illness, but always becomes depressed and never succumbs to a manic episode. In this case the patient is usually described as having a unipolar depressive illness.

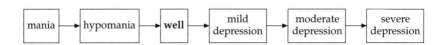

Figure 7.1   *The spectrum of mood disturbance*

The alternative is a bipolar illness where the patient may switch from depressive illnesses to manic ones and vice versa. It is a little more difficult to classify people who have repeated episodes of manic or hypo-manic illness. These people are usually classified as having bipolar illnesses and this is both because of genetic evidence linking the aetiology of recurrent mania to bipolar illness and also because of the expectation that, in time, those who have episodes of mania only will get depressive episodes too. The ratio of mania to depression is often higher early in the course of illness, and depression becomes more prominent later.

It is also important to recognize that there is also a condition called 'mixed affective psychosis', in which patients can have features of both mania and depression present at the same time. This is much more common than is often realized, because we find it difficult to accommodate the notion that people can have both elevated and depressed mood simultaneously.

The remaining group is rare but attracts a great deal of interest, and is made up of people often called 'rapid cyclers'. No, this is not an Olympic event; it describes people who move so rapidly from mania to depression and vice versa that it is difficult to keep up with them. Some people can change their mood daily, and have attracted a great deal of attention because they appear to have true endogenous mood disorders which change from mania to depression and vice versa. This is often predictable and independent of external circumstances. However, intensive study of this group of people has not really helped in understanding the other forms of mood disorder.

Depressive illness

The depressed patient first and foremost has an abnormality of mood. 'Affect' is a sophisticated word for 'mood', hence the term 'affective disorders'. Someone who asks (often somewhat pompously) if there is an 'affective component' to a disorder is merely using the jargon for 'is depression or mania present'? In depressive disorder the patient usually complains of low mood. However, if the patient denies this or cannot respond appropriately to questions, there is usually objective evidence on examination of low mood, as reflected in the patient's appearance and behaviour. Severely depressed individuals tend to sit hunched forward in their chairs, with a miserable, frowning expression and poor eye contact. Movement and activity may be increased indicating agitation, or reduced with minimal movements and absence of gestures. Similarly, speech is usually slowed and unspontaneous, and the content of speech reduced. These features together constitute *psychomotor retardation* in which there is poverty of movement and speech.

The most severe form of psychomotor retardation is depressive stupor in which the patient is conscious but shows little or no movement what-soever. This nowadays is thankfully rare but can still represent a severe diagnostic and management problem. There are other forms of stupor as well as those caused by depression, including (paradoxically) manic stupor, in which the person is so overactive they have come to a full stop. A form of schizophrenia, catatonic stupor, and a rare form of conversion disorder, hysterical stupor, can also present in the same way. These have to be separated from stupor due to physical conditions, of which the most common is a lesion of the midbrain that leads to a similar state commonly called *coma vigil*, in which the person appears to be taking notice of everything going on in their surroundings but makes no response to it whatsoever. It is hoped that the community mental health worker will not often be put into the position of having to make a differential diagnosis of stupor; it is usually only possible by talking to someone who has been with the patient and who can describe how the patient has been before the state of stupor has begun.

Most patients with depression have thoughts that tend to revolve around negative aspects of their life. Their thinking may be quite distorted in that they remember only the bad things that have happened to them and expect that the future will be just as grim, or even worse. Hopelessness, pessimism, low self-esteem, self-reproach, guilt, anhedonia (the inability to enjoy anything), loss of interest and energy, poor concentration, suicidal thoughts and homicidal thoughts (usually linked to suicide) are all features of depression. In the most severe cases patients do not just think about death and dying but start to consider harming themselves and ultimately turn to thoughts of suicide. Ideas may then be translated into actions and a suicide attempt made.

It is an unfortunate fact that many depressed patients often commit suicide when they are in the process of improving or have apparently got better. This is because they now have the energy and motivation to carry out the suicide intent that they developed earlier. There is recent evidence that patients who are discharged from psychiatric hospitals are 200 times more likely to kill themselves in the first few weeks after discharge than an average person of similar age (Goldacre et al., 1993). Many such patients have significant depressive disturbance and it is often the community mental health worker who is in the best position to pick up the warning signs of suicide intent. This subject must never be avoided with those who may be at risk and the warning signs listed in Table 7.1 should heighten awareness of the dangers in community practice.

Table 7.1   *Warning signs of suicide intent*

Behaviour	Reasons for concern
Past history of frequent suicide attempts	Past behaviour is one of the best predictors of future behaviour
Patient complains of having no reason for living	Personal or medical circumstances give little reason for hope (e.g. incurable illness, long-term unemployment, no close relationships)
Alcohol or drug abuse	Factors inhibiting suicide tend to be removed when the person is under the influence of alcohol or drugs
Sudden cessation of repeated threats of suicide	If the patient's clinical state has not improved this may indicate that a serious suicide attempt is being planned or is about to be executed

The somatic symptoms of depression are what used to be called the biological or endogenous symptoms, and are listed below. They are considered to be of importance in predicting a good response to treatment with antidepressant drugs.

- Poor sleep characterized by broken sleep and early morning wakening (waking 2 hours earlier than usual).
- Diurnal variation in mood, with depressed mood worse in the mornings.
- Reduced appetite with weight loss.
- Reduced libido.
- Amenorrhoea (cessation of monthly periods) in women.
- Loss of emotional responsivity to surroundings.
- Lack of interest and enjoyment.

Psychotic symptoms are often present in the more severely unwell patients. These include both delusions and hallucinations and in this respect the symptoms overlap with those in schizophrenia. However, in most instances the psychotic features are consistent with the mood disturbance. For example, depressed patients may feel that they have no money and are a burden on their relatives, even though they are well off (delusions of poverty). Such delusions are often described as 'mood congruent' delusions.

Mania

Patients with a manic illness also have a primary disturbance of mood, and this is characteristically elated or excited. However, manic patients may also be irritable and suspicious because they are annoyed with other people for not agreeing with their grandiose or impractical ideas. There is also an increase in activity, both mental and physical, which is often described as psychomotor acceleration (as opposed to psychomotor retardation in the depressed patient). Patients think quickly, speak rapidly and seem always to be on the move. They are restless, agitated, disorganized, with an apparently decreased need for sleep and rest. Although their appetite may be increased, they usually lose weight owing to their disorganized, haphazard approach to meals and their sustained levels of overactivity.

In contrast to the depressed patient, manic individuals often have an excessive self-regard and frequently over-reach themselves when putting ideas into action. This manifests itself in self-important attitudes and grandiose ideas or delusions concerning their abilities and roles. Socially they may be disinhibited, make poor judgements and consequently behave recklessly, particularly with regard to sexual and financial matters. However, the psychotic beliefs do not just revolve around grandiosity, and manic patients (just like patients with schizophrenia and other delusional illnesses) can experience distressing persecutory beliefs. Hallucinations also occur and may be in a number of modalities, although auditory hallucinations are the most common. Patients may also experience a heightened sense of perception and especially remark on the vividness of colours and sounds.

Aetiology

Much research has been undertaken over the years to examine the causes of mood disorders. At one end of the spectrum are the biological, genetic and biochemical theories of causation, and at the other end are the social and anthropological causes. In reality, mood disorders usually arise from a combination of these factors rather than from either one or the other. Certainly most mental health workers now feel that in order to treat the depressed or manic patient properly both biological and social aspects of their care should be considered.

Biological factors

Genetic factors are relevant in bipolar affective disorder but much less so in unipolar depressive disorder. It is also now accepted that depression is associated with altered function of certain brain transmitters called monoamines. Noradrenaline and more recently serotonin activity has been shown to be reduced and most of the antidepressants appear to act, at least in part, by increasing the functional response to these substances in the brain (Lader and Herrington, 1990), (see Chapter 2).

Social factors

Loss of a loved person or object is a very common reason for depression. Such 'exit events' are more common in people immediately before they become depressed. There is also some evidence that depression is more common after loss events (e.g. bereavement, redundancy, divorce) than others, and also more common in social classes 4 and 5 in whom there is often greater vulnerability to life events. Life events probably bring episodes of illness forward in time in individuals who are vulnerable to becoming ill at some point anyway. This suggests that the life events act as a trigger rather than a cause.

A well-known and often-quoted piece of research is that of Brown and Harris (1978) concerning vulnerability factors to depression. These authors studied a sample of the female population in Camberwell in south London, and defined four factors that increased vulnerability in women. These were loss of mother before the age of 11 years, three or more children less than 15 years old, lack of a confiding relationship, and lack of employment outside the home. These factors alone were not felt to be sufficient to cause depression, but increased the chance of a woman becoming ill in the presence of some kind of precipitating life event. It should be added that although these factors seem logical and reasonable, they have not been exactly replicated in subsequent similar research projects.

Treatment

There are many different treatments available for patients with affective disorders and there can never be a substitute for a careful assessment by members of a multidisciplinary team. Each patient is an individual and the treatment protocol must be tailor-made to suit their own personal requirements. Having said that, there are guidelines that can be used to help mental health workers navigate their way through the maze of different approaches. Psychological methods of treatment are discussed first, but most of this chapter relates to drug therapies. This is not meant in any way to minimize the importance of psychological therapies, and readers are encouraged to refer to a more detailed book for additional information. It should also be added that none of the drug treatments precludes the use of any of the psychotherapies, and indeed in clinical practice much benefit can be gained by combining treatments, (see Chapter 3).

Psychological treatments

Psychological treatments can be summarized as:

- supportive
- behavioural
- cognitive
- analytic.

Case vignette 7.1

Nigel, a 22-year-old man was referred to a community mental health team by his general practitioner because of depressive symptoms. No apparent cause for his depression was known but his parents thought it followed an argument. After assessment by a psychologist and a nurse in the team it was realized that the problem was more complex. After several interviews Nigel admitted that he had been depressed because a friend of his had died. He and several of his colleagues had been taking amphetamines, LSD and other drugs of abuse. They had taken these drugs after late-night parties and after one of these his friend had collapsed and died. He had not disclosed this to anybody else but had become increasingly guilty about his friend's death, feeling himself to be partially responsible. He was treated by a programme of cognitive and behavioural therapy which emphasized that his attribution of responsibility for his friend's death was not the only possible explanation of the events, and more constructive thinking led to improvement in function. He steadily improved and was ready to return to work when he was formally told that he had lost his job because of prolonged sickness. After this he became much more depressed and was unable to respond to further psychological therapy.

He was seen by the psychiatrist in the team and prescribed lofepramine 140 mg daily increasing to 210 mg daily after he failed to respond after 3 weeks. He gradually improved and after 6 weeks was back to his normal self. He was maintained on the antidepressants but 3 weeks later became suddenly overactive, believed he had won £5000 and sold many of his personal possessions for very low prices, believing that he was making a large profit on each transac-

tion. When assessed again he was overactive and disinhibited, tried to sell what remained of his belongings to the psychologist and then offered to give them away when this was refused. He was diagnosed as having a hypomanic episode, antidepressant therapy was stopped and he was treated with the antipsychotic drug haloperidol in doses up to 40 mg daily. Although he was close to being admitted to hospital, his family gave him considerable support and the episode was treated entirely at home. After a further 7 weeks he was back to his normal self again and agreed to take the mood-stabilizing drug, lithium carbonate. Nigel remained well, moved out of the family home into a new flat with his girlfriend and shortly afterwards married her. Two years later Nigel felt he no longer needed the lithium and it was agreed that this could be stopped, despite some reservations; at the time his wife was pregnant, and it was felt that he might have difficulty in coping with the responsibilities of fatherhood. After the birth of his daughter he did indeed have some difficulty in adjustment, but this was overcome by further counselling sessions without the need for any more intensive psychological treatment and without the need for drug therapy. One year later he remained well and on no therapy.

This account illustrates how patients can move from minor mood disturbance to much more severe illness (in this case bipolar affective psychosis) and then return ultimately to the premorbid state of health without any mental impairment. You will note that the treatment followed the range of mood disturbance shown in Figure 7.1. Initially psychological treatment (cognitive and behaviour therapy) was used and appeared to be of benefit. Subsequently a more severe depressive episode supervened, and as this was followed shortly afterwards by a manic episode, it seems likely that the patient had bipolar affective psychosis. This was treated accordingly, initially with antipsychotic drugs and then with lithium. However, because of the past history of drug misuse there is always the possibility that this could have been a triggering factor in the mood disturbance. During the severe depressive phase and the hypomanic phase of illness, drug treatment was the mainstay. The psychological treatments again came into their own at the end of the episode when the difficulties were clearly reactive to childbirth. It is even possible that the drug treatment could have triggered off the episode of mania because antidepressants may precipitate mania in predisposed individuals. However, the important adjective is 'predisposed'; the episode of hypomania would not have been triggered in a person who did not have the tendency to develop bipolar affective psychosis.

The important lesson to be learnt from this type of case is that it is wrong to be rigid about treatment at any one time in an individual's problem. It was also impossible to see at the outset that the patient would develop a manic episode. He had never had any episodes previously and there was no family history of depression or mania. What was unusual was that the whole episode was treated successfully at home and this was probably because a good therapeutic relationship had been built up in the earlier stages of the mood disorder.

Physical treatments

Electroconvulsive therapy

Although the decision to give electroconvulsive therapy (ECT) is seldom made by a community mental health worker it is important to know the indications for treatment, not least because if they are present in someone being treated in the community then admission to hospital and assessment for ECT should be considered urgently. Although sounding a barbarous treatment, ECT is safe and highly effective at treating not only severe depressive illness but also some forms of acute schizophrenia, particularly when catatonic features are present (see Chapter 6). Because ECT requires general anaesthesia, albeit for less than 20 minutes, consent is required and this may have to be obtained through a relative and a medical second opinion if there are difficulties in obtaining informed consent from the patient. The advantages of ECT for severe depression are that the treatment works quickly, usually with some response after two treatments, although this is not usually developed into consistent improvement until after four to six treatments; and ECT may also work when antidepressants have failed, and so can be an indication for resistant severe depression. In cases of severe depression in which the suicidal risk is great, or in which there is a danger to the person's health (e.g. depressive stupor with refusal to eat or drink), ECT may be given because of its rapid action. Sometimes a delay for up to 4 weeks while antidepressants began to work may be considered unduly risky, and every mental health worker will have experienced frustration and anxiety while waiting for depressed patients to respond to drug treatment.

Because of the advances made in treating depression in recent years, with both drug and non-drug treatments, the use of ECT is diminishing, and most patients with mood disorders, even with the severe ones, do not require its use.

Psychosurgery

Psychosurgery, like ECT, has aroused a great deal of controversy. It involves the cutting of fibres linking the rest of the brain to the frontal cortex, either through physical division (using the surgeon's knife), or by indirect means, including destruction by radioactive particles (the best-known substance being yttrium) or by focusing sublethal beams of radioactive particles to a point where they kill the pathways at the point at which they converge. The two major procedures, stereotactic limbic leucotomy and subcordate tractomy, are still used occasionally in cases of resistant depression and also in some cases of resistant obsessive-compulsive disorder and phobic anxiety. However, only two centres in the UK now carry out such operations and, without some major break-through in the near future, it is likely that this form of treatment will become extremely rare.

Pharmacological treatments

Antidepressant drugs

A number of different types of drugs are used to treat patients with depression. The term 'antidepressant' refers only to the therapeutic effect of a drug rather than a particular class, and so antidepressants are a heterogeneous group which vary widely in both chemical structure and mode of action. There are three main classes of antidepressants: the tricyclic antidepressants, the monoamine oxidase inhibitors and newer antidepressants. This last group includes many compounds of which the selective serotonin reuptake inhibitors (SSRIs) are the most important. It is worth mentioning at this point that there is very little difference between these groups in terms of general efficacy, and the choice of drug is determined more by their side-effect profiles than by any other factor.

In order to understand how antidepressants relieve depression it is necessary to know something about the biochemistry of depression. Where one nerve cell meets another there is a gap called a synapse. When the electricity, which constitutes the nerve impulse, travels down the cell and reaches the nerve ending it is unable to jump across this synapse. Instead it causes the release of a chemical neurotransmitter substance which passes across the gap to the nerve cell on the other side. In other words the nerve impulse is translated first into chemical energy, and then back into electrical energy. The transmitter released into the synapse is then cleared away ready for the next time by the process of reuptake (see Chapter 2).

In depressive disorders the amount of transmitter substance available at some synapses may be reduced. Most of the transmitter substances are amines, and in the case of depressive illness, two amines – noradrenaline and 5-hydroxytryptamine (5-HT, serotonin) – are the most important. In depression these amines are probably reduced and antidepressants appear to work by increasing the amount or effectiveness of amines available in the synaptic cleft for transmission. The tricyclic antidepressants and the SSRIs prevent the reuptake of amines from the synapse and consequently help to maintain high concentrations so that they increase the efficiency of synaptic transmission. Monoamine oxidase inhibitors produce a similar effect by preventing the breakdown of amines by enzymes (monoamine oxidases) after they are released into the synaptic cleft. Thus, in summary, antidepressants are all thought to work by increasing the amount of noradrenaline and 5-HT available at the nerve endings, but they do this in slightly different ways (Figure 7.2).

- Tricyclics prevent reuptake of both noradrenaline and serotonin transmitter amines.
- Serotonin reuptake inhibitors are more selective and preferentially prevent serotonin reuptake.
- Monoamine oxidase inhibitors block the metabolism (breakdown) of the transmitters once they have been released into the synaptic cleft.

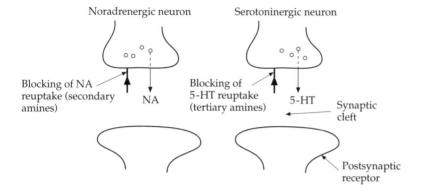

Noradrenergic neuron   Serotoninergic neuron

Blocking of NA
reuptake (secondary   NA
amines)

Blocking of
5-HT reuptake   5-HT
(tertiary amines)

Synaptic
cleft

Postsynaptic
receptor

Figure 7.2 *Mechanism of action of antidepressants (5-HT, 5-hydroxytryptamine; NA, noradrenaline)*

Drugs used in treating mood disorders

Tricyclic antidepressants and related drugs

Most of the tricyclic antidepressants were developed in the 1950s. They are called 'tricyclics' because of their chemical structure which consists of three benzene rings (i.e. three cycles). The first antidepressant to be marketed was imipramine and, like many discoveries in psychiatry, it was found by accident during research on the antischizophrenic effects of chlorpromazine. Imipramine is in fact an analogue of chlorpromazine. Since then many similar compounds have been developed, differing mainly in the degree of sedation and toxicity they produce.

The choice of tricyclic antidepressant depends largely on the degree of sedation needed (Table 7.2). An agitated patient is more likely to need a sedative drug than a retarded depressed patient. Those who are having major difficulty in sleeping may also benefit from a sedative antidepressant. However, most of the sedative antidepressants are more dangerous in overdosage and so if there is a strong suicide risk it may be wiser to forgo the advantages of sedation and to chose clomipramine or lofepramine.

A decision also has to be made about whether to put the patient on a full dose immediately. In general it is wiser to start on a low dose and increase to full dosage after 1–2 weeks. It is an unfortunate fact that most patients treated with antidepressants in the community do not receive a full antidepressant dosage. This is due to a combination of factors: the delay in onset of significant benefit (up to 4 weeks after treatment is given in full dosage); the spectrum of side-effects of these drugs (see below); and apparent improvement on low dosage. This last factor may be accounted for by people improving spontaneously, but it is also fair to note that the sedative effect of these drugs occurs early and for some depressed people this is of considerable benefit. Choosing which antide-

Table 7.2   *The commonly used tricyclic antidepressants*

Drug	Typical daily dose (mg)	Main features
Imipramine (Tofranil)	150	The original antidepressant; also effective in phobic and anxiety disorders
Amitriptyline (Tryptizol)	150	The second ticyclic anti-depressant to be discovered, similar to imipramine but produces much more sedation
Doxepin (Sinequan)	150	Similar to amitriptyline in most respects
Dothiepin (Prothiaden)	150	The most popular anti-depressant in the UK over the past few years. Similar to amitriptyline but slightly less sedating
Trimipramine (Surmontil)	150	Probably the most sedating of the tricyclic antidepressants, best given at night for agitated patients
Protriptyline (Concordin)	30	Provides very little sedation. Similar to nortriptyline
Nortriptyline (Allegron)	100	Little sedation, but in other ways similar to amitriptyline
Desipramine (Pertofran)	150	Less sedative than imipramine, toxic in overdosage
Clomipramine (Anafranil)	100–150	Partial SSRI (i.e. preferentially inhibits the uptake of 5-HT). Less dangerous in overdosage than other tricyclic antidepressants apart from lofepramine. Also used in treatment of phobias and obsessive-compulsive disorder
Lofepramine (Gamanil)	140–210	The safest tricyclic anti-depressant; produces very little sedation

pressant to use is therefore an important task, and the community mental health worker can help by asking the set of questions set out in Table 7.3.

Table 7.3 *Questions to be asked before prescribing a tricyclic antidepressant*

1. Is the patient at risk of suicide?	Clomipramine or lofepramine (or an SSRI) should be chosen if suicide is considered to be a major risk
2. Is the patient physically well?	Tricyclic antidepressants can slow down conduction in the heart and in the presence of pre-existing heart disease can cause complications
3. Is the patient taking any other medication?	Some interactions between tricyclic antidepressants and other drugs can be dangerous; in particular, some drugs taken for hypertension (ganglion blockers) and monoamine oxidase inhibitors should generally be avoided except under special circumstances (see combined antidepressant therapy below)
4. Has the patient taken antidepressants before?	Previous response is almost the best indication of likely response on this occasion. If a patient has responded well to an antidepressant before it may be wise to give that drug again in the first instance

Side-effects

Common side-effects include postural hypotension, cardiac toxicity and symptoms due to interference with the function of the autonomic nervous system – this is the system concerned with the response to stress and danger, under the influence of adrenaline and noradrenaline. However, the autonomic nervous system also controls more vegetative functions such as sleep and eating, and the neurotransmitter involved in these functions is called acetylcholine. Tricyclic antidepressants have an antagonist effect at these nerve endings and cause the following symptoms:

constipation
tremor
urinary hesitancy and retention
dry mouth
blurred vision
agitation and delirium.

These side-effects are worse in the elderly who can often only tolerate lower doses. Fortunately the elderly may also only need small doses for a successful therapeutic outcome and this is related to differences in the way the body handles and metabolizes the drugs as well as to an increased sensitivity to the drugs. In young children tricyclics are seldom used because of cardiotoxicity, although they are being used more frequently in teenagers.

One of the main difficulties in making an assessment of side-effects is the close similarity between the side-effects of tricyclics and the somatic symptoms of depressive illnesses. Considering the patient's condition prior to starting pharmacotherapy may help to distinguish between the two.

Lastly, it is necessary to mention the effects of taking tricyclic anti-depressants in excessive amounts as may happen in an overdose. Most of these drugs are potentially fatal in overdose because of their toxic effects on cardiac tissue, but lofepramine and clomiprimine are relatively free of this danger. Patients who do take an overdose are usually drowsy and are at risk of developing dangerous disturbances of heart rhythm. The issue of dangerousness in overdose is particularly important when the patient is known to be actively suicidal or to have expressed suicidal ideations. Previous episodes of self-harm are also relevant since these are strong predictors of further attempts. Indeed, it has been demonstrated that about 10% of people who self-harm will commit suicide eventually. For high-risk patients tricyclic antidepressants may be an ill-advised choice since in prescribing them the patient is also being given a lethal amount of medication. However, there are ways around this particular problem if the staff in the multidisciplinary team are motivated and have enough time and resources. Strategies to counteract the risk of overdose include giving the patient only a week's supply of medication at a time, assuming that community mental health workers can visit these clients regularly to supervise the administration of weekly prescriptions. Other coping strategies include hospitalization where the administration of medicine is closely supervised, and the use of some of the newer antide-pressants such as the SSRIs which are less dangerous in overdose.

Selective serotonin reuptake inhibitors

Selective serotonin reuptake inhibitors work in a similar way to the tricyclic antidepressants, but instead of inhibiting the reuptake of both noradrenaline and serotonin, they very selectively inhibit the reuptake of serotonin alone. It is this specificity that sets them apart. The first SSRI was introduced in 1982 and was called zimelidine; it was subsequently withdrawn owing to rare but serious adverse reactions. Since 1989 five other SSRIs have been marketed: fluvoxamine, fluoxetine, sertraline, paroxetine and citalopram. All have been shown to be effective in the treatment of depressive illnesses. None has been shown to be more effec-tive than the tricyclic drugs, though they have been useful in patients with refractory depression not responsive to tricyclics. This poses the question of whether patients should receive a tricyclic antidepressant or an SSRI when they first present with a depressive illness. This question is particularly pertinent in an age of cost-cutting, since SSRIs are currently considerably more expensive than tricyclics. At present there are no firm guidelines for indecisive clinicians, but some of the following issues are relevant to this dilemma.

- The side-effect profile of the SSRIs is better than that of the tricyclics, with virtually none of the autonomic effects such as dry mouth and constipation, although they do sometimes interfere with sexual functions, e.g. delaying ejaculation.
- However, SSRIs do cause mild nausea, diarrhoea and occasionally vomiting. In a minority of patients these effects are severe enough to warrant changing to a different drug.
- The SSRIs are extremely safe in overdose and although they can cause seizures, very few deaths attributable to SSRI overdose have been reported.
- Cardiotoxicity is extremely rare which makes these drugs safe to use in the elderly and those with specific cardiac disease.
- Fluoxetine has been associated with the kind of side-effects usually associated with antipsychotics, e.g. motor restlessness (akathisia) and parkinsonian effects.
- The SSRIs do not generally have sedating effects and some have been reported to be 'mildly activating'. Drugs such as fluoxetine should therefore be prescribed in the morning as they may cause insomnia.

There have been reports that fluoxetine causes an increase in suicidal behaviour and other impulsive behaviours. This has not been confirmed in controlled studies, and to date the only evidence is anecdotal and seems to be projected mainly by the media.

The SSRIs may precipitate mania in some individuals. However, all other antidepressant drugs can have a similar effect.

Side-effects

Side-effects of SSRIs include:

   racing thoughts, anxiety, nervousness, tremor
   insomnia, headache
   nausea, diarrhoea, vomiting, mild/moderate weight loss, constipation
   delayed ejaculation, anorgasmia
   blurred vision, dry mouth (rarely).

Drug interactions can also occur with SSRIs. Occasionally these drugs can be associated with the syndrome of restless movements (akathisia) discussed in Chapter 6 and therefore should be taken with care in combination with antipsychotic drugs. There can also be interactions with lithium and monoamine oxidase inhibitors, possibly due to excessive levels of serotonin being present in the brain. The 'serotonin syndrome' is characterized by racing thoughts, pressured speech, elevated or depressed mood, confusion, high pulse rate, high blood pressure, fever, tremor, slurred speech, lack of co-ordination, bloating, and abdominal cramps and diarrhoea.

Monoamine oxidase inhibitors

Monoamine oxidase inhibitors (MAOIs) were the first antidepressants to be used in 1957 and were shown to be more effective than the other agents available at that time. However, they were replaced rapidly by the tricyclic antidepressants as the latter were found to be more effective in treating typical depressive symptoms. Evidence for this was unsatisfactory; MAOIs are effective when given in higher dosage and are also sometimes more effective than other antidepressants in treating anxiety syndromes associated with depression including phobias. Many of the patients who respond well to MAOIs are described as having atypical depression, which is an unsatisfactory term implying that people are depressed but do not necessarily appear so. Such patients often have increased rather than reduced sleep and an excessive appetite associated with weight gain. Many of these symptoms are related to anxiety, which often appears to be the more prominent feature (Puri and Tyrer, 1982).

The MAOIs became even less popular after the demonstration in 1963 that an unusual adverse effect was created by certain foods (the so-called 'cheese reaction'). All the foods concerned (e.g. cheese) contain high levels of tyramine or dopamine (Table 7.4), which when present in the circulation can raise blood pressure and increase the risk of strokes due to cerebral haemorrhage. Normally the monoamine oxidase enzymes in the gut prevent these amines from entering the blood stream because the amines are deactivated before they are absorbed. However, with the monoamine oxidase inhibited by the drug there is no such removal and so the amines can enter the blood stream and thence the nervous system, which can create sudden and catastrophic rises in blood pressure.

Table 7.4   *Foods containing tyramine and dopamine which can create the hypertensive 'cheese reaction' in patients on monoamine oxidase inhibitors (MAOIs)*

Dopamine	Broad beans (when eaten as small whole pods)
Tyramine	Most cheeses (but not mild ones such as cottage cheese)
	Certain red wines e.g. Chianti
	Seasoned game
	Pickled herrings
	Some strong beers (but not most commercial varieties)
	Meat and vegetable extracts (e.g. Marmite)

When interactions were also demonstrated between MAOIs and certain cough or cold cures containing amines (phenylephrine, ephedrine, pseudoephedrine) and opiate analgesics (e.g. pethidine), as well as some antidiabetic drugs, it was felt by many psychiatrists that

MAOIs should be abandoned altogether. However, these drugs have always retained some adherents, and the introduction of some new compounds has reawoken interest in them. These new compounds are reversible inhibitors of monoamine oxidase (sometimes called RIMA).

These RIMA compounds do not create the 'cheese reaction' to nearly the same extent as the traditional MAOIs because monoamine oxidase is only temporarily inactivated by the RIMA and quickly returns to normal levels when tyramine and dopamine are present. Evidence to date suggests that normal quantities of foods containing tyramine and dopamine are safe when taken at the same time as a RIMA drug. The best-known of these compounds is moclobemide (Manerix) given in a dosage of 300–600 mg daily.

The older MAOIs include isocarboxazid (Marplan) (10–40 mg daily), phenelzine (Nardil) (30–90 mg daily) and tranylcypromine (Parnate) (10–30 mg daily), also sometimes prescribed in combination with trifluoperazine (Parstelin). (Combination tablets are not usually a good idea because they preclude dose adjustment of each component separately.) Because some patients often are only treated with these drugs after they have failed to respond to all others, they tend to remain on them for long periods once they have responded. This should always be borne in mind when the prescription of another medication is being considered or when there are some unusual or unexplained clinical reactions. The community mental health worker should remember this when faced with any reaction that may be related to diet or drug interaction and check whether any other drugs – particularly MAOIs – are being taken.

Care should be taken when starting or stopping MAOIs. Sometimes the patient will have been treated unsuccessfully with a tricyclic or SSRI first and will then be given an MAOI as a second-line antidepressant; in these cases it is necessary to allow a 'wash-out' period of at least three weeks between stopping the tricyclic and starting the MAOI, to allow the first drug to be fully removed from the patient's system. When changing from an MAOI to a tricyclic or SSRI there should always be a period of at least 3 weeks before the change is made, because starting either of these types of drugs while the MAOI is still active can be dangerous.

Combined Antidepressant Therapy

Combined antidepressant therapy comprises monoamine oxidase inhibitors in combination with tricyclic antidepressants. As mentioned earlier there can be serious problems with the serotonin syndrome when SSRIs are combined with MAOIs, but there is some evidence that certain combinations, particularly amitriptyline (a tricyclic) and phenelzine (a traditional MAOI) may be safe and actually protect patients from the 'cheese reaction'. Combination therapy, which is always begun with a tricyclic antidepressant followed by gradual addition of the monoamine oxidase inhibitor, is used in cases of severe resistant depression or in other forms of resistant neurotic disorder. Because MAOIs and tricyclic antidepressants exert their action in slightly different ways, the combination therapy may add something that neither drug alone can deliver.

Case vignette 7.2

Olga was a 44-year-old woman who had suffered since adolescence with anxiety, fears and depression. She had even received ECT as an adolescent because of depressive symptoms. She was seen initially by a community mental health nurse and referred for day hospital care because of persistent agoraphobia. Although she partially overcame this by taking up cycling as she found this more congenial than travelling by public transport, she continued to suffer severe anxiety. Although she cycled to the day hospital and back and carried out her responsibilities towards her two young children without apparent difficulty, she found that each of these activities made her more anxious and she eventually had to stop coming to the day hospital because of the strain. She did not respond to either amitriptyline or, at a later stage, phenelzine, despite receiving these drugs in full dosage. It was decided at a joint meeting of all team members that further psychological treatment would be likely to be of limited value because over 20 years of illness she had received hundreds of hours of input with only limited gain. It was decided to treat her with combined antidepressants, amitriptyline and isocarboxazid, and she improved dramatically after 4 weeks of treatment. Olga lost her high level of background anxiety, improved in self-confidence and obtained a job as a shop assistant, where she rapidly progressed to more senior positions in the chain. Whenever either drug was withdrawn or reduced she became anxious again and so it was decided to maintain the combination treatment long-term. Seven years later she remains extremely well and has no symptoms, but only by taking regular supplies of both drugs.

Lithium

Lithium is a metal but exists in nature as salts contained in inorganic ores. In psychiatry its main use has been in the treatment of bipolar affective disorder. It is used in patients with manic-depressive disorder to prevent relapse, or where this is not possible to reduce the frequency of episodes of illness. It is an effective treatment for mania and more recently it has been shown to have a useful role to play in the acute treatment of depression as well, especially when given to augment the effect of an antidepressant drug. It is still unclear how lithium actually works. Many patients whether in hospital or in the community will be taking lithium, and it is important for community mental health workers to have a good grasp of the principles underlying treatment.

Lithium is prescribed either as a citrate or a carbonate. It is an oral preparation and patients should only need to take a single daily dose – often at night to reduce the impact of side-effects. Side-effects even when mild may distress the patient, and it is important that the patient be afforded a regular opportunity to discuss any problems. Common side-effects include fine tremor, nausea and vomiting, thirst, increased production of urine, and weight gain. Despite these, most patients seem to adapt well to being on lithium, and even initially marked side-effects often reduce in severity with time.

Any patient due to be started on lithium should have a full physical examination and blood tests to exclude renal and thyroid disease. This is important as there are reports of lithium causing impairment of renal and thyroid function, although these effects are not usually serious or irreversible. It is now thought that renal impairment occurs much less frequently than was previously thought, usually after prolonged lithium treatment over a matter of decades. Even then it seems to cause minimal damage which only sophisticated tests of renal function can detect. However, this is a controversial subject and some people believe that lithium can cause severe impairment in a small number of patients. Whatever the truth, it seems sensible at this stage to recommend that patients on lithium should have their renal function assessed at 3-monthly intervals.

Lithium can cause hypothyroidism (underactivity) and also – although less commonly – hyperthyroidism (overactivity). Both conditions will be detected if thyroid function is checked at 3-monthly intervals. Should thyroid dysfunction occur the patient will not necessarily have to stop lithium therapy but should be referred to a physician with an interest in thyroid disorder for further advice. In the elderly or any patient with a history of cardiovascular disease an electrocardiogram should be performed prior to lithium treatment.

After screening the patient is usually started on a relatively low dose of lithium carbonate, often 400 mg given at night. Five to six days later the serum lithium level should be measured at a standard time after the last dose, and the dose adjusted accordingly. Usually the dose will need to be increased further, often to 800 mg or more daily. The clinician should aim to keep the lithium level within the therapeutic range of 0.6–1.0 mmol/l when measured 12 hours after the last dose. Regular blood testing should be carried out – weekly at first, then every 2 weeks, and when the clinician is satisfied that the patient has a stable serum level the testing can be carried out as infrequently as every 3 months. The interval should not usually be longer than this.

Mental health workers need to be aware that lithium toxicity, although not common, can be particularly dangerous. Lithium is absorbed quickly from the gut and rapidly finds its way into the blood stream. From here it passes slowly into nervous tissues as well as other organ systems. As the lithium passes through the kidneys it is filtered into the urine along with other chemicals, drugs and waste products. When the concentration of lithium in the blood rises to a critical level (e.g. owing to increased intake or reduced removal by the kidneys), the patient starts to experience symptoms of toxicity. Factors leading to toxicity include the following.

- Dehydration due to fluid deprivation, persistent nausea and vomiting, and diarrhoea commonly occurs when patients have bouts of gastroenteritis or some other infectious illness, particularly if associated with fever. Similarly in psychiatric patients, acute depressive illnesses may be associated with a poor diet and restricted fluid intake. Early detection is important in order to treat the depression as well as to avoid lithium toxicity.

- Concurrent treatment with diuretic drugs tends to increase urine output and potentially raise serum lithium levels.
- Pregnancy has a marked effect on body biochemistry and radically alters the concentration of many drugs including lithium. Lithium should not be prescribed to pregnant women since it can have harmful effects on the developing fetus.

Symptoms of lithium toxicity are different from other unwanted side-effects which may persist when the lithium level is within the therapeutic range. Toxic symptoms include the following:

coarse tremor
ataxia – stumbling, unsteady gait
dysarthria – slurred speech as if intoxicated with alcohol
gut disturbance – diarrhoea.

Carbamazepine

When a patient with a bipolar depressive illness fails to respond to anti-depressant medication or to prophylaxis with lithium, the clinician has the option of adding carbamazepine as an additional or replacement treatment.

Carbamazepine is an anticonvulsant and its primary use is in the treatment of epilepsy and a related condition, trigeminal neuralgia (severe episodic pain in the distribution of the main nerve to the skin of the face). The role of carbamazepine in bipolar disorder was discovered more recently. It has now been shown to be effective in both the prophylaxis of mania and depression and in the treatment of resistant mania (Post et al., 1983, 1986). There are some reports of its usefulness in treating unipolar illnesses (depression only), but this is more controversial.

The mechanism of action is not clear, although it seems to particularly affect an area of the brain known as the limbic system which is an area associated with mood and arousal. Carbamazepine also seems to have important stimulant effects on benzodiazepine (BDZ) receptors which are found throughout the brain. This helps to explain its anticonvulsant properties (the benzodiazepines are also used to raise the seizure threshold).

Carbamazepine is taken as an oral preparation. It has a tendency to affect the white cells in the blood, reducing their numbers (neutropenia), and possibly reducing immunity to infection. For this reason it is impera-tive that any patients receiving carbamazepine should have regular blood tests to monitor their white cell numbers. In a small minority of patients carbamazepine is associated with hepatitis and so liver function should also be monitored.

As with all drugs carbamazepine does have some side-effects. These tend to be mild and include nausea, dizziness, sedation and unsteadiness of gait. To avoid these unwanted effects patients should initially be prescribed a small dose which can then be increased gradually.

Tryptophan

Tryptophan is an amino acid found in many foodstuffs such as milk, and particularly in beef steak. Amino acids are the building blocks for protein synthesis, and tryptophan, like many other amino acids, is used by the body in a number of synthetic reactions after its absorption from the gut. In terms of brain function, tryptophan has a vital role to play since it is one of the precursors of the important neurotransmitter, serotonin. Since serotonin levels are thought to be low in patients with depression it is logical to assume that the administration of tryptophan may alleviate the mood disorder by raising serotonin levels. The theory behind this treatment rests on the hypothesis that the serotonin levels are low because not enough is being produced. If more precursor tryptophan is made available then in theory the production system can be saturated and the maximum amount of serotonin produced. In practice the biochemistry is probably much more complicated than this, with many different transmitters interacting to cause depression. However, some studies have shown that tryptophan has a valuable role to play in the treatment of depression, mainly by boosting the action of antidepressant drugs.

In the past tryptophan therapy has had a rocky ride and there have been significant prescribing problems. For many years tryptophan was prescribed for the treatment of resistant depressive illness, often in tandem with an antidepressant drug (Pare, 1985). However, more recently there have been reports of tryptophan causing an uncommon but serious adverse effect resembling an allergy affecting the blood, muscles and nervous tissue. For this reason, in the UK tryptophan is nowadays used only on a 'named patient' basis for people with severe, resistant depression.

Further reading

Lader, M. and Herrington, R. (1990). *Biological Treatments in Psychiatry*. Oxford University Press.
Leonard, B. E. (1992). *Fundamentals of Psychopharmacology*. Chichester: John Wiley.
Paykel, E. (ed.) (1988). *Handbook of the Affective Disorders*, 2nd edn. Edinburgh: Churchill Livingstone.

8

Drugs in neurotic and stress-related disorders

Although 'neurosis' is not a popular term among diagnostic experts nowadays, it is still extremely useful when assessing patients, particularly in community settings. Whoever is involved with assessing the patient realizes early on that most of their complaints or symptoms do not require any fancy language to describe them in detail. Whether the person is complaining of feelings of nervousness, physical symptoms, the need to repeat things over and over again, or perhaps a list of unpleasant emotions and feelings that have only been experienced since a major personal catastrophe or accident, the type of problem is usually all too clear to the therapist. The person with the problem is not 'out of touch with reality'; their mental function has not disintegrated in the same way that it often seems to do in conditions such as schizophrenia.

This does not mean that the person's distress is always easy to understand, or that there are not diagnostic difficulties. The conditions formerly described as 'hysteria' are also included in this group. In these disorders physical symptoms and syndromes are unconsciously simulated by the patient so that initially the person presents with a problem such as memory loss, paralysis, convulsions or other conditions that clearly seem to be outside the realm of mental inquiry. It is only when one examines the circumstances under which they occur that one can suspect that all is not what it seems.

It is with the neurotic disorders above all others that people argue so much about the place of drug treatment. Neurotic symptoms are exaggerations of normal experiences that are noted by everybody at various times in their lives, therefore, so the argument goes, it would be wrong to treat them with drugs that can have major effects on mental function.

There is an opposite argument, that people who suffer from these disorders suffer enormously, and because their experiences are rooted so deeply in reality one could argue that these people suffer more than those with more severe forms of mental illness. If we have the means of relieving these symptoms it would be callous and possibly even sadistic to withhold them from suffering people because they do not fit in with a purist scheme of things.

In current practice, drug treatment is widely used in the treatment of neurotic disorders (Balter *et al.*, 1984). It is difficult to tell if it is overused, but certainly one could argue that if the full range of psychological treatments were available to all those who are currently receiving drugs then the overall response to treatment might be better. However, psychological treatments, the best-known being *cognitive therapy* and *anxiety management training*, although often very effective are also time-consuming and need skilled practitioners to administer them. Although we are moving fast in training our practitioners there are still far too few to meet the needs of these patients. Even if all these practitioners were available when needed, it is important to realize that people with the severe forms of these conditions are not able to function well enough to follow a complicated psychological treatment programme and therefore drug treatment may still be necessary, at least initially. As we have explained many times already in this book – and although this can get tedious it is still worth repeating so that the message does strike home – drug and psychological treatments do go well together in most instances and this certainly applies to the neurotic disorders. However, there is one possible exception which we will come to shortly.

The major symptom in the neurotic disorders, anxiety, is at the heart of much of human experience and a large part of mental pathology, but it is only in this group of conditions that, peacock-like, it displays its many features in all their magnificent colours. The variety and novelty of these features may sometimes fool the assessor into thinking that anxiety is not the main feature. Indeed, it may not be present at all on the surface, but it does not need much digging beneath the surface to identify the common syndrome of fear (about something real or something unidentified), uncertainty about the future and a feeling of dread. It is therefore necessary to discuss the main drugs for treating anxiety as a symptom before moving on to the different disorders that share anxiety as an important defining feature.

Benzodiazepines

Benzodiazepines are the most commonly prescribed psychotropic drugs in the world and everyone involved in community mental health practice will have heard of them. What they will also be aware of is the different perception of benzodiazepines over the years. Initially they were regarded as 'wonder drugs' that could be used to replace barbiturates and other dangerous drugs of dependence, and from the time of their introduction in 1960 to the late 1970s their prescribing increased so rapidly that concern was expressed that the total population of the planet might be treated by the year 2012. In fact, many more of these drugs might have been prescribed if advice had been followed from certain quarters. A report by the Office of Health Economics, whose impressive title disguised the influence of pharmaceutical companies in its presentation, suggested in 1975 that tranquillizers such as the benzodiazepines should be regarded as suitable for use in the area of self-medication, at least in so far as this would place them in an intermediate position between 'medical' and 'social' drugs, and so tend to preserve the independence of the user and protect him or her from the 'social side-effects of medicalization'. In short, if benzodiazepines were freely on sale we should all be happier.

With this constant hymn of praise it was not surprising that these drugs were regarded rather like Aldous Huxley's 'soma', the drug that was given to everyone in his *Brave New World* so that everyone could live satisfying and pain-free existences. Unfortunately, this ultimate 'happy pill' let us down. It was realized that dependence was a problem with benzodiazepines in the late 1970s and since then there has been continued concern about this side-effect.

In order to put this into context, and to understand benzodiazepines in relation to other antianxiety drugs, we need to look at the way these drugs work. They act by reinforcing the effects of gamma-aminobutyric acid (GABA), which is one of the most powerful inhibitory neurotransmitters in the nervous system (see Chapter 2). Thus when GABA systems are activated there is a general calming effect on nerve cell activity. Benzodiazepines are rather like alcohol, barbiturates and other sedatives in possessing this effect of enhancing GABA activity. Where they differ is that they also have special places where they act in the nervous system, called benzodiazepine receptors. As described in Chapter 2, the receptor is a useful concept to describe how a drug will work in one setting but not in another. Like a lock, which will only respond to the action of a key that fits the lock exactly, a drug will only act on a receptor when it too fits (or binds to) the receptor exactly. In fact, the benzodiazepine receptor is not as precise a selector of keys as many other receptors in the nervous system, and drugs that are not benzodiazepines but are similar to them, can bind to these receptors and so affect brain cell activity.

The ability of benzodiazepines to bind to the benzodiazepine receptors allows them to have a special influence on the cells possessing GABA receptors which is denied to other drugs. This means that they act at lower doses and are generally much safer than other compounds such as alcohol and the barbiturates.

However, when benzodiazepines are withdrawn after regular long-term use there can be problems. The GABA system becomes used to constant activation by benzodiazepines when given regularly, so that when they are withdrawn there is a state of GABA underactivity. This, as you may imagine, leads to symptoms opposite to the effects of GABA, such as agitation and excitation. Thus, some patients become anxious and unwell when benzodiazepines are reduced or withdrawn, and these problems may be worse than the original symptoms for which the tablets were prescribed. The natural tendency is to go back to taking benzodiazepines again, and indeed many patients do this, but it does not solve the problem as it only postpones the problems to a later date when drug withdrawal or reduction is tried again.

Clinical use

The clinical use of benzodiazepines has been dramatically affected by concern over the risk of dependence in recent years. However, this concern has mainly been over the use of benzodiazepines prescribed for the relief of anxiety. By far the most well-known drug in this group is diazepam (Valium). When concern over possible dependence with the

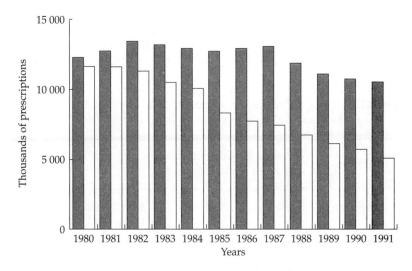

Figure 8.1 *Changes in numbers of prescriptions of benzodiazepines in England prescribed primarily as hypnotics (dark bars) and those prescribed for anxiety (light bars) over 12 years since concern was first raised over dependence problems with benzodiazepines (data reproduced by permission of the Department of Health). Separation (insomnia/anxiety) of benzodiazepines is as in Table 8.4*

benzodiazepines became prominent in the UK in the early 1980s, heightened by popular television programmes (e.g. *That's Life, The Cook Report*), this highlighted drugs such as diazepam and lorazepam (Ativan) to a much greater extent than others. However, all benzodiazepines are similar, and dependence on one can easily be transferred to another, a phenomenon known as *cross-dependence*. Rational prescription of benzodiazepines should have led to a reduction in the prescription of all benzodiazepines once concern over dependence was pointed out. In fact, reductions were shown mainly for benzodiazepines used for the treatment of anxiety, with much less change in those used for sleep disturbance (Figure 8.1).

The indications for benzodiazepines have therefore altered, mainly because of concern that long-term use of benzodiazepines (and by long-term we mean anything in excess of 4 weeks continuous treatment) makes people more likely to become dependent (see below).

The main uses of benzodiazepines are illustrated in Table 8.1. Even this list is not exhaustive, because clearly anxiety can be present in a wide range of other disorders (e.g. schizophrenia, early dementia) and treatment with benzodiazepines in these conditions may be considered appropriate for short periods. However, for the community mental health worker, the use of benzodiazepines in the treatment of stress disorders, insomnia, generalized anxiety and panic, phobias and treatment of alcohol and drug dependence are the most important. There are some general rules that apply to all these indications and these are summarized in Table 8.2.

Table 8.1   *Clinical indications for benzodiazepines (for convenience the dosage of diazepam alone is given for all indications)*

Disorder	Usual daily dosage	Recommended duration	Comments
Stress reactions	5–10	1–3 days	May be used in IF dosage for up to 2 weeks
Insomnia	5–10	IF	
Anxiety states (neuroses)	5–20	IF	Similar dosage used for treatment of secondary anxiety and other psychiatric disorders
Agoraphobia and social phobias	2–20	IF	To be taken before exposure to phobic situations
Hypochondriacal states	5–15	IF	Use only when symptoms clearly related to anxiety
Neuromuscular disorders	5–10	For duration of disorder	Dependence may be a necessary evil if control of the disorder is successfully achieved by drugs
Epilepsy	10–30	Variable depending on control of seizures	Best used for short periods, particularly valuable in status epilepticus
Drug and alcohol withdrawal	5–40	7 days	See Chapter 9 for further details
Anaesthesia premedication	5–20	Preoperatively	Produces anterograde amnesia, thereby giving special advantages

IF, intermittent flexible dosage determined by patient up to an agreed maximum.

Table 8.2   *General principles of treatment with benzodiapines*

Principle	Preferred benzodiazepine groups
Intermittent flexible dosage	All
Anticipation of symptoms	Short-acting group
Prophylaxis	Long-acting group

Intermittent flexible dosage

The term, 'intermittent flexible dosage', which is quite a mouthful, is better than the more common prescription 'as required' or 'pro re nata' (p.r.n.). It describes three prescribing instructions rolled into one:

- Take this drug only when necessary.
- Do not take more than a certain amount at any one time.
- Do not take more than a certain maximum in each day (sometimes week).

This is particularly important when prescribing a benzodiazepine because the risks of dependence are much greater when a drug is taken in regular dosage and, more importantly, the attitude of the patient towards the benzodiazepine tends to be a much more positive and effective one if a drug is used flexibly (Winstead *et al.*, 1974). The community mental health worker is often involved in treating anxiety with both psychological and drug treatments (of which by far the most common group is the benzodiazepines).

If people think of benzodiazepines as drugs to be used in emergencies and that the main treatment will be psychological, they are much more likely to use the drug sensibly and avoid attributing too much of any improvement shown to the drug. It has been shown in research studies that when patients attribute most of their improvement to a drug treatment rather than to themselves, then they are much less likely to be able to stop the drug without relapse and probably less likely to improve with psychological treatments (Basoglu *et al.*, 1994). This goes back to the common problem of prescribing and taking drug therapy. Taking drugs is a passive process and requires much less work than any other form of treatment. If patients get into the lazy way of behaving and always take a benzodiazepine whenever they feel anxious it is easy to see how this habit can grow inexorably to dependence. If, however, the drug is only taken as a first-aid measure at times when anxiety is intolerable it is more likely to be used sensibly and sparingly. More importantly, because tolerance (the loss of a drug's effect with repeated dosage) occurs early after taking benzodiazepines the emergency value of medication will be much less in someone who has been taking a drug more or less regularly compared with another person who is taking it only intermittently.

The simple instruction 'take as required' tends to encourage greater consumption than intermittent flexible dosage. The mental health worker is in an excellent position to explain to the patient these principles and, when done well, this prevents a great deal of unnecessary prescription and later problems.

Anticipating symptoms requiring drug treatment

Anticipation of symptoms is linked to intermittent flexible dosage. Although patients can obviously take a drug at time of maximum symptomatology it is much better if they can anticipate symptoms by taking the drug in advance of the symptoms reaching their peak. Benzodiazepines start working (on an empty stomach) after about 15 minutes and their maximal effect is at about 1 hour, although this varies for different compounds. If it is possible to anticipate the situations where symptoms of anxiety will be most prominent, so that a benzodiazepine can be taken about 1 hour beforehand, a great deal of suffering can be prevented rather than treated. The best example of predictable anxiety is the phobia. As phobias are situational anxieties they can be anticipated if the situation can be predicted accurately. Thus, for example, a vicar who only feels anxious when giving his Sunday sermon can be helped greatly by taking a benzodiazepine a short time before his sermon is about to start so the maximal effect of the drug is when he expects to feel anxious. Even in other forms of anxiety it is possible to predict to some extent when symptoms are going to be worse. It is sometimes helpful for patients to keep diaries of their levels of anxiety because there are often certain times of the day when anxiety levels are predictably high.

Short-acting benzodiazepines are normally preferred for warding off predictable symptoms. It is important for the useful effects of the drug to wear off as quickly as possible, and if a long-acting compound is used this may not be achieved. The person will only feel sedated after the peak of anxiety has worn off. Diazepam is one of the best drugs for using when anticipating anxiety because it is relatively short-acting in acute dosage and also is quickly absorbed into the brain, it is superior in this respect to most other benzodiazepines (Leonard, 1992).

Prophylaxis

Prophylaxis is long-term prevention. Benzodiazepines are sometimes used for this purpose, for example to prevent epileptic seizures in patients who are withdrawing from alcohol after being dependent, and also similarly in some patients with epilepsy who only respond to benzodiazepines (which are excellent anticonvulsants). There is also some evidence that benzodiazepines are helpful in the treatment of tardive dyskinesia (see Chapter 7) and for the treatment of this condition they also have to be given regularly. The regular use of benzodiazepines in this way contradicts the principles of short-term use mentioned above; however, although these are rare exceptions, they are important ones, and the community mental health worker should be aware of them. The authors have come across several occasions in which doctors have stopped a benzodiazepine on the grounds that it could be causing dependence given in regular dosage, when it is in fact being given perfectly properly for one of these conditions.

Benzodiazepine dependence

Chapter 9 describes the problems of drug abuse and its management, including that of benzodiazepine abuse. However, benzodiazepine abuse is usually a secondary consequence of drug abuse rather than a primary problem. Those who abuse drugs usually do so because of their immediate euphoric or pleasure-inducing (hedonic) effects; benzodiazepines only have these properties to a minor degree. (If you want to construct a league table of the euphoriant effect of drugs of abuse in your area, find out the street value of each drug; the most euphoriant will command the highest price.)

However, most people who are dependent on benzodiazepines have had them prescribed in good faith and have become dependent by accident. They have found they cannot stop their drugs without unpleasant withdrawal reactions. It is these withdrawal symptoms, together with the phenomenon of tolerance, that constitute most of benzodiazepine dependence. Tolerance, the phenomenon of reduced drug effects with repeated use, is well demonstrated with the acute effects of benzodiazepines but is not usually a serious problem in long-term dosage for anxiety and sleep disorders. Someone who slept well on 5 mg of nitrazepam (Mogadon) in 1980 often sleeps just as well on the same dose now.

Withdrawal symptoms are the main feature of what is now described as *low-dose dependence* and avoidance of these remains the major reason for continuation of drug treatment. Approximately 35% of patients prescribed benzodiazepines for longer than 4 weeks are likely to develop a significant degree of dependence inasmuch as they are unable to stop the drug after an appropriate period of time because of withdrawal symptoms (Tyrer, 1986). You may like to read that again: yes, the figure *is* only 35% – most people can take benzodiazepines and stop them without any problems. It is sometimes hard to believe this after reading about the subject in the popular press, in which dependence on benzodiazepines has been described as 'worse than heroin'. It is also important to realize that the immediate concern has created a negative perception in the minds of both doctors and patients with regard to benzodiazepines. This is another example of the nocebo effect ('I will harm') described in Chapter 1, and means that many patients develop apparent withdrawal symptoms which are not genuine ones (Tyrer *et al.*, 1983).

It is extremely important to identify the symptoms of identifying benzodiazepine dependence as soon as possible because the condition, once fully developed, is extremely difficult to treat (Table 8.3).

Table 8.3   *How to recognize dependence on benzodiazepines*

Stage	Description	Clue to detection
First stage	Tolerance	Patient notices, and often complains, that the tablets 'don't work as well as they used to' Requests doctor to increase dose to produce previous beneficial effect – benefit of tablets does not last as long as it did initially
Second stage	Searching for more	Patient runs out of tablets before next prescription is due Visits doctor more frequently complaining of more severe symptoms Visits other partners in the practice to obtain additional tablets Complains to doctor that a stronger tablet is needed
Third stage	Withdrawal syndrome	Increase in anxiety symptoms (e.g. panic) when there is an interruption in the supply of tablets Presence of new symptoms such as excessive sensitivity to noise, light and touch, buzzing in the ears, itching sensations, unsteadiness Symptoms all improved quickly by taking the tablets again
Fourth stage	Illicit purchase	Devious methods to obtain additional drugs (e.g. registering with another doctor, pretending that prescription has been lost, taking other people's supplies) Purchase of additional supplies of tablets (or other benzodiazepines) without prescription

The first thing to emphasize is that dependence on benzodiazepines is not inevitable. Some people can take them for years without ever showing any signs of dependence and can stop them at any time. Others can take them for as little as 4 weeks and find it extraordinarily difficult to stop them after this time because of withdrawal symptoms. Two examples illustrate the variations.

Case vignette 8.1
Quentin suffered from agoraphobia in his early 30s and was treated with chlordiazepoxide (Librium) by his general practitioner and subsequently by a psychiatrist. He improved but continued his tablets. Fifteen years later he was concerned that he might not need the tablets and saw the psychiatrist again. It was felt that he probably no longer needed the Librium and it was reduced extremely gradually over 12 weeks. Quentin was warned about the dangers of withdrawal symptoms and was advised to stop reducing tablets if he experienced any untoward effects. He reduced his medication as planned and did not experience any symptoms during withdrawal. Three months later he remained perfectly well and could not understand why others of his acquaintance had had so much difficulty in reducing benzodiazepine tranquillizers.

Case vignette 8.2
Renée was a 50-year-old woman who had always been a worrier but had never taken any treatment for her symptoms. One of the reasons for this is that she was frightened of doctors and would not consult them if at all possible. However, she needed to have several teeth removed and it was felt that this ought to be carried out under general anaesthesia and that she should stay in hospital for a short time. The operation went fairly well but she lost more blood than expected and was kept in hospital for 5 days altogether and during this time she was prescribed nitrazepam (Mogadon) in a dose of 5–10 mg as required at night. Because she was so nervous about the operation she asked to have two tablets and this was maintained throughout her admission. Because she felt better with the medication she was discharged taking 5 mg at night and continued this from her general practitioner for 3 weeks. At the end of this time it was felt she should no longer need the tablets but when they were stopped she experienced a severe attack of panic, accompanied by shaking all over her body. She was put back on her tablets (5 mg at night) and asked to reduce them gradually. Unfortunately this also led to panicky symptoms, together with severe problems in sleeping. After persisting on only 2.5 mg at night she became depressed, could not concentrate and felt at the end of her tether. It was only after referral to a psychiatric day hospital and regular attendance there for 3 months that she was able to stop her Mogadon entirely.

If we could identify people who are dependence-prone, we could prescribe freely for as long as considered necessary for the majority who would not become dependent. Although we cannot do this satisfactorily at present, we know something about the special risks of dependence, and these are worth discussing separately.

Choice of benzodiazepine

There are around fifty benzodiazepines available world-wide, but in the UK these have been restricted to eight available on prescription (diazepam, chlordiazepoxide, temazepam, nitrazepam, lorazepam, oxazepam, loprazolam and lormetazepam) with two others, clobazam and clonazepam, only available on prescription for the treatment of epilepsy. An approved drug name ending in *-pam* almost always indicates it is a benzodiazepine. Whilst sharing many therapeutic properties, these drugs vary in their potency (in this sense the dosage needed to produce a required drug effect), their speed of absorption, metabolism and excretion from the body. They are classified into *short-acting* and *long-acting*, according to the duration of their effects in the body. The long-acting drugs have effects lasting more than 24 hours, and most short-acting benzodiazepines have effects lasting for 12 hours or less.

There is much evidence, none of it conclusive, that short-acting, high-potency benzodiazepines are more likely to induce dependence. The major benzodiazepines in clinical use are listed in Table 8.4 and, of these, triazolam (Halcion), alprazolam (Xanax) and lorazepam (Ativan), all potent benzodiazepines with relatively short half-lives, have been associated with many more problems with dependence than the other compounds (partly as a consequence of this triazolam is no longer available on NHS prescription).

Dosage

Dependence is normally considered as being of two types, high-dose and low-dose dependence. High-dose dependence typically involves the use of drugs in higher than therapeutic dosage, usually obtained illegally and involving the 'drug-seeking behaviour' typical of addicts (Chapter 9). Sometimes benzodiazepines are prescribed in high dosage in anxiety and, perhaps not surprisingly, this is more likely to produce dependence than when low dosages are used. Low-dose dependence occur in therapeutic practice when patients are unable to stop treatment because of withdrawal problems.

Duration

It is also predictable that patients who have taken benzodiazepines for a long time are more likely to become dependent than those who have taken it short-term. We still do not know the shortest time that a benzodiazepine can be taken safely without risking dependence. However, we do know that when people take therapeutic doses of benzodiazepines for 4–6 weeks and then stop suddenly, *rebound anxiety* and *rebound insomnia* occur frequently. These rebound symptoms are similar to the withdrawal syndrome that happens after longer use (Tyrer, 1986).

Once patients have taken benzodiazepines for 6 weeks or longer it would be wrong to assume that the dependence risk is directly related to the duration of treatment (a common statement made mainly by self-help groups). In fact, the severity of withdrawal symptoms when stopping after 5 years is little different from stopping treatment after only 1 year (Tyrer, 1986; Holton et al., 1992).

Table 8.4 *Summary of the main features and uses of the most widely used benzodiazepines, listed in order of potency*

Drug (Trade name)	Available on NHS prescription	Normal daily dosage (mg)	Speed of action	Type of drug	Main clinical use
Triazolam (Halcion)	No	0.125–5	Fast	Short-acting	Insomnia
Lormetazepam	Yes	0.5–1.5	Fast	Short-acting	Insomnia
Alprazolam (Xanax)	No	0.75–4	Medium	Short-acting	Panic
Loprazolam (Dormonoct)	Yes	1–2	Fast	Short-acting	Insomnia
Lorazepam (Ativan)	Yes	1–5	Fast	Short-acting	Anxiety
Clonazepam (Rivotril)	Yes	1.5–10	Medium	Long-acting	Epilepsy*
Diazepam (Valium)	Yes	4–30	Fast	Short-acting (but long-acting in chronic dosage)	Anxiety epilepsy muscle spasm
Nitrazepam (Mogadon)	Yes	5–15	Medium	Long-acting	Insomnia
Clobazam (Frisium)	Yes	10–30	Fast	Long-acting	Epilepsy*
Temazepam (Normison)	Yes	10–30	Fast	Short-acting	Insomnia
Chlordiazepoxide (Librium)	Yes	10–60	Medium	Long-acting	Anxiety alcohol withdrawal (see Chapter 6)
Oxazepam (Serenid)	Yes	30–90	Medium	Short-acting	Anxiety

*Prescription in NHS only permitted for treatment of epilepsy.

Personality

There has been debate for years over whether certain people have 'addictive personalities'. The problem is that those who abuse drugs clearly develop personality characteristics that are typical of addiction, but it is not known whether these features were present before they started abusing drugs. The same could be said of personality in the field of benzodiazepine dependence. However, in our own work we have found that personality is the most important single factor predisposing an individual to dependence. In particular, patients with 'dependent personality characteristics' are at special risk of becoming dependent.

People with dependent personalities are extremely common amongst those with neurotic and stress-related disorders, and terms such as the 'general neurotic syndrome' have been proposed to describe a combination of dependent (and to a lesser extent, obsessional) personality disorder with both anxiety and depressive symptoms (Tyrer, 1985). So it is to be expected that many who present to doctors with anxiety symptoms also have dependent personalities. However, many more do not, and if evaluation of the anxious person (a task admirably performed by many community mental health workers) reveals no evidence of such personality disorder (or the antisocial and borderline features of other personality disorders associated with drug abuse) then there should be less concern about the prescription of benzodiazepines.

The benzodiazepine withdrawal syndrome

For the benzodiazepine withdrawal syndrome to be diagnosed the following features are necessary:

- Symptoms must always follow drug reduction or withdrawal (usually within 5 days).
- There may be an increase in the previous symptoms of anxiety and/or emergence of new symptoms that have not been experienced before.
- Some improvement should occur after the first 14 days of reduction.

The common symptoms of the benzodiazepine withdrawal syndrome are shown in Table 8.5. It is important to realize that there could be many other explanations for each of these symptoms (although this is less true for the uncommon ones), and the fact that someone has two or more of the symptoms in the left-hand column may only indicate that they are more anxious than usual for an entirely different reason from stopping or reducing a benzodiazepine drug. Nevertheless, as the early symptoms of withdrawal are identical to those of anxiety, it is necessary to pay attention to the important symptoms of anxiety as well.

Helping people to stop benzodiazepines

There are many ways in which carers and community health workers can help patients who have problems in giving up benzodiazepines.

Table 8.5   *Symptoms experienced in benzodiazepine withdrawal*

Common (more than 50%)	Uncommon (less than 5%)
Panic	Getting confused
Shaking	Memory loss
Stomach churning	Getting abnormally suspicious (paranoid) about people
Feeling sick	Epileptic seizures (fits)
Blurred vision	Twitching of muscles
Sounds appearing very loud	Hallucinations (either visions or noises, often voices, or tactile
Itching sensations	hallucinations)
Runny nose	
Depression	
Panicky feelings	
Pins and needles	
Feeling physically ill as though with flu	
Feeling cut off from reality	

Sometimes the problem may not be genuine symptoms of the benzodiazepine withdrawal syndrome, but rather fear of developing these symptoms before they have occurred. Help can be considered in three stages.

Stage one

- Choose a time when the patient's life is fairly settled and there are unlikely to be any additional stresses.
- Always reduce the tablets gradually. The rate of reduction can depend on personal preference but a rate of about 10% on each occasion of reduction is about the most that should be attempted (e.g. week one, 20 tablets; week two, 18 tablets; week three, 16 tablets, and so on).
- Advise the patient to avoid taking other stimulants such as caffeine-containing drinks (e.g. cola, coffee, strong tea).
- Try to have a carer or relative available to give extra support during the time of withdrawal, should it be needed.

Stage two

- Try to produce a greater sense of calm and relaxation by any combination of anxiety control techniques such as yoga, meditation, relaxing in a hot bath, doing more of something that leads to relaxation (but do not use alcohol for this purpose).

- Obtain more formal treatment for anxiety such as going to an anxiety management group.
- Advise getting a self-help book from the library and following the instructions carefully.

Stage three (possible additional drugs to help with symptoms)

The drugs used to aid withdrawal are shown in Table 8.6, and the procedure for introducing them is normally as follows:

- Change to another benzodiazepine which can be reduced more slowly (e.g. diazepam, which comes in 10 mg, 5 mg and 2 mg tablets, each of which can be split in half).
- If bodily symptoms such as tremor and palpitations are a problem then beta-blocking drugs such as propranolol in low dosage (e.g. 20–40 mg a day) may be helpful.
- Take another antianxiety drug that is not addictive (if a doctor approves) and reduce the benzodiazepine under cover of the drug. The most popular of the drugs used are buspirone (a non-addictive drug which acts in a different way from benzodiazepines and which is discussed below) and the antidepressants, which may also treat any underlying depression experienced as a withdrawal symptom. However, research studies have not shown much benefit from either of these drugs in standard practice (Ashton *et al.*, 1990; Tyrer *et al.*, 1996).

Table 8.6　*Drugs sometimes used to help people to stop benzodiazepines*

Main withdrawal symptom	Drug treatment
Bodily symptoms of anxiety (e.g. tremor, palpitations, flushing)	Propranolol (20–80 mg) for duration of symptoms
Insomnia	Short course of 2–4 weeks of a hypnotic (non-benzodiazepine) drug such as chloral hydrate or promethazine
Depression	Sedative antidepressants may help in subsequently withdrawing from the benzodiazepines provided that they have been taken for a sufficient time before withdrawal begins. After withdrawal has been completed the antidepressant (e.g. trimipramine, dothiepin) can be reduced gradually (Tyrer *et al.*, 1996)
Epileptic fits	This is a rare event and more than one fit is unusual. A short course of phenytoin or carbamazepine may sometimes be needed

Long-term management after successful drug withdrawal

A few people may experience continued symptoms to a greater or lesser degree for many months after stopping their benzodiazepines. Although this looks on the surface as though it cannot be a benzodiazepine withdrawal syndrome, it may be related. It is sometimes described as a 'post-withdrawal' syndrome that includes not only anxiety symptoms but a general feeling of illness, difficulty in concentration and irritability. It is possible that this could be a consequence of benzodiazepine dependence even though it may persist long after the last molecule of drug has left the body. It is difficult to know how best to help such people apart from following the general principles described above. However, in many cases the problem does get better over several months and advocating patience may often be the best policy.

Other sedatives and hypnotics

Most of the other sedative drugs that are used for anxiety are similar to benzodiazepines in that they act on the same neurotransmitter system, GABA. These drugs include chlormethiazole (Heminevrin), the barbiturates (which nowadays should never be prescribed for anxiety), glutethimide (Doriden), compounds containing chloral hydrate or similar salts (Noctec, Welldorm) and meprobamate (Equanil). In general these drugs are not as effective as the benzodiazepines but still carry the same risk of dependence because they act in roughly similar ways. However, some of these (particularly the drugs containing chloral compounds) still have a place, particularly in helping people to sleep. They are sufficiently different from the benzodiazepines for them to be used sometimes as benzodiazepine substitutes in helping to treat patients who are going through the withdrawal syndrome. However, they should not be used for more than a few weeks under these circumstances as they can cause dependence in their own right. They are also much more toxic in overdose than benzodiazepines.

Buspirone

Buspirone drug is a member of a new group, which also includes compounds such as gepirone and ipsapirone, which may become available for the treatment of anxiety or depression in the future.

Buspirone has one major advantage over the benzodiazepines; it does not produce dependence, and so there is no reason in principle why it should not be continued for several months or even longer (although its main indication is for treatment of short- and medium-term anxiety). Despite this obvious advantage it has not proved to be a particularly popular drug. This seems to be mainly because it takes several days before its full effects are shown (unlike the benzodiazepines which act almost immediately). It also tends to make people feel a little unwell and generally discontented, and as these effects appear before its beneficial ones this does not help compliance.

Buspirone, given in dosages between 5 mg and 20 mg daily, is useful in the treatment of some patients with anxiety. If there is good evidence that the person has the risk factors mentioned earlier in this chapter, or is (or has recently been) dependent on alcohol, then the drug may be preferred to others.

Because the drug does not act on GABA receptors but on receptors for serotonin (5-HT), it is very different from the benzodiazepines, barbiturates, alcohol (another dangerous sedative drug which would not be allowed on the market these days if it was being introduced for the first time) and the other sedatives mentioned above. Therefore buspirone provides an important alternative to these drugs in the treatment of some patients with anxiety. However, it is important for any community mental health worker seeing patients being treated with buspirone to emphasize that the benefits are a little delayed and it would be unwise to stop treatment too early.

Zopiclone (Zimovane) and zolpidem (Stilnoct) have also been introduced for the treatment of insomnia. They are not benzodiazepines but have somewhat similar actions, and act on sites close to the main benzodiazepine receptor. Although some advantages have been claimed for them over the benzodiazepines, particularly in terms of reduced dependence potential, these remain to be confirmed in practice, and it is reasonable to regard these drugs as having the same risk of dependence as benzodiazepines until it is definitely proved otherwise.

Antidepressants

Some may think it odd that these drugs are being described in this chapter. However, the name 'antidepressant' is somewhat misleading. All the drugs in this group help anxiety to a greater or lesser degree, and they may also help many of the other symptoms of neurotic disorder, including obsessional and phobic symptoms (Hudson and Pope, 1990).

These drugs probably act in a similar way in these disorders as in depression. There is always a delay before the full benefits of treatment are shown (although in very anxious patients the sedative actions of these drugs occur immediately), symptoms of depression, anxiety and other disorders all tend to resolve at around the same time, and the benefits and risks are roughly the same. The main advantage of antidepressants over other drugs used to treat anxiety is that they do not carry the risk of dependence to any significant degree, and certainly not to the same extent as benzodiazepines and other sedatives. If long-term treatment is being considered (which can usually be decided from knowledge of the patient's previous symptoms when first assessed) then it is reasonable to choose an antidepressant if the symptoms are sufficiently handicapping.

This is an important decision and has many implications. Once someone is treated with an antidepressant the expectation is that it will be taken for at least 4 weeks (preferably 6) in the first instance before its benefits have been fully evaluated and, if improvement has been shown, treatment is likely to continue for a period of between 6 months and many years. If people have been struggling with disabling symptoms for several years before they consider antidepressants then this decision may be a fairly easy one, but if the symptoms are of recent origin and related to obvious events, it would be much less appropriate to give antidepressants. If, as so often happens, the obsessional, phobic or anxious symptoms are accompanied by depression to a greater or lesser degree, then the decision to give antidepressants may be more obvious.

Antihistamines

Antihistamines have certain important differences from the other drugs mentioned in this chapter; they are available without prescription for both sedation purposes and the treatment of allergies and sea-sickness. They include promethazine (Phenergan) and diphenhydramine (Nytol). They have a low risk of dependence, which has been shown to occur only in those who are prone to abuse drugs of any sort. When large quantities are taken at one time there can be some pleasurable sensations mixed with the unpleasant ones of oversedation. In ordinary practice, however, there is not really any problem with these compounds. They are mild sedatives and are often used in low dosage in liquid form (elixirs) for the sedation of children of any age. Taken occasionally in this way they are valuable and have no effect on growth or other aspects of child development.

Their only common adverse effects are a dry mouth and sometimes a hangover effect when they have been taken at night (i.e. it is difficult to wake up the next morning and get moving). The main advantage is that their consumption can be controlled by the patient without having to see a doctor. This may be particularly helpful for people who like the freedom to pursue self-help approaches in anxiety.

Case vignette 8.3

Sean had always been an anxious person and at certain times in his life, such as when applying for jobs and getting married, he has been extremely nervous about the formal occasions involved. He presented for help for the first time at the age of 45 because he was afraid that he would become redundant from his job in a packing factory. He found he could not stop thinking about this, often could not concentrate adequately, and felt tense and anxious most of the time.

He was felt to have a problem involving generalized anxiety rather than any other disorder and different methods of treatment were prescribed for him, including self-help using yoga and other exercises and also the possibility of drug therapy for short periods.

He decided that self-help would be the most appropriate method but was concerned that at times when he was extremely anxious he might need to take tablets of some sort. He was interested that antihistamines could be taken without the need for prescription and decided he would get some from the pharmacist and test out their effects.

Sean was not seen again for another 6 months. At that time he was a great deal more confident, had been to his local library, read and subsequently purchased books on medication, and had joined a small group. He still became anxious at times but found that taking promethazine 25 mg occasionally (never more than three times a week) took the edge off his symptoms and made it easier for him to meditate and relax. He was discharged from further care at the clinic.

Drug therapy in different neurotic disorders

So far in this chapter we have not discussed the different diagnoses that make up the disorders of neurosis (a term now regarded as outmoded in many quarters but which we feel is still very useful). This is because we wanted to explain the principles behind each of the drug treatments beforehand, as these are often more helpful than trying to match each specific diagnosis with a drug treatment. This is partly because the classification of neurotic disorders remains a controversial issue and there are many mixed syndromes.

Stress and adjustment disorders

In stress and adjustment disorders the cause of the anxiety, depression, panic and other symptoms is all too obvious. Before the experience of a clearly stressful event the person concerned was usually well and most or all the symptoms have followed the event. The mainstay of treatment of stress and adjustment disorders is psychological. The person has to adjust to the consequences of the external stress and, whilst time itself is a great therapist, its effects can be accelerated by a combination of sympathetic listening, more active counselling and sometimes intensive psychological treatment (both cognitive and psychodynamic) to promote the resolution of the problem. Most of you reading this will be living in a part of the world in which earthquakes are rare; however, if you imagine the impact of an earthquake destroying our ordered lives and wrecking our towns and cities, you have a good parallel with stress and adjustment disorders. If the damage is small, the disaster is easier to accept; we are anxious and distressed at first but try to compensate for the disruption and repair the damage. If the damage is more extensive we may have difficulty in taking it all in. We may *deny* the extent of this at first, and, if our lives have been completely disrupted in such a way that all we have worked for is completely ruined by the damage, we may maintain this denial for months or years. Psychological treatment is largely concerned with promoting acceptance and helping to rebuild our lives again. The extent to which treatment needs to be prolonged or intensive depends on the degree to which we can accept the disaster and its implications.

Unlike an earthquake, the damage caused by its mental equivalent is less obvious because much of it is internal. The distress at first leads to symptoms of anxiety, panic, depression, social withdrawal, anger, despair and mixtures of these and other emotions. At this stage drugs may be requested to relieve the distress, or thought to be appropriate by a carer because of the degree of suffering and severity of symptoms. Drug treatment is perfectly appropriate, provided *it is not continued after the acute phase is over*. Although benzodiazepines may appear the obvious choice for this task, it is important not to continue them for more than about 3 weeks at the most and to keep the dosage low. One of the less appreciated adverse effects of benzodiazepines is *anterograde amnesia*, or memory loss occurring during the time of administration of the drug. This can be a problem with all the sedative drugs that act through GABA transmission, and is well demonstrated by the best known of these, alcohol. Too much alcohol leads to blackouts, after both acute and long-term administration, which are excellent examples of anterograde amnesia.

Memory loss need not be important or a disadvantage, particularly if it helps to remove unpleasant images from a nasty experience. However, if it is necessary to retain memory in order to come to terms with a person-ally significant stress (e.g. the death of a close relative), a drug that produces amnesia may promote the development of denial and create the circumstances that psychological treatment is designed to prevent. For this reason it is better to take benzodiazepines, chloral hydrate or drugs such as chlormethiazole if insomnia is a major problem, in doses that are sufficient to relieve symptoms but not great enough to 'blot out' the experiences.

Post-traumatic stress disorder, the most severe form of adjustment reaction, occurs after exceptionally severe stress that is beyond normal experience (e.g. exposure to death of a loved one in an accident, witnessing a murder or a major disaster such as the loss of the *Herald of Free Enterprise* after it overturned in the sea off Zeebrugge in Belgium). Unfortunately, in some parts of the world and in some professions the dangers of existence are such that post-traumatic stress disorder is quite common. In hostile environments such as the north of Norway or in high-risk occupations such as firefighting, more than half the population endure experiences that would qualify in diagnostic terms for post-trau-matic stress disorder. In many instances the symptoms may be delayed and can last for many years, with repeated anxiety, depression and panic, inability to work and frequent flashbacks of the experiences.

With such prolonged distress it is often necessary to combine psycho-logical treatment with drug therapy, and in addition to antianxiety drugs such as the benzodiazepines and buspirone it may be necessary to take antidepressants (either the tricyclic ones such as amitriptyline or lofepramine, or the SSRIs such as paroxetine and fluoxetine) (Friedman, 1988). When the condition becomes persistent it is often difficult to distin-guish the major symptoms of post-traumatic stress disorder from moderate or severe depression, or agoraphobia with or without episodes of panic. It is only the characteristic onset of symptoms after the major stress that gives the clue to diagnosis.

Case vignette 8.4

Yono was a waitress aged 22 years who worked in a restaurant. She had never experienced any psychiatric disturbance before her presen-tation to a community mental health nurse as an emergency. She had been present when an argument had broken out between two of her male colleagues. This became violent and ended with one of the combatants running after the other with a machete and killing him by almost severing his head from his body. Yono had to run for help past a river of blood as the man lay dying on the concrete floor of the kitchen. Although everyone congratulated her on her composure after the assault she found she could not stop thinking about it, had severe difficulties in sleeping and had recurrent nightmares of the final stage of the assault when she remembered blood spurting from the carotid artery in her colleague's neck before he died. At this point in the nightmare she always woke up in a sweat believing she was being attacked as well. She was treated by gradual and gentle recalling of the events of the assault and her feelings (debriefing), and further counselling about her fears. It was felt appropriate to ask her to see the psychiatrist in the team, who considered that a sedative antidepressant was appropriate for a period of around 4 months to help her insomnia and help to relieve her morbid fears and depression. After 3 weeks treatment with dothiepin 100 mg at night she was much improved and able to achieve more in her counselling sessions. After 3 months she was completely free of symptoms and it was thought appropriate to withdraw the antidepressant gradually over a 4-week period. She remained well and has had no further psychiatric contact since.

Generalized anxiety disorder and mixed anxiety depressive disorders (cothymia)

Generalized anxiety disorder and the mixed anxiety depressive disorders are the most common mental disorders. A recent UK national survey carried out by the Office of Population Censuses and Surveys (OPCS) showed that over 9% of women and 5% of men had the mixed disorder – 'cothymia' is a shorter term suggested by one of the authors (P.T.) in 1989 for this syndrome – and 3.5% of women and 2.6% of men had generalized anxiety disorder (Meltzer *et al.*, 1994). It is worth reflecting on these figures before considering drug treatment, as it is doubtful whether the National Health Service administration, community pharmacists or general practitioners could cope with the demand if most of these people received a prescription for drug therapy. For this reason alone, self-help psychological treatments should always be considered first (Lader *et al.*, 1992).

Unlike the adjustment disorders (which probably overlapped with these conditions in the OPCS survey) these two conditions are often persistent and also overlap with the enduring condition, anxious personality disorder, discussed in Chapter 10. Because of this it is generally unwise to treat cothymia and generalized anxiety disorder with benzodiazepines and other sedative drugs except for specific short-term emergencies. If treatment is linked to psychological management such as anxiety management training, self-help approaches or relaxation therapy, the drug is less likely to be relied on than when it is the sole form of treatment.

When symptoms are persistent it is sometimes appropriate to prescribe one of the 'non-GABA' drugs such as buspirone (e.g. 5–20 mg daily) or low doses of antipsychotic drugs (e.g. thioridazine 25–75 mg daily). These have the advantages of carrying virtually no risk of dependence (almost every drug carries some risk, as even placebo tablets can lead to a dependence syndrome), and so therefore can be considered for treatment in the longer term. Care has to be taken to monitor patients for parkinsonian symptoms such as tremor or stiffness when using antipsychotic drugs because some people are sensitive to these low doses. There is also a very slight risk of tardive dyskinesia (see Chapter 6) with antipsychotic drugs even in this dosage. Although this adverse effect is extremely rare, it is best to remove the risk altogether by not prescribing these drugs for longer than 6 months in regular dosage for either of these anxiety disorders.

Antidepressants may also be considered for the treatment of generalized anxiety disorder, *even when there is no evidence of depressed mood*. This is still an issue that arouses debate, because it is possible to argue that even if depression is not present on the surface it may be hidden amongst the other symptoms. The decision to prescribe antidepressants should not be made lightly, but if symptoms are not only severe but also handicapping a wide range of functions then it is possible to argue the case for prescribing antidepressants if psychological approaches alone are ineffective. As with other forms of anxiety, both old and new antidepressants are effective, although there is increasing evidence that the SSRIs may be more effective than the tricyclic antidepressants in alleviating the symptoms of anxiety after the latent period between first administration of the drug and clinical response (3–5 weeks) has passed. It is important to stress this latent period to people taking these drugs, and the tricyclic antidepressants have one advantage in this respect; they induce sedation immediately and, although this is not the ideal form of anxiety relief, it can nonetheless be extremely valuable to an agitated and desperate patient.

Panic disorder

Panic disorder is often regarded as fundamentally different from generalized anxiety disorder and other neurotic diagnoses. Its fundamental component is the panic attack: sudden attacks or paroxysms of anxiety, fear or terror, occurring in the absence of an obvious cause. Although there has long been awareness that panics were an intrinsic part of the spectrum of anxiety – indeed, the importance of the symptoms was described over a century ago by Sigmund Freud – there is less agreement over the status of panic disorder as a separate condition.

Interestingly, its diagnosis is closely related to drug treatment. Donald Klein, a respected and highly influential psychopharmacologist in the USA, found in 1962 that antidepressants in the form of the tricyclic antidepressant, imipramine, was effective in treating what he described as *endogenous anxiety*. This condition would now probably be described as agoraphobia with panic attacks, as it comprised marked phobic symptoms as well as panic. Klein argued that whereas generalized anxiety disorder responded to sedative drugs such as the benzodiazepines, panic disorder did not respond and that this condition should be treated with antidepressants. If a treatment can be selected entirely on the basis of diagnosis it is of excellent value and so Klein felt justified in arguing that panic disorder was a new and worthy diagnosis (Klein, 1967).

Subsequent work has not shown support for the argument that tricyclic antidepressants selectively *blocked* panic attacks as Klein argued. Benzodiazepines, particularly the drug alprazolam, which has been specially marketed for the treatment of panic disorder (despite the absence of evidence that it is superior to other benzodiazepines such as diazepam), are effective in treating panic, and, as mentioned in the section on generalized anxiety disorder above, antidepressants of all kinds are effective in this condition as well as in panic.

Nevertheless, the diagnosis of panic disorder has become established, at least for the immediate future, and has to be considered on its merits. It is certainly a more severe form of anxiety than generalized anxiety disorder, and it often develops into agoraphobia. One problem is deciding where agoraphobia begins and panic disorder ends, and Isaac Marks (one of the leading critics of the diagnosis of panic disorder) has argued that panic is just one of many features that make up the syndrome of agoraphobia and does not deserve special diagnostic mention.

For the therapist, the main problem of panic as a symptom is its unpredictability and its speed of onset. Most panic attacks develop from the earliest symptom of mild discomfort to the peak of frightened distress in the space of a few minutes with severe bodily complaints of palpitations, dizziness, sickness, choking sensations and shaking, and no treatment has yet been devised that can halt a panic attack in its tracks and prevent its expression once started. (This is a topic of current research; new drugs similar to the benzodiazepines are being tested which could be absorbed under the tongue and act sufficiently quickly to abort the attack.)

Most treatment is therefore directed at *preventing the next panic attack* and, if effective, all subsequent ones. Antidepressants, both tricyclic antidepressants and SSRIs, are effective in this respect but only after the 2–5 week latent period when the drug is creating the biochemical changes in the body that lead to the treatment effect. If the panic attacks are occurring every day then there are likely to be many more episodes before the drug will begin to show its effects. Benzodiazepines, as discussed earlier, act much more quickly, and so it is reasonable to give a drug such as diazepam in a dosage of 2–20 mg daily to give more rapid benefit. This ten-fold difference in drug dosage may seem too great a range, but panic attacks come in a variety of shapes and sizes and a few people respond to a very low dose of benzodiazepine.

It is also perfectly reasonable to prescribe a combination of benzodiazepines and tricyclic or other antidepressants, with clear instructions that the benzodiazepines will be stopped after a few weeks, by which time the antidepressants should have started to show their benefit. Other drugs, such as buspirone, are relatively ineffective in the treatment of panic disorder and are not usually given.

Combined psychological treatment and drug therapy are very common in panic disorder and, in choosing the timing and nature of the combination, the community mental health worker should remember the relationship between the effects of psychological and drug treatment shown in Figure 4.2. Drug treatment is ideal at first if symptoms are severe, but if it is relied on too much there is a danger that it will become the only treatment. The person taking the pills is likely to attribute most or all of any improvement shown to the drugs and to feel that a healthy life without their support is impossible. Some of the nonsense created by the media over the drug fluoxetine (Prozac) is a consequence of doctors (who should know better) and journalists (who will often distort and manipulate to get a good story) attributing all the changes that happen after drug prescription to the drug alone. We all have minds of our own, and even minds that are addled by silly stories in the press should be able to distinguish changes that are a direct consequence of the drug from those that are part of our repertoire of attitudes and behaviour which are quite independent. It is one of the most important tasks of the community mental health worker to emphasize to people with the neurotic disorders in particular that their free will is not being removed by drug therapy, and that the drug concerned is only being given in most cases as a temporary support while other forms of resolution, including time itself, are being introduced.

Cognitive and behaviour therapy is as equally effective in panic disorder as in generalized anxiety disorder and can be of great help in preventing panic symptoms from spiralling out of control (Hawton *et al.*, 1989; Tyrer, 1989). It can be combined with drug therapy without any difficulty, provided that the community mental health worker emphasizes that changes in thinking about panics are independent of the effects of drugs and should be developed even if the symptom is (temporarily) better through the effects of drug therapy.

Phobias

Of the three main types of phobia – agoraphobia, social phobia and simple or specific phobias – the last can be dealt with most easily. The word 'phobia' describes both the fear experienced in, and subsequent avoidance of, certain situations, and the three groups of phobias describe the important situations which usefully separate the cause and treatment of the conditions. Simple phobias are those of clearly circumscribed situations such as exposure to dogs (canophobia), cats (felophobia), high buildings (acrophobia), spiders (arachnophobia), in which the acute fear or anxiety is precipitated by the presence or sight of the phobic object, and should not be treated by drug therapy. Such phobias are very common, particularly in children and young women between the ages of 15 and 20 years, where they can affect 5–10% of the population, but are rarely a severe handicap. The preferred treatment, if one is required (most people do not seek professional help) is gradual exposure to the phobic stimulus, preferably in a graded way (Marks, 1987).

However, there is one form of simple phobia, that of fear of public performance by a musician or actor, in which drug treatment may be of value. Such fears are more like acute stress than a true phobia, because most people feel nervous when asked to perform in front of an audience. Treatment with a beta-blocking drug in low dosage such as propranolol 10–40 mg is an excellent way of reducing the anxiety and tremor involved in public speaking (and most clearly in playing a musical instrument such as a violin) without the risk of reducing performance generally through sedation, a common risk with other antianxiety drugs.

Social phobias are irrational fears and avoidance of social situations. These can range from formal events such as weddings, funerals and job interviews to informal ones such as merely sitting in a public house having a few drinks. In the most severe forms of the condition the person concerned avoids all social contacts apart from those of his or her immediate family and there is great restriction in lifestyle. People with social fears are particularly concerned with being observed or scrutinized by others and are often convinced that they have some obvious blemish of their appearance or behaviour that shines forth like a beacon and makes them an object of observation, and by implication, ridicule. Thus a fear of blushing can lead to a total refusal to enter situations in which embarrassment could be shown, and, since social occasions are noted for their unpredictability it is not surprising that complete withdrawal from social contact could follow.

As with all phobias, treatment by gradual exposure is one of the essential ingredients of progress, but as it is difficult to predict the nature of many social occasions it is difficult to introduce the person steadily from short informal contacts along the pathway to long, formal occasions. Drug treatment may therefore be necessary at times to break down the barriers to progress. Benzodiazepines help the anxiety of phobias as much as the anxiety of generalized anxiety disorder, but they have a major snag; they can interfere with the behaviour therapy involved in gradual exposure and may compromise its effectiveness. For this reason it is best not to combine the two treatments simultaneously although they can each have their place (see case vignette 8.5).

If benzodiazepines are used they may often be given at a fixed time in the day to cover the phobic exposure and so the dose may be kept at a much lower level than in less predictable anxiety. Antidepressants, both tricyclic antidepressants and SSRIs, are also effective in reducing the anxiety of persistent social phobia. More recently, the reversible monoamine oxidase inhibitor moclobemide (Manerix), in a dosage of 150–300 mg daily, has been used with benefit in social phobia, although whether it is superior in its effects to other antidepressants remains to be established.

Case vignette 8.5

John had just been appointed vicar to a new parish. He was keen to create a good impression and increase the size of his congregation. He spent a great deal of time preparing his sermons but found he became increasingly anxious just before he was about to deliver them. His anxiety about his performance increased and eventually he had a panic attack during one of the sermons. He was unable to continue and spluttered to a premature halt in such a way as to reassure his congregation that he was in control even though they were surprised he had finished so early. This experience shattered his self-confidence and he presented for help via his general practitioner in a distressed state, fearing that he might have to give up his job.

He was treated at first with anxiety management by a community mental health nurse, including relaxation training, exercises and a cognitive component to avoid 'catastrophizing' thoughts when he was preaching. Although this was effective to some extent in that he felt much more confident about coping with his panics, he still experienced great anxiety every Sunday morning and often used to dread this time approaching each week. At this stage he was treated with diazepam, 5 mg initially during a normal working day to test its effects, and later 2 hours before going to the church on Sunday. He found this had a significant effect on his anxiety level and was greatly relieved that he could predict this effect with some confidence. He continued to take 5 mg of diazepam a week for the next 3 years, after which time he felt sufficiently confident about his ability (and his congregation) to stop treatment. He was able to do this without difficulty and now remains well on no therapy.

Agoraphobia

Agoraphobia is literally a phobia of the market-place, but as this covers open and closed spaces, crowds, busy streets, shops, supermarkets and public transport it encompasses a great deal. The common feature is that speedy withdrawal or escape from these situations is difficult. It is usually the most severe form of phobia and can be severely handicapping. As with social phobia, the most enduring and effective treatment is gradual exposure to the phobic situation, at first accompanied and later alone. Although this is often entirely efficacious, there are many people who manage to face their phobic fears consistently but who still do not become confident and calm in these situations. Panic attacks can also compromise progress in many instances and can sometimes unravel months of progress in a few distress-laden minutes.

For this reason additional treatment with drugs is often considered. The drug treatment of agoraphobia is very similar to that for social phobia. Benzodiazepines may be helpful in reducing the acute and severe anxiety symptoms but care should be taken not to continue these drugs for too long as dependence can be common. Many people with agoraphobia have anxious or dependent personality structures and are more prone to develop benzodiazepine dependence. If regular treatment is deemed to be necessary for more than 4 weeks, as it usually is, then the possibility of antidepressant treatment, again with any of the three major groups (tricyclics, SSRIs and MAOIs) should be considered. In this context it is worth stressing that many people with agoraphobia become depressed and may need treatment for this as a separate problem. Just as an antidepressant, if effective, is preventive against the next panic attack, it may also prevent the next episode of depression.

There is the same concern with combining behaviour therapy and benzodiazepines as for social phobia, and in general the combination should be avoided. In some instances it may be justified to continue anti-depressant therapy long-term or almost indefinitely, and provided this is planned rather than just accepted, this can be a reasonable policy.

Alcohol and anxiety

People with all types of neurotic disorder may complicate their problems by using alcohol, which the Royal College of Psychiatrists reminds us is our favourite drug, as a mainstay of treatment. This can be justified in the emergency treatment of an adjustment or stress disorder but rarely in other circumstances. Alcohol dependence will always follow regular heavy consumption, and there is a strong danger of this in agoraphobia, social phobia, panic and generalized anxiety.

Drugs such as the beta-blockers, propranolol and oxprenolol, and buspirone may be used to relieve anxiety and can be taken safely with alcohol in a reducing programme. Benzodiazepines, mainly chlordiazepoxide, can also be used in the detoxification of those with alcohol dependence as described in Chapter 9. However, the idea that such medication can be quickly stopped after alcohol has been with-drawn is often a notional one only. Many people continue to take exces-sive alcohol, or sometimes amounts within the normal range, after a detoxification programme. At this stage, what should the doctor and community mental health worker do? In practice, when it has been shown that drug treatment modifies alcohol consumption it is hard to justify stopping drugs immediately, and for a limited time both drugs and alcohol may be taken together. This is nonetheless a potentially harmful combination and clear limits should be set on its duration – usually no more than a matter of a few weeks.

In exceptional cases it may also be justified to prescribe benzo-diazepines long-term, even if dependence is likely to be (or has already been) created, if the alternative is the much more serious alcohol dependence (see p. 235). Benzodiazepine dependence has sometimes been claimed to cause cognitive impairment and memory loss, but the evidence is not strong and certainly the greater danger of cirrhosis of the liver, oesophageal varices (distorted veins close to the stomach which may often rupture), alcoholic dementia (Korsakov's psychosis), and vitamin B_1 deficiency make long-term alcohol use much more serious.

Obsessive-compulsive disorder

Obsessive-compulsive disorder, also called obsessional neurosis, is one of the most serious of the neurotic disorders in terms of severity and duration. Obsessions are repeated thoughts (ruminations) or actions (rituals) that are resisted by the sufferer and recognized to be inappropriate or silly, but nonetheless have to be carried out. If they are resisted and not carried out then there are often intolerable levels of anxiety. For this reason obsessional disorders are often regarded as anxiety disorders, although they are very different from some of the milder forms. It is also important to note that minor degrees of obsessional symptoms are common in all forms of neurotic disorder and also in depression. Indeed, obsessional symptoms are extremely common in depressive disorder and usually improve as depression improves, and in such instances the treatment of the depression is the main consideration.

There is considerable argument between the promoters of drug therapy and behavioural therapy as to which is the preferable treatment of obsessive-compulsive disorder. This depends to some extent where the therapist starts with regard to Figure 4.2. Drugs, mainly antidepressants in this condition, are easy to administer and are more rapidly effective than the main forms of behaviour therapy, response prevention (encouraging the person to resist the ritual or rumination) and gradual exposure. However, unlike drug treatment, once behaviour therapy has been used and shown to be effective, relapse is much less likely to occur even after treatment is withdrawn completely.

The decision whether to invest in behaviour therapy which is more difficult to implement but more long-lasting, or drug therapy, which sometimes may have to be semipermanent to prevent relapse, is to some extent artificial. Patients will often choose one type of treatment and refuse another, and so the choice is often only theoretical. The advantages of combining drug and psychological treatments are great in obsessive-compulsive disorders and so the argument about type of treatment should not be 'either/or' but rather 'if and when'.

Drug treatment mainly consists of antidepressant therapy. Benzodiazepines may be given short-term as part of a focused treatment of anxiety in connection with the obsessions, and low doses of antipsychotic drugs may also be appropriate at times. Of the antidepressants the SSRIs currently appear to be the most effective at relieving obsessional symptoms, but there is little evidence that clomipramine (a tricyclic antidepressant which is also a partial SSRI) is any less effective than the newer SSRIs, fluoxetine, paroxetine, sertraline, fluvoxamine or citalopram (all given in the same doses for obsessional disorders as for depressive ones). The issue of cost is important here as clomipramine is twenty times cheaper than the average SSRI, and if long-term treatment is considered these differences can be large.

Case vignette 8.6

Nobby worked as a gas-board meter reader. He preferred an ordered life and was pleased when he was appointed to this post. Unfortunately he developed obsessional symptoms after 5 years. He had doubts about whether he had recorded the meter readings accurately and kept worrying about this. He took to writing the meter readings on his hands and on many different forms but was still not satisfied he had always been accurate. His anxiety levels increased and at times he had episodes of panic. He was treated by a community team with a combination of response prevention (to avoid writing on his hands), anxiety management (to reduce the crescendo of anxiety that sometimes followed the avoidance of his rituals) and clomipramine in a dose of 100 mg at night (as he also had some insomnia and preferred the sedative effect at this time). He improved steadily and after 3 months was almost symptom-free. His clomipramine was reduced but he continued attendance with the psychologist once a month. Over the following 3 years he had minor setbacks, one of which required 3 months of clomipramine treatment, and currently he is very well.

Eating disorders

Although eating disorders are not included in the neurotic and stress-related disorders in ICD-10 they are closely related. The place of drug treatments is limited in these disorders but nonetheless important. Obesity, anorexia nervosa and bulimia nervosa are the main conditions in this group.

Obesity

Obesity is a major public health problem quite independent of mental health services. A significant minority, even a majority in some age groups, of the population is overweight. Because many of the drug treatments in psychiatry – antipsychotic drugs, tricyclic antidepressants (but not SSRIs) and MAOIs – stimulate the appetite, this problem is perhaps more prevalent in mental health services.

Two forms of drug treatment are available: bulk additives such as methylcellulose (Celevac) and sterculia (Prefil) which expand the stomach and give a sense of fullness, and the appetite suppressants. Neither of these is very satisfactory. The effects of bulk compounds can be simulated by eating bran and low-energy, high-bulk foods such as salads, and there is not much more that can be gained by the drugs. Of the appetite suppressants, fenfluramine in two forms (Ponderax and Adifax) is undoubtedly effective but *relapse is almost universal* when the drug is withdrawn. Other appetite suppressants such as dexamphetamine (Dexedrine) should not be used as they are highly addictive.

Anorexia and bulimia nervosa

An important treatment is now available for anorexia and bulimia nervosa, the symptoms of which include fear of gaining weight (sometimes described as the relentless pursuit of thinness), bingeing followed by guilt and induced vomiting or taking laxatives, and their physiological consequences, which in the case of anorexia nervosa include amenorrhoea (in women), severe weight loss and malnutrition to the point of death.

Bulimia nervosa is associated with depression and personality disturbance but in most people does not lead to severe weight loss. In most cases treatment with an SSRI is often appropriate, and fluoxetine in particular has been evaluated for this condition. It is about as effective as when used in depression; sometimes higher doses (e.g. 40–60 mg daily) are needed, and as it will treat associated depression, it can have combined value.

Treatment of anorexia nervosa involves a limited role for drug therapy. Antipsychotic drugs such as chlorpromazine used to be advocated, partly because they increase appetite (although despite its name, appetite reduction is not a prominent feature in the condition). Because these can lead to hormonal disturbance and amenorrhoea as part of their adverse effects, they have a limited role. The tricyclic antidepressants, which also stimulate the appetite, may sometimes be useful if there is depression coexistent with the anorexia nervosa, but these drugs are rarely likely to be effective when given in the absence of depressed mood or significant anxiety disturbance.

Although the treatment of eating disorders in hospital (particularly when there is severe malnutrition) can encompass a wide range of drug treatments, these are seldom going to be important in community management; psychological therapy, particularly collaborative approaches such as cognitive therapy and self-care manuals (Schmidt and Treasure, 1993; Treasure et al., 1996), is likely to become the mainstay of treatment.

Further reading

Cookson, J., Crammer, J. and Heine, B. (1994). *The Use of Drugs in Psychiatry*, 4th edn. London: Gaskell/Royal College of Psychiatrists.

Lader, M., Beaumont, G., Bond, A. *et al.* (1992). Guidelines for the management of patients with generalised anxiety. *Psychiatric Bulletin*, **16**, 560–565.

Marks, I. M. (1987). *Fears, Phobias and Rituals*. Oxford University Press.

Tyrer, P. (1986). *How to Stop Taking Tranquillisers*. London: Sheldon Press.

Tyrer, P. (1989). *The Classification of Neurosis*. Chichester: John Wiley.

9

Substance abuse

Nicholas Seivewright MB ChB, MRCPsych

Consultant Psychiatrist in Substance Misuse,
Community Health Sheffield NHS Trust

Drug abuse

Prescribing drug treatments to drug abusers is clearly different from prescribing in other psychiatric conditions. Although some drug abusers only use 'street' drugs such as powdered preparations of heroin or cocaine, many use pharmaceutical products of some description – for instance dihydrocodeine, dextromoramide (Palfium) or methadone. In some cases these are illicitly obtained as part of a pattern of varied drug abuse, whilst other individuals may be taking the same drugs reliably and properly as their prescribed medication in a treatment programme (especially methadone). Pharmaceutical drugs may be present in the drug scene as a result of burglary from pharmacies, but also prescribed medication intended for one individual may be illicitly diverted to another, the so-called 'grey market'. This diversion of medication prescribed to drug abusers can give drug services a bad name, the most cynical view being that 'everybody just sells their methadone to buy heroin'. Clearly this is not the case, but it is up to drug services to mini-mize diversion of supplies and to employ drug treatments in a respon-sible way, given their abuse potential. Huge benefits can be brought about by the proper use of substitute drugs such as methadone, both for the individuals concerned if it enables them to remove themselves from heroin use, and for the wider community through the attendant reduc-tion in crime, and this effectiveness needs to be recognized, as does the fact that some diversion of supplies is probably inevitable if such treat-ments are to be provided at all.

It is often thought that drug treatment has no place in the treatment of drug abuse, but this is wide of the mark. Although the causes of drug abuse may be many, and include more social and environmental ones than constitutional causes, the major problem in treating drug abuse is that those who abuse are 'tuned in' to taking drugs to relieve unpleasant symptoms, and therefore are much happier taking other drugs as treat-ment than undergoing psychosocial or psychological treatments. Although many of the drug treatments available are far from ideal they are certainly better than nothing and the notion of *harm reduction* is a key element of this (Department of Health, 1991).

Substitute and non-substitute drugs

The upshot of these various considerations is that drug treatment of drug abusers is not always a simple exercise, but in theory the principles are straightforward. Drug treatment is dominated by methadone, which is the drug we will consider in most detail. Methadone is the main example of a 'substitute' drug, one that is given to directly replace an individual's drug of addiction (usually heroin), bringing the benefits of being on a clean, legal pharmaceutical medication. The next step with a substitute drug is to reduce it gradually until the individual is off drugs altogether, although this is not always done – see below. In addition to the use of substitute drugs, there has been much research into medications that may help addicts in other ways. Table 9.1 outlines the possible indications for the range of drug treatments in drug abuse.

Table 9.1   *Uses of drug treatments in drug abuse*

Substitute drugs
Detoxification
Maintenance

Non-substitute drugs
Detoxification
Alteration/nullification of drug effects
Reduction of drug craving

As indicated, substitute drugs may either be used in short reducing courses, referred to as *detoxification*, or as more prolonged courses usually at the same dose, referred to as *maintenance*. For instance, an individual may be given a methadone course which starts at, say, 60 mg per day and then reduces in increments of 5 mg in the daily dosage, say every 2 weeks, down to zero. This may be done by a clinic as an outpatient procedure or in general practice, or quicker detoxification may be achieved by hospitalization of the drug user. Alternatively, an individual may be started at 60 mg per day in an arrangement that continues for the foreseeable future, if it is not anticipated that the drug user will be able to reduce successfully without relapsing into using street drugs. Clinical decisions about whether a person will be able to detoxify or will require ongoing treatment, or reinstating ongoing treatment if a detoxification course fails, occupy a large amount of treatment services' time and activity, and this issue is considered in more detail in the section on methadone.

Table 9.1 also outlines the use of drug treatments other than substitute drugs. Drug services are naturally extremely interested in medications that are effective in controlling drug abuse but are not themselves related substitutes with high abuse potential, because of the problems of security and diversion involved in issuing drugs such as methadone. There have been some important developments in this area, and the aspects of drug abuse that may be treated in this way are indicated. Thus there are medications that can reduce the symptoms of drug withdrawal states without themselves being substitutes from the same drug group, which are useful in the process of detoxification. The most important development in this category is lofexidine for opiate withdrawal, considered below. Secondly, some medications appear to be able to alter the subjective effects of the drugs of abuse, rendering them less appealing or euphoriant. None with that effect is yet in routine use, but an important separate development has been naltrexone, again in opiate abuse. This is a so-called antagonist of opiates, in that if naltrexone has been taken in tablet form, any opiates such as heroin which are subsequently taken are rendered completely ineffective. This is extremely useful in people who have undergone detoxification from opiates. The final way in which non-substitute medications may act is to reduce craving for drugs of abuse. Research is at an early stage, but the main possibilities are indicated in the following review. Because the prescribing of drugs, particularly substitutes, to drug abusers is a contentious issue, the broader arguments about the subject are discussed first.

The general issue of prescribing substitute drugs to drug abusers

Some find the idea of prescribing substitutes such as methadone to drug abusers at best peculiar, at worst repugnant. We are giving a substance closely related to the very one that they are using problematically, and in the case of methadone are replacing one drug of addiction with another. If we do this for the drug users, why don't we give alcohol abusers cans of beer? I once heard a strong advocate of maintenance prescribing to addicts say to that last point, that 'if the alcoholic had just sold the shirt off his back and robbed his grandmother to get alcohol, I probably would prescribe him some', implying that the inherent crime involvement added extra reasons to remove someone quickly from street drug addiction. Certainly the reasons for which one prescribes substitutes go far beyond the purely medical; one of the strongest single benefits is removing drug users who are committing acquisitive crime from the immediate need to do so, and it has been suggested that methadone programmes should partly be paid for by crime prevention funding, or even by neighbourhood projects.

It has to be accepted that even though one might have ideological reservations about methadone, prescribing it is the single most effective way of quickly removing an individual from the physical, psychological and social problems of street drug use, and recently there has been increased support for maintenance prescribing following the advent of human immunodeficiency virus (HIV) infection among drug users. Apart from the risks posed to drug users themselves, injecting drug users form the route through which HIV will most commonly spread to the general heterosexual population, and HIV policy recommendations have included the expanded provision of methadone programmes. It is now being increasingly recognized that achieving some of the intermediate goals of drug abuse treatment, although by definition not abstinence from all drugs, is almost too easy with methadone maintenance, and the methadone becomes an 'inhibitor of change', with many individuals 'stuck' on methadone with little prospect of removing themselves from it, possibly until middle or even old age. Once again it seems that benefits in some individuals cannot be obtained without disadvantages in others.

Although disagreement is certainly possible, most medical opinion has held that substitute prescribing is justified in cases of opiate dependence, but not in cases where the main drug of abuse is a stimulant such as amphetamine or cocaine. The reasons that lie behind this consensus of opinion are summarized in Table 9.2.

Table 9.2 *Rationale for prescribing substitute drugs to drug abusers*

	Opiates	*Amphetamines and cocaine*
'Social' reasons – reduce crime, stabilize lifestyle, etc.	Yes	Yes
Attraction into treatment	Yes	Yes
Physical dependence	Yes	?
Drug type has acceptably safe effect	Yes	No
Long-acting version available to prescribe, enhancing stability	Yes	No

There are two arguments that could in theory favour prescribing of both opiates and stimulants, and probably a range of other drugs as well. These are the 'social' reasons – prescribing amphetamines may well in some cases reduce crime and stabilize the lifestyle of individuals obtaining amphetamines illicitly – and the fact that a prescribing programme would undoubtedly engage users in treatment, which is another priority that has been identified in HIV policy recommendations, as engagement in treatment means that users can regularly collect clean injecting equipment and receive 'harm reduction' advice. However, conventional medical opinion requires more than that, and Table 9.2 indicates three reasons why amphetamine prescribing is not favoured in the same way as prescribing to opiate users. First, amphetamines are not physically addictive (although many see the distinction between physical and psychological addiction as both unhelpful and inaccurate, since psychological symptoms are produced by physical, i.e. neurochemical, means). Secondly, stimulant drugs probably have inherently more destabilizing effects, including a significant risk of psychosis, and it is generally considered unjustifiable to reproduce these effects through prescribing. Finally, even if one overcomes these reservations about prescribing stimulants, there is no pharmaceutical substitute that has benefits equivalent to those that methadone has for opiate users, such as a long duration of action which enhances stability. Although some treatment centres are experimenting with amphetamine prescribing in a small number of cases, there is no support for it at present from the various advisory bodies in drug abuse (Department of Health, 1991).

Although the matter of prescribing to drug abusers therefore becomes invested with certain wider issues, there are treatments indicated for various forms of drug abuse, and these are reviewed below and also elsewhere for interested readers (Seivewright and Greenwood, 1996). Opiate abuse is by far the most common problem to present to most treatment services, not because it is the most prevalent, but because opiate abusers tend to develop more severe degrees of the range of problems that drug abuse brings, and because the provision of methadone, as well as other pharmacological treatments, tends to be viewed as an immediately useful form of treatment in the way that counselling-based treatments for other forms of drug abuse are not.

Heroin abuse

Substitute drug treatment

The routinely prescribed substitute drug treatment for heroin abuse is *methadone*. This is a synthetic opiate which is considered the preferable substitute for heroin abusers because, as well as conferring the general advantages of transferring to a legal pharmaceutical supply, there are three advantages of a more clinical nature. First, methadone is effective by mouth, which heroin is not (heroin has to be injected or smoked). Thus being able to convert an injecting heroin user to oral methadone is a great step forward, as it is the injecting itself that causes a substantial proportion of the problems of drug abuse. The second advantage is that methadone is long-acting, so that an individual can achieve a stable effect from just one, or possibly two, doses per day, in contrast to the much shorter-lasting effects of heroin. Thirdly, methadone is relatively non-euphoriant, which means that the user is less likely to be tempted to use a large part of their supply in one go. Various preparations of methadone are available, the most commonly used being methadone mixture (1 mg in 1 ml), a liquid preparation which is usually green in colour. For some reason even experienced addicts persist in mistakenly referring to this as 'linctus', but the linctus is in fact a different strength liquid preparation (2 mg in 5 ml). There are also methadone 5 mg tablets, but drug services are usually reluctant to prescribe these as they can be more easily abused by injection. Finally, methadone also comes in the form of ampoules, i.e. glass phials of liquid prepared for injection. We have just mentioned that one of the main advantages of methadone is that it is given by mouth, but in some intractable cases, where individuals seem unable to avoid injecting, the injectable form of methadone is sometimes given, the rationale being that this is at least one step up from injecting street drugs. This would usually only be done by specialist services with a clear treatment contract having been drawn up with the individual concerned.

Methadone may be prescribed in either a reducing detoxification course or as maintenance treatment. Agreed maintenance, with both doctor and client agreeing that there is no requirement for the dose to be reduced, would nearly always be a late stage in treatment, and again usually the province of specialist services. Most initial courses of methadone are for a gradual reduction, over a period of approximately 3–12 weeks, although there is no 'correct' exact rate. This may routinely be done by general practitioners, as (contrary to popular belief) there is no licence required to prescribe methadone to drug users. In view of relapse rates further methadone courses are often required, while it is highly desirable if other aspects of a client's personal situation can be addressed by a community drug team, as clearly methadone treatment cannot be effective in isolation.

It is common for a drug user on a reducing course to progress well initially on methadone treatment but then to relapse into street drug use when the dose has substantially dropped. Such individuals may need to be given maintenance treatment, or else have their methadone temporarily increased to the dose that seems to prevent them relapsing, before trying again. One problem that can develop is that the longer a methadone reduction course lasts, the more uncomfortable it often becomes, producing a particularly pervasive version of the opiate withdrawal syndrome. This is probably related to the long-acting nature of methadone, the very feature that makes methadone a good drug for maintenance making it an unsatisfactory drug for detoxification (Ghodse and Maxwell, 1990). The withdrawal effects from methadone are much complained about by addicts, and lie behind the allegation that 'methadone is more addictive than heroin'.

The main beneficial effect of methadone is enabling drug users to extricate themselves from use of street drugs, and treatment needs to be structured so that as far as possible this is made a condition of treatment. This is the reason for regular urine testing, in which use of other drugs can be detected. Broadly speaking, it is not as easy to set up treatment contracts and monitoring in general practice as it is in specialist clinics which solely deliver drug addiction treatment, and there is little doubt that so far the best results of methadone treatment have been achieved in structured programmes in specialist settings. However, the sheer scale of drug use means that methadone must be provided in different settings, and it is likely that the earlier cases will tend to be treated in general practice and the more intractable cases in clinics.

Methadone should not be the first line of treatment for the early stages of experimental heroin abuse. This would risk creating an addiction in an individual who was not addicted before treatment, and non-opiate drugs such as lofexidine are much more suitable in such cases. There is some research interest in developing other substitute drugs that may be more appropriate in early cases, but this is a development for the future.

Finally, some drug addiction specialists claim that methadone is an inherently unsuitable substitute drug for heroin abusers, as many such individuals simply cannot make the adjustment from the euphoriant effects of heroin to the very different experience of methadone. This explains the use in some clinics of morphine or heroin itself as the substitute treatment, including experimental use in the form of cigarettes (to avoid injecting). Some of the arguments brought to bear can be persuasive, but so far there is not enough evidence to justify a major change from methadone as the standard substitution treatment.

Non-substitute drug treatment

The advantage in being able to manage drug abuse by medications that are not related substitutes has been referred to. Although this can apply in any treatment setting, it is particularly relevant in some, such as police custody, prisons, some residential facilities and general practices who do not feel that they can offer controlled drug prescribing. For many years the main alternative to using an opiate in opiate detoxification has been clonidine (Ghodse and Maxwell, 1990). This medication acts on the opiate withdrawal symptoms that are related to overactivity of the noradrenaline system, and has been a moderately effective alternative to methadone. It does, however, have one major disadvantage, which is its effect on blood pressure. This can reduce during treatment (clonidine is used as a medication for reducing high blood pressure), or rise sharply after treatment, both effects sometimes being to dangerous levels, and this has virtually made clonidine unsuitable for outpatient treatment. A significant development therefore has been the recent introduction of lofexidine, a related drug to clonidine which is similar in its effects on opiate withdrawal symptoms but without the effects on blood pressure. Although its relationship to clonidine makes at least an initial blood pressure reading advisable, lofexidine is safe for use in outpatient treatment. Some doctors use lofexidine (or clonidine) as an additional aid in the course of a methadone detoxification, but probably the best use is simply on its own as an alternative to methadone. If an individual has been on high levels of heroin or methadone, a reduction on methadone to a more moderate level may be necessary before lofexidine is then instituted. Although experience with lofexidine is still being collated, it is a most promising development and seems set to become used routinely as the main non-opiate method of detoxification from heroin or methadone.

Another drug introduced in recent years which may have a major place in management of opiate abuse is naltrexone. Its use is in relapse prevention, as an aid to psychological or counselling strategies. After detoxification, an individual who has been off opiates for 10 days can be put on naltrexone, a tablet medication which if taken daily completely blocks the effects of any opiates subsequently taken. Provided compliance with naltrexone has been reliable, this acts as a strong disincentive to relapse into taking heroin, as no effect will be achieved. To achieve the all-important aspect of daily compliance a family member can be involved, and naltrexone has even been used compulsorily as a condition of a court order as an alternative to custody. Once again naltrexone has the potential to become a routinely used medication, and probably should be, given the limited effectiveness of psychological relapse prevention strategies. It is important to have clear confirmation, including urine testing, that the individual has definitely been free of opiates.

The other main area in which medication may be able to help control drug abuse is in reduction of drug craving. Naltrexone may have this effect as well as its more direct effect referred to above, while reduction of craving may be a secondary effect of some psychiatric medications which are mainly used for other purposes. There are pointers to two of the newer antidepressants, fluvoxamine and fluoxetine, having this effect to some extent, but more evidence is required before they can be considered clinically indicated for that effect alone.

Other opiate abuse

Some illicit drug abusers regularly use pharmaceutical opiates, such as dextromoramide (Palfium) or dipipanone (Diconal), along with heroin, and therefore have a combined form of opiate dependence. In terms of substitution treatment, such individuals should be prescribed methadone except in rare cases. It is virtually impossible to achieve stability using the pharmaceutical opiates mentioned, especially as they tend to be highly prized by addicts and used very unreliably, including by injection. Other treatments are indicated as for heroin abuse, although it is notable that individuals who have substantially abused pharmaceutical opiates are often particularly difficult to manage.

A group who are less involved in the street drug scene are those individuals who abuse minor pharmaceutical opiates such as co-proxamol (Distalgesic), dihydrocodeine or codeine. Tranquillizer and alcohol abuse are sometimes associated features, and often such individuals have other long-standing personal problems. Drug services sometimes try to convert such opiate usage to methadone, but this is often resisted because of the perceived associations of methadone with street users. It can sometimes be preferable to prescribe a reducing course of dextropropoxyphene, which is the opiate half of Distalgesic and thus avoids the paracetamol component which incurs liver damage.

Case vignette 9.1

Alan was a 25-year-old man who had started abusing Distalgesic after breaking up with his girlfriend. He worked in a power station operating sensitive machinery and was suspended from work after he fell asleep one day after heavy use of the drug. After admitting abuse of Distalgesic to his general practitioner (who had initially prescribed it to him for headaches), he saw a drug dependence specialist and was prescribed a reducing dose of dextropropoxyphene. This was combined with couple therapy carried out by a community mental health nurse. The therapy went well and during its course Alan and his girlfriend learnt better ways of coping with their frequent violent arguments that did not involve escaping into drug abuse. By the end of the reducing course of dextropropoxyphene (2 months) the couple were reconciled and Alan returned to work. One year later he remains well and is married.

Amphetamine abuse

The reasons why substitute prescribing is not usually supported in this group have been analysed above. Amphetamine abuse is one of the stronger elements of the early evidence for fluoxetine treatment in drug abuse, in that prescription of fluoxetine can help some amphetamine users to stop or cut down. Because of the potential problems of combining a stimulant drug with any psychoactive medication, such a trial of treatment should always be closely monitored.

Amphetamine abuse, unlike opiate abuse, can create a paranoid syndrome indistinguishable from paranoid schizophrenia. The community mental health worker needs to be aware of this before deciding that any new schizophrenia-like pathology is actually due to schizophrenia.

Unfortunately drug abuse often goes hand in hand with schizophrenia, particularly in inner cities. There is much argument over whether the schizophrenic symptoms are precipitated by the drug abuse, particularly by amphetamines, or whether those who are predisposed to schizophrenia are more likely to experience psychotic symptoms when they take such drugs. The important thing is always to be aware of this problem in clinical practice.

Case vignette 9.2

Stephen was a young Afro-Caribbean man who was diagnosed as having schizophrenia at the age of 22 years. He developed the idea that he had special abilities and was also a millionaire. He could not understand why others did not appreciate his talents and abilities and became paranoid about their refusal to accept his inflated views about himself. He also believed that his mind was being controlled by a microchip inside his brain which gave him instructions (by auditory hallucinations) at regular intervals.

He rapidly responded to treatment with low doses of antipsychotic drugs in hospital and afterwards was discharged on a small dose of flupenthixol decanoate (Depixol) 40 mg every 4 weeks. He was seen by an occupational therapy member of a community mental health team, both before discharge at the day hospital and subsequently. Although he was coping extremely well before discharge on the same dose of medication, he relapsed within a month and had to be readmitted. Again he responded well and was discharged a month later. On this occasion it was arranged that he should attend the day hospital every weekday to keep a close eye on his progress. Three weeks after discharge he suddenly became more paranoid, accused the occupational therapist of making assessments so she could sell them to others who wanted to copy his great abilities and maintained that the microchip had been inserted back into his brain.

The occupational therapist had daily records of his progress and there was no evidence that any external stresses had contributed to Stephen's relapse. On discussion with the clinical team it was felt that, despite Stephen's insistence he did not take drugs, drug abuse might have been a factor. Urine testing confirmed that he had recently taken amphetamines and when this result was presented to Stephen he admitted that he had been lying. It was estimated that he had been taking the equivalent of 50 mg of amphetamine daily and this explained his paranoid symptoms. When this was explained to Stephen he was quite surprised that his drug use, which he regarded as recreational and quite independent of his therapy, was indeed related to his symptoms, and he subsequently stopped using amphetamines entirely.

Cocaine abuse

Cocaine abuse is the subject of great concern to drug services in the UK at present, as cocaine, particularly in its 'crack' form, can produce states of extreme disturbance, often characterized by severe distress and sometimes violent behaviour. Cocaine is not exactly physically addictive in the usually accepted sense of the term, but an acute psychological withdrawal, including intense craving, occurs in some users. This appears to be sometimes an almost unbearable state which leads to repeated compulsive use of large quantities.

There is virtually no support for substitute prescribing in this group, and most efforts have been directed towards finding a medication that effectively relieves these withdrawal features. A number of medications have proved moderately effective, but none is in routine usage, certainly not outside hospital.

Cocaine use appears common in some areas in patients on methadone treatment, and there is even suspicion that it is particularly tempting to use cocaine in this situation, because of the effect that the combination of the two drugs produces. Broadly the same range of medications have been tried to reduce additional cocaine use by methadone patients, but again nothing conclusive has been demonstrated.

Benzodiazepine abuse

The benzodiazepine tranquillizers are most closely associated with a group who would not usually be called drug abusers, that is individuals with minor psychiatric problems who have been prescribed these drugs in ordinary therapeutic dosage. Many such people have been helped to withdraw from tranquillizers, although there are others who have become so strongly dependent that there is little alternative to them staying on their medication. Benzodiazepines are, however, also substantially used by illicit drug abusers, particularly temazepam, capsules which can be abused by injection (despite a recent change in manufacture). Benzodiazepine abuse in this group is nearly always secondary, for instance to heroin or amphetamine abuse, but substantial problems can result, again particularly from temazepam abuse (Darke, 1994).

The only clinical situation in which prescribing benzodiazepines to abusers could actually be recommended is in states of acute withdrawal, but claims of this are not always straightforward, and such prescribing may often be unwise in a community setting.

No separate drug treatments have been shown to directly influence benzodiazepine abuse. However, it may be that some individuals on low doses of prescribed methadone abuse benzodiazepines to enhance the effect of their methadone, which is a recognized chemical effect. There may therefore be some cases in whom an increase in methadone eliminates benzodiazepine abuse, but such a strategy can only be tried in a closely monitored situation. With the established role of methadone it is certainly better for the patient to be on an adequate dose of methadone and avoid other drug abuse – benzodiazepines, amphetamines or cocaine – than to be prescribed an inadequate dose of methadone and attempt to enhance its effects with other drugs.

Other drug abuse

The recent phenomenon of methylenedioxymethamphetamine (MDMA, Ecstasy), appears to be producing a range of psychiatric ill-effects rather in the way that lysergic acid diethylamide (LSD) can do, including psychosis, flashback experiences, panic disorder and depression. Antipsychotic drugs and antidepressants may be necessary for some of these complications, the latter probably preferably being a 5-HT reuptake inhibitor (SSRI), as this is the main neurochemical affected by the drug.

Alcohol abuse

The pharmacological treatment of alcohol abuse is a little more straight-forward than that of drug abuse, as there is not a range of different substances involved with possible different drug treatment indications, and there is also not the complicating issue of the provision of substitute treatments. However, there are some similar pitfalls to those in drug abuse, including the commonly encountered unsatisfactory situation of alcohol abuse continuing along with abuse of prescribed medications such as tranquillizers. There are a small number of medications for which there are 'proper' indications in the treatment of alcohol abuse, and these are reviewed in turn, starting with those used to enable withdrawal (detoxification) from alcohol, and then the ones used to try to prevent relapse.

Chlordiazepoxide

Chlordiazepoxide is the main drug used to reduce the physical with-drawal symptoms from alcohol, which include tremor, sweating, nausea, high pulse rate and blood pressure, confusion, and epileptic fits. It is a benzodiazepine tranquillizer (i.e. it belongs to the same drug group as diazepam, nitrazepam, etc.), and as such has sedative, tranquillizing and anticonvulsant actions. The other benzodiazepines would also work for the same condition, but chlordiazepoxide has become established in the treatment of alcohol withdrawal, and it has the benefit that among the benzodiazepines it appears to have a low potential for dependence and abuse. Usually doses of 60–100 mg per day are prescribed in acute alcohol withdrawal, with the dosage then gradually reduced.

Using chlordiazepoxide to treat alcohol withdrawal is likely to be most satisfactory with the patient in hospital, where dosage can be controlled and there can be some certainty that the individual is not taking alcohol. In an outpatient or community setting there is less control over both of these aspects, and it is easy to see how a well-intentioned outpatient detoxification programme can merge into a situation where both alcohol and chlordiazepoxide are being taken in various unreliable combinations, which is dangerous because of the combined sedative effects. Although chlordiazepoxide is low in abuse potential the potent tranquillizing effect is still there, and alcohol abusers are often particularly attracted to abusing tranquillizers because the effects are broadly similar. A healthy scepticism is therefore required regarding any outpatient treatment with chlordiazepoxide, since a straightforward detoxification is only rarely achieved, and often a 'double abuse' situation may be occurring.

There are, however, some individuals in whom chlordiazepoxide successfully eliminates alcohol drinking not only during the stage of withdrawal, but also afterwards if prescription is continued. There are differing opinions about how satisfactory a situation that is – there has been an epidemic of individuals with minor psychiatric disorders such as anxiety becoming dependent on benzodiazepines, which has rightly been the source of much concern, but on the other hand it is no doubt preferable to be dependent on 20 mg of chlordiazepoxide a day than dependent on alcohol, in terms of side-effects such as liver damage. Prescribing tranquillizers long-term, if it definitely enables an alcohol abuser to stop drinking, is perhaps the nearest situation we have to the use of substitution treatments in drug abuse, and it should probably be acknowledged that this may be beneficial in some cases, provided the prescriber is certain that double abuse is not occurring.

Chlormethiazole

Chlormethiazole is undoubtedly an effective treatment for alcohol withdrawal symptoms, but its use in alcohol abusers has become problematic and is the subject of controversy. Chlormethiazole is a tranquillizer with similar actions to the benzodiazepines, although it is chemically different. When it first became available, its use in treating alcohol abuse was heavily promoted and it has gained a reputation for being almost specific for that disorder. It is often used on medical wards if alcohol abusers are admitted for withdrawal, a particular advantage being that it can be administered intravenously in the acute stages. However, it is unfortunate that chlormethiazole has become so associated with alcoholism treatment in this way, as it is probably no better than chlor-diazepoxide, and has a number of disadvantages. The two main disadvantages are that the drug is particularly dangerous in overdosage, especially when combined with alcohol, and it is frequently abused by alcoholics if they obtain it for outpatient treatment. All tranquillizers are abused by some individuals, but chlormethiazole appears highly prized by this group, probably because of the euphoriant effect that can be achieved if it is taken with alcohol in moderate dosage. It is now the opinion of most specialists who treat alcohol abusers that chlormethiazole is unsuitable for this group outside hospital.

A number of other drugs, including the beta-blocker propranolol, have been investigated in the treatment of alcohol withdrawal symptoms, but none is considered suitable for routine use.

Other medications

Vitamin treatments are often required in alcohol abusers, especially when definite alcohol dependence (alcoholism) has developed. There are a number of reasons why alcoholics become specifically deficient in vitamins, especially the vitamin B group, including dietary factors and impaired absorption because of the damage alcohol causes to the stomach lining. Many readers will be familiar with the use of Parentrovite in detoxification from alcohol, which is a high-dose injection preparation of vitamins B and C. This used to be administered routinely in hospital alcoholism treatment units, but it has recently fallen from favour because of the risk of allergic reactions. Oral vitamin treatments should be used unless for some reason that is impossible, and nowadays a combined high-dose tablet preparation of the vitamins is the usual choice. The reason replacing vitamins is important is that vitamin B deficiency, particularly that of vitamin B_1 (thiamine), is thought to be part of the reason for some of the complications of alcoholism, including the typical brain damage which occurs in severe cases.

Alcoholics often give a history of having had epileptic fits, which can be a feature of the alcohol withdrawal syndrome. They may therefore have been prescribed anticonvulsants such as phenytoin or carbamazepine, either as ongoing treatment or else just during detoxification. All anticonvulsants require careful monitoring, often including regular blood testing to detect whether circulating drug levels are adequate, and so such treatment can soon become unreliable if an individual relapses into drinking. As with all medications in this patient group, their safe and effective use virtually relies on abuse of alcohol having stopped.

Preventing relapse

Disulfiram (Antabuse)

There is one drug of established importance that is used to prevent relapse in alcohol (ethanol) dependence, disulfiram, commonly described by its trade name Antabuse. Disulfiram is an important medication, which if suitably used can be one of the most effective interventions for treating alcohol abuse, but the nature of the treatment means that great care is required. The principle of treatment derives from the fact that disulfiram and alcohol produce a marked chemical reaction if taken together, causing not only symptoms such as sweating and flushing, but effects on pulse and blood pressure, which can even be fatal if combined doses are high enough. The disulfiram-ethanol reaction is therefore to be avoided at all costs, and the object of treatment is that an individual on disulfiram will be deterred from drinking alcohol through fear of this potential interaction. This is something of a balancing act, but properly used in a motivated individual the medication can be an effective deterrent. It may be argued that this kind of treatment undermines the personal willpower needed to refrain from alcohol, but unfortunately neither willpower nor clinical psychological treatments are usually effective enough to prevent relapse in alcohol abuse, and disulfiram should definitely have a place in treatments offered by a specialist service (Ghodse and Maxwell, 1990).

There are a number of practical considerations to be addressed in disulfiram treatment. It used to be common practice for a disulfiram-ethanol reaction to be induced in controlled circumstances in hospital by administering a small amount of alcohol, but this has become less usual and treatment now relies on a clear explanation of what the reaction would be. A problem with disulfiram treatment is that the individual may simply stop taking it if they are determined to drink alcohol, and (as with the similar naltrexone treatment in opiate abuse) it is preferable to recruit someone such as a family member or spouse who can assist in ensuring compliance. Even when disulfiram is taken, it is not uncommon for alcohol abusers to test it out by drinking some alcohol to see if they can 'get away with it' without any ill-effects, and in fact if the standard dose only of disulfiram is used, this is quite often successful! Higher dosages may therefore have to be used to effectively prevent drinking, while at the other extreme some individuals appear particularly suscep-tible to disulfiram and experience a reaction even from the small amounts of alcohol used for example in cooking. Despite these considerations, a proportion of alcohol abusers derive great benefit from treatment with disulfiram. If significant amounts of alcohol are taken by someone on disulfiram and a disulfiram-ethanol reaction occurs, this constitutes a medical emergency and immediate medical treatment must be sought.

There has been much research interest in the potential of medication to reduce relapse by reducing craving for alcohol, as there has been in relation to drugs of abuse. One medication, acamprosate, has recently been introduced for this purpose in detoxified alcohol abusers. The newer SSRI antidepressants fluvoxamine and fluoxetine may be able to reduce craving for alcohol, and alcohol consumption, in some individuals. Antidepressants in general are frequently prescribed to alcoholic patients, usually because there has been evidence of clinical depression at some stage. Certainly depression is very common among alcohol abusers, for a whole range of reasons including the direct effects of alcohol, distress at declining personal situations, or underlying personality disorder, and self-harm attempts are also frequent. However, for every alcohol abuser who is deriving significant clinical benefit from an antidepressant, there are probably several others who have simply attracted prescription of an antidepressant at some stage and are using or abusing them to no good effect, especially if alcohol abuse has continued.

Detection of drug and alcohol abuse

Drug and alcohol abuse are both extremely widespread and it is important for all mental health workers to be able to detect when abuse may be contributing to an individual's problems. The standard advice on drug abuse that appears for instance in leaflets for parents, such as being suspicious when a young person develops a new network of friends of a particular type, loses interest in previous hobbies, shows a general change in attitudes and behaviour or a decline in school or college work, is sometimes maligned but is probably reliable. Similarly, an older person developing an alcohol problem may simply appear increasingly generally unwell, and work performance may decline.

There are, however, more specific signs of drug and alcohol abuse, although perhaps not as many as one might expect. All drugs of abuse produce some kind of intoxication not totally dissimilar from that produced by alcohol, and the person may be witnessed in such a state, acting peculiarly or talking in a slurred or incoherent way. The stimulant drugs such as amphetamines, Ecstasy or cocaine produce overactivity and agitation, whilst heroin, tranquillizers and cannabis produce drowsiness and sedation, the person sometimes falling asleep after use. If usage of virtually any drug becomes heavy there is a general decline in health and weight loss – in fact it is this feature that drug users tend to notice about each other, so that they can usually tell when somebody is 'in a mess' with drugs, and weight tends to increase when somebody is successfully established in treatment. Some of the relatively few specific signs are reddening of the eyes caused by cannabis, small pupils by heroin, reduction in sleep and appetite in those taking stimulants; alcohol has a characteristic smell, and often causes a mild tremor in people who are in the early stages of developing a drinking problem. Solvent abusers sometimes have a characteristic rash on the face if they have been used to inhaling glue or other substances from plastic bags. If someone is injecting there will be injection marks, but these are not always easy to spot, and there may be attempts to conceal them by wearing long-sleeved clothes.

In any clinical setting, use should be made of two straightforward tests to detect drug or alcohol abuse. All that is needed to detect drugs of abuse is an ordinary sample of urine collected in a plain container obtained from the hospital laboratory. Most of the commonly used drugs are detectable in urine, although each laboratory can advise on their own particular system. This is therefore an easy method, and the only problem in a general community mental health setting may be whether a worker feels able to ask for a urine sample, if they have more of a counselling than an investigative role. Sometimes giving advance notice is a good thing, with the worker indicating that at the next appointment a routine urine sample should be taken (there may be some occasions where it is not suitable to mention that this is for drug screening, but usually such concealment is not necessary). The consequent delay in obtaining the sample is usually of no great importance, since many of the drugs of abuse remain detectable in urine for several days, and most drug abuse is ongoing; whilst if it has been stopped specially in order to provide a drug-free urine sample at the next appointment, that may be all to the good! Although alcohol is detectable in urine, a blood test for alcohol level is preferable, partly because a liver function blood test can be done at the same time to detect any liver impairment. Of the liver function tests, the gamma-glutamyl transferase level is of most interest, as this is raised in a high proportion of alcohol abusers, and it is relatively specific – i.e. there are not many other causes for an abnormal result. As with the urine test for drug screening, some advance warning to the patient is often appropriate.

Further reading

Department of Health (1991). *Drug Misuse and Dependence: Guidelines on Clinical Management*. London: HMSO.

Ghodse, A. H. and Maxwell, D. (1990). *Substance Use and Dependence: An Introduction for the Caring Professions*. London: Macmillan.

Seivewright, N. A. and Greenwood, J. (1996). What is important in drug misuse treatment? *Lancet*, **347**, 373–375.

10

The place of drug treatment in personality disorder

The diagnosis of personality disorder is not a happy one. It invokes a set of negative ideas: that such patients are difficult to get on with, sighs of resignation about taking them on for treatment, the expectation that they have persistent problems in relationships of all kinds, and pessimism that these conditions are ingrained and will continue without any change for the better. This, as we hope to demonstrate, is an unfair summary, but it is true that personality disorders are much more difficult to treat than most other conditions in psychiatry.

In understanding this issue it is important to separate personality disorder from the other conditions described in this book, which together can be described as 'mental state disorders'. The latter may arise in certain vulnerable people, but, just like a medical illness such as pneumonia there is usually a time both before and after the illness when the person is free of the disorder entirely. Of course there are some medical conditions, like congenital heart disease, that may persist throughout life, but even here there is an obvious localized area of pathology that can be separated clearly from the rest of the 'normal' body. Mental state disorders are also concerned with symptoms and behaviours that can be recognized on clinical examination and which together make up the clinical discipline of phenomenology: the delineation of specific mental events that helps to make diagnostic divisions (e.g. auditory hallucinations spoken like a commentary are typical of schizophrenia).

Personality disorder is different. It describes characteristic ways of behaving, and persistent attitudes and thinking patterns. Here we are not looking at the state of the person at a single moment in time but at a long-standing pattern of usual behaviour (Tyrer and Stein, 1993). In short, we are looking at the whole function of the individual, not just a segment. This possibly explains the difficulty that many professionals have in dealing with people who have personality disorder. Whereas we can forgive people with schizophrenia, manic-depressive illness or dementia when they carry out a whole range of antisocial, inconsiderate or stupid actions, we have much more difficulty with those who have a personality disorder. The first group are seen as ill; they are acting differently from their normal selves and they often feel extremely sorry for what they have done afterwards. Those with personality disorder have no such excuse; their deficiencies and insufferabilities are with them always, holding them back like a metaphorical ball and chain which is a permanent drag on their lives. Under these circumstances it is much easier to blame these people to a much greater extent than we do those whom we would regard as more 'genuinely' ill.

We all have personalities and the variation amongst these is so great that each one has a unique stamp like a fingerprint, even if we are identical twins (as is one of the authors). Most of us have personalities that adapt us to the kind of lives we lead in spite of occasional problems. In personality disorder the blend does not work so well. Persistent personality characteristics interfere and intrude on our day-to-day function to such an extent that they create persistent problems to others around us, sometime to society in general, and ultimately to ourselves. Normal personalities help us to adapt to situations; abnormal personalities prevent us from adapting.

It may be thought that drug treatment has no part to play in the treatment of such a condition. After all, despite the widespread action of drugs throughout the body, it is difficult to conceive of one that would have a long-term effect and change the person's personality in any significant way. Surely personality disorders would be more appropriate to treat by psychological means, if at all? This rhetorical question has no answer yet but it seems likely that drugs may have some role to play, even if only as extras in a long therapeutic drama.

Diagnosis of personality disorder

It is far from easy to identify personality disorder. Many people have criticized the concept of the diagnosis because, at least in the past, those receiving the label appeared to have it more as a judgement than as a diagnosis, and in particular because their therapists disliked them in some way. This dislike may have been due to conflict in their interview, antipathy to their lifestyle or attitudes towards past and current events, or a myriad of other ways in which the person did not conform to the expectations of the interviewer. Fortunately this view is now redundant and no longer can be justified in any psychiatric service. Personality disorder shows itself by persistent problems with relationships and with adjustment to normal situations in life. It is not defined by the personal views of the interviewer but by the consequences of persistent attitudes and behaviour.

The main problem in defining personality disorder is finding out whether the personality presenting at the time of illness (assuming there is a separate illness) is the same as the personality before illness, the *premorbid personality*. Often there can be confusion. It is all too easy to say that the angry psychiatric patient who is detained unwillingly is suffering from a paranoid personality, that the expansive manic patient is demonstrating a histrionic personality, and that the indecisiveness and procrastination of the depressed person indicates obsessional (anankastic) personality functioning. For this reason it is always a good idea to get additional information about the person's premorbid functioning. Often this can be obtained from patients themselves (except when they lack insight), but this should be supplemented by information from relatives, friends and other professionals if sufficient sources are not available.

Good general practitioners often know the personality of patients they have been seeing for many years without always being able to formalize it in specific terms, and the same may apply to housing workers, landlords and a host of other people who see the individual regularly. One of the advantages of working in the community is that workers can often have access to this useful body of information, enabling a good personality assessment to be made. A long-term carer or relative with good knowledge of human relations is an even better judge. Such people should always be listened to carefully when trying to distinguish the nature of the patient's personality before their illness began.

Psychiatrists have long argued over the value of making a diagnosis of personality disorder. This is partly because they have found the diagnosis to be unreliable (i.e. there is poor agreement between psychiatric assessments of personality). One of the problems in making the diagnosis of personality disorder is that it is only after prolonged contact that an assessor has a good idea what constitutes the patient's usual personality and what might be temporary aberrations as a consequence of illness. The community mental health worker may often have a much better idea of this distinction because of more frequent contact with the patient in a variety of different settings. There is therefore a good case for those who have the most contact with a particular patient providing the most useful information which enables the correct diagnosis of personality status to be made. Some knowledge of the classification of personality disorder is the important next step.

Classification of personality disorder

The classification of personality disorder is far from ideal (Tyrer et al., 1991). Once an individual is felt to have some degree of personality disorder (i.e. a persistent abnormality of attitudes or behaviour which is independent of any abnormality of mental state), it is useful to separate this abnormality by time and degree. The main types of personality disorder are shown in Table 10.1. Because there is a great deal of overlap between these terms it is often useful to separate the different personality disorders into three main groups, and these are also indicated in the table.

The major psychiatric classifications (DSM-III-R (the revised 3rd edition) and DSM-IV (the current 4th revision) in the USA and ICD-10, the latter being the International Classification) make no distinction between different grades of personality abnormality. People are classified as either having a personality disorder or not having a personality disorder, even though there is abundant evidence that this does not reflect the range of personality disturbance. It is therefore often helpful to introduce an intermediate term, 'personality difficulty', to indicate that someone has some degree of personality problems that do not constitute a disorder in the full formal sense.

Drug treatment of personality disorder

There is much argument about the place of drug treatment in this group of conditions, which are regarded by many as untreatable and by others as only treatable by psychosocial methods. It is also important to realize that because so many of the personality disorders are associated with other mental illness, drug treatment may be given for the illness part of the condition independently of the personality component. It is also worth stressing that research on the treatment of personality disorder is extremely difficult because of the long time-scale of the condition. Short-term treatment trials have been carried out and have shown some encouraging results, but it is much more important to know whether the gains made by treatment are maintained and whether drug treatment needs to be continued long-term. We do not yet have the answers to these questions, but as the subject is so important it cannot be ignored. We shall therefore be discussing in this part of the chapter the 'state of the art', a somewhat pompous phrase which is often used to describe our best guess in a subject in which there is little information that can be relied on absolutely.

Rather than discuss the individual personality disorders, which overlap considerably with each other, discussion is confined to the three major groupings of personality disorder: the flamboyant, the withdrawn, and the anxious or fearful. These disorders are not often seen in pure form in clinical practice, but drug treatment is discussed at first for the disorders alone and then in relationship to the common mental state conditions that coexist with personality disorder.

Flamboyant personality disorder

Antipsychotic drugs

The most convincing evidence of the effectiveness of drugs in any form of personality disorder is that for relatively low doses of antipsychotic drugs in impulsive and borderline personality disorders (Table 10.2). Several research studies have shown that dosages of antipsychotic drugs in the low range – e.g. chlorpromazine 100–150 mg daily, haloperidol 5–7.5 mg daily, injections of fluphenazine decanoate (Modecate) 12.5 mg every 4 months – are effective in controlling some aspects of antisocial behaviour (Tyrer and Seivewright, 1988). It is still far from clear how these drugs exert their action in these conditions, but it is likely that they have a positive effect on impulsive behaviour.

Impulsive behaviour is often a central element of the antisocial group of personality disorders, particularly in those commonly described as borderline (impulsive personality is a related diagnosis in ICD-10) (Table 10.1). Such people not only fail to 'look before they leap' but often leap without thinking either. This impulsiveness shows itself in many ways: repeated acts of physical aggression when frustrated, impulsive theft when the opportunity arises (e.g. shoplifting), injudicious use of alcohol and other drugs, gambling and other forms of financial irresponsibility,

Table 10.1 *Comparison of current classifications of personality disorder*

Group	ICD-10 Description	Code	DSM-III-R Description	Code
Odd/withdrawn	Paranoid – excessive sensitivity, suspiciousness, preoccupation with conspiratorial explanation of events, with a persistent tendency to self-reference	F60.0	Paranoid – interpretation of people's actions as deliberately demeaning or threatening	301.00
	Schizoid – emotional coldness, detachment, lack of interest in other people, eccentricity and introspective fantasy	F60.1	Schizoid – indifference to relationships and restricted range of emotional experience and expression	301.20
	No equivalent		Schizotypal – deficit in interpersonal relatedness with peculiarities of ideation, appearance and behaviour	302.22
Anxious/fearful	Anankastic – indecisiveness, doubt, excessive caution, pedantry, rigidity and need to plan in immaculate detail	F60.5	Obsessive–compulsive – pervasive perfectionism and inflexibility	301.40
	Anxious – persistent tension, self-consciousness, exaggeration of risks and dangers, hypersensitivity to rejection, and restricted lifestyle because of insecurity	F60.6	Avoidant – pervasive social discomfort, fear of negative evaluation and timidity	301.82
	Dependent – failure to take responsibility for actions, with subordination of personal needs to those of others, excessive dependence with need for constant reassurance and feelings of helplessness when a close relationship ends	F60.7	Dependent – persistent dependent and submissive behaviour	301.60

Table 10.1 (*continued*)

	Dissocial – callous unconcern for others, with irresponsibility, irritability and aggression, and incapacity to maintain enduring relationships	F60.2	Antisocial – evidence of repeated conduct disorder before the age of 15 years	301.70
	No equivalent		Narcissistic – pervasive grandiosity, lack of empathy, and hypersensitivity to the evaluation of others	301.81
Flamboyant/dramatic	Histrionic – self-dramatization, shallow mood, egocentricity and craving for excitement with persistent manipulative behaviour	F60.4	Histrionic – excessive emotionality and attention-seeking behaviour	301.50
	Impulsive – inability to control anger, to plan ahead, or to think before acts, with unpredictable mood and quarrelsome behaviour	F60.30*	Borderline – pervasive instability of mood and self-image	301.83
	Borderline – unclear self-image, involvement in intense and unstable relationships	F60.31*		
	No equivalent			

*Included under heading of emotionally unstable personality disorder.

Table 10.2 *Summary of drug treatment in flamboyant personality disorders*

Drug group	Typical example	Clinical indications (if any)
Antipsychotic drugs (low doses)	Flupenthixol 1–3 mg daily	Definitely effective in the short term, probably by reducing impulsive behaviour
Tricyclic antidepressants	Amitriptyline 100–150 mg daily	No specific indications. In patients who are depressed and have this group of disorders there is a risk of suicide attempts, and these antidepressants may be contraindicated because of their greater toxicity (except for lofepramine and clomipramine)
Other antidepressants (including SSRIs)	Fluoxetine 20 mg daily	Some slight evidence that they may be effective in the short term; mechanism of action uncertain
Lithium salts	Lithium carbonate 600–1200 mg at night	Some slight evidence that they may be effective in reducing alcohol intake in flamboyant personality disorders who are prone to alcohol dependence
		Are also effective in what used to be called 'cyclothymic personality disorder' but is now regarded as a mild form of manic-depressive psychosis
Monoamine oxidase inhibitors	Moclobemide 150 mg daily Phenelzine 45 mg daily	No real indications Less effective than tricyclic antidepressants in personality disorder
Benzodiazepines	Diazepam 5 mg twice daily	No clinical indication. May sometimes be contraindicated in patients who have an anxiety disorder in addition to this personality disorder because of the risk of abuse
Other sedative / hypnotics	Chloral hydrate 1000 mg at night	No specific clinical indications
Other drugs	Disulfiram 200 mg o.m. to aid abstinence from alcohol	Probably unwise to give drugs with potential dangers such as disulfiram because of the unpredictability of behaviour in these disorders

and reckless sexual behaviour. The antipsychotic drugs in low dosage reduce this impulsivity, not by general sedation, which could be achieved more effectively by higher dosages or with different drugs, but by delaying impulses in a more subtle way. The people concerned are both more reflective and able to exercise better control over their emotions.

Although much of the evidence for the effectiveness of these drugs has come from open studies (which often overstate the benefits of a treatment), randomized controlled trials have also demonstrated that these relatively low doses of antipsychotic drugs significantly improve impulsive and irritable behaviour. The research studies have normally treated patients for up to 12 weeks but not longer and it is not known if the improvements are maintained. However, even if improvements were maintained, there is concern about the possibility of important side-effects, including not only akathisia (subjective and motor restlessness) in both its acute and chronic forms, but also the slight risk of developing tardive dyskinesia (see Chapter 6). Although this sometimes seems to be a theoretical risk and although tardive dyskinesia is much less common in younger people (who would normally be treated for this purpose) and the doses used are not large, it is still an important issue. We need to have excellent evidence of benefit before we can justify the risk of such an unpleasant adverse effect as tardive dyskinesia. For this reason there are no current recommendations to continue treatment with antipsychotic drugs for more than 3–4 months. Despite this, some psychiatrists have used depot injections of drugs such as fluphenazine decanoate (Modecate) for long periods in the treatment of these personality disorders with no adverse effects. However, this practice cannot be recommended at present.

It is often important for the community mental health worker to make it clear to other professionals, as well as to the patient, that prescription of low-dose antipsychotic drugs for personality disorder alone does not suggest in any way the patient has a schizophrenic process. It is particularly important to explain this to general practitioners because sometimes there will be a tendency for the dose of the antipsychotic drug to be increased into the antipsychotic range if the patient presents at the surgery for another reason.

Antidepressant drugs

It may be thought that antidepressants would be particularly helpful in these personality disorders as depression is so often part of the syndrome. However, this depression differs markedly from that of most depressive illnesses in that the mood changes dramatically from day to day and mainly shows itself in subjective depression (low mood) rather than the biological (somatic) accompaniments of the disorder. Short-lived depression of only a few days is now separately diagnosed as brief recurrent depression in ICD-10; antidepressants are usually all ineffective in this group (Montgomery et al., 1994).

Tricyclic antidepressants such as amitriptyline are of little value and are less effective than the antipsychotic drugs, which suggests that the depression of the flamboyant personality disorders is quite different from the depression of the mood disorders discussed in Chapter 8. There is also the fear that the greater toxicity of these antidepressants may lead to a fatal overdose in those who are concurrently depressed with a mood disorder at the same time as having a flamboyant personality disorder. For this reason there are arguments against using these antidepressants in those who have flamboyant personality disorder unless close supervision of the patient can be ensured (e.g. as an inpatient). This does not apply to those tricyclic antidepressants that are safer in overdosage, such as lofepramine and clomipramine.

The new antidepressants, which are generally much safer, are now sometimes used in personality disorder although their evidence for their efficacy remains somewhat thin. Much of the publicity surrounding the use of fluoxetine (Prozac) in the USA includes claims that 'it changes people's personalities'. However, there is little evidence that the underlying personality structure is altered by treatment with this antidepressant, although there is no doubt that when a chronic depression is treated successfully by a drug the underlying personality may appear to change. In fact, what is often happening is that the underlying personality is being allowed to express itself because the depression is no longer inhibiting behaviour.

Although lithium carbonate has no obvious place in the treatment of personality disorder there is some evidence that in people with mood disorders who also drink excessively, it may reduce alcohol intake and settle antisocial behaviour as well as reducing alcohol intake. It is difficult to know whether this is due to an effect on the personality; it is more likely that any benefit, if confirmed, is related to a property of lithium in reducing alcohol craving.

Monoamine oxidase inhibitors do not have a clear place in the treatment of personality disorders although there have been one or two reports to suggest that they may be effective in some patients with borderline personality disorder (Cowdry and Gardner, 1988). As discussed earlier, it is always difficult to tell what is going on when a treatment appears to help in borderline personality disorder, as the condition includes so many components, only some of which are long-standing personality ones.

Despite these encouraging signs it is difficult to know if there is any long-term place for drug treatment in personality disorders of this kind. In general patients tend not to be compliant and, as the drugs that are the most effective antipsychotics are the least attractive to consume, it is a major problem to maintain a therapeutic plan. However, as the following vignette indicates, it can sometimes be of considerable value.

Case vignette 10.1

Andrew, aged 34 years, was referred to a community mental health team because of his increasing concern about his episodes of anger. These were much more frequent on Friday night after he had been paid and had gone off to drink with workmates in a pub. The frustrations he felt during the week often exploded into violence after alcohol and he had been arrested on two occasions for assault. He had always had difficulty in controlling his temper and had frequently been violent with his family.

At first he was treated with anger control techniques, (avoiding confrontation, identifying warning signs in advance and role-playing to promote constructive and conciliatory responses) but this had only limited effect, mainly because of his alcohol use. Because his alcohol intake was intermittent it was not considered appropriate to consider treatment with disulfiram, also because of concern over the dangers of drinking while on the drug (see Table 10.2) but he was prescribed thioridazine in a dose of 50–100 mg per day to be taken in the latter half of each week and certainly on Fridays. He found this made him feel calmer (the benefits might have been due at least as much to the sedative effect of thioridazine as to any effect it had on impulsive behaviour), and confined his prescription to Thursday and Friday evenings. Although he was not always reliable in taking this he found that on the occasions he did take the drug he was more settled, drank less (again partly because of advice about the dangers of drinking too much with thioridazine) and his violent episodes were much less frequent. A year later he was still taking thioridazine in a dosage of between 50 mg and 100 mg each week and in view of this low dosage it was felt safe to continue. However, it had been agreed that this would not continue beyond a second year as by then we hoped to have other strategies available to control his anger. The psychological approaches were maintained and have become more effective since his alcohol consumption has fallen.

Withdrawn personality disorder

Antipsychotic drugs

There is no good evidence that drug treatment is effective in this group of personality disorders (Table 10.3). The only condition that has been shown to respond to some extent is schizotypal personality disorder, a condition that is not recognized as a personality disorder in ICD-10 but instead is included amongst the schizophrenic illnesses. It would be surprising if this condition failed to respond to antipsychotic drugs, if it is a variant of schizophrenia.

In the schizoid and paranoid personality disorders the most important effect of the disorder is to inhibit compliance. Paranoid patients tend to be suspicious of all medication unless they can be certain of exactly what has been put into it, and schizoid patients have little motivation to take medication as their aims are often different from those of the therapist.

In those who have withdrawn personality disorders the chief task of the community mental health worker is to establish a working relationship with the patient. It would be misleading to call this a therapeutic alliance as the relationship is unlikely to be close or beneficial enough to merit this term. However, over the course of contact, positive relationships can develop and the patient may continue to collaborate with treatment because there are some rewards in continuing the association.

Table 10.3 *Summary of drug treatment in withdrawn personality disorders*

Drug group	Typical example	Clinical indications (if any)
Antipsychotic drugs (low doses)	Flupenthixol 1–3 mg daily	Good evidence of efficacy but this is mainly confined to studies based on the American diagnosis of schizotypal personality disorder (a condition regarded as similar to schizophrenia in other countries). Compliance may be a serious problem
Tricyclic antidepressants	Amitriptyline 100–150 mg daily	No specific clinical indications but no problems with treatment of coincidental depression with these disorders
New antidepressants (including SSRIs)	Fluoxetine 20 mg daily	No specific clinical indications
Lithium salts	Lithium carbonate 600–1200 mg at night	No specific clinical indications
Monoamine oxidase inhibitors	Moclobemide 150 mg daily	No specific clinical indications
Benzodiazepines	Diazepam 5 mg twice daily	No specific clinical indications but possibly less risk of dependence
Other sedative and hypnotic drugs	Chloral hydrate 1000 mg at night	No specific clinical indications
Other drugs	Central nervous stimulants (e.g. dexamphetamine 5–10 mg daily)	Occasionally recommended to activate those with schizoid personality disorder so that they integrate better with society. Not recommended because of abuse potential

Antidepressant drugs

There is no evidence that antidepressants have any part to play in treating this group of personality disorders. However, if significant depressive episodes occur during the course of the personality disorder there is no reason why antidepressants should not be prescribed, and the response is no different from that of similar patients who are depressed without these personality problems. It often takes much longer to establish treatment successfully; the following vignette illustrates this.

Case vignette 10.2

Bob was a 45-year-old university graduate who had worked as a teacher in the past and had special skills in music and in art. Unfortunately he had been handicapped in his work and other activities by a serious bipolar affective psychosis. Since the age of 18 he had had over 25 admissions to hospital, mainly with manic or hypomanic episodes, and for the last 10 years had been unemployed. He had always been a suspicious person who had no close friends and had a detached attitude towards the human race. He regarded himself as slightly superior to other people and could not understand why others could not appreciate his talents. On each of his admissions to hospital he was prescribed antidepressants (for a depressive episode) and antipsychotic drugs (for manic episodes) and improved fairly quickly in hospital. Unfortunately when he left hospital he was reluctant to attend outpatient clinics and invariably became lost from care. After periods varying from 4 months to 24 months he relapsed and again had to be admitted to hospital because of self-neglect or manic behaviour.

He was referred to the community mental health team early in the course of one of the relapses and it proved impossible to prevent admission to hospital. However, one of the health workers, a psychologist, maintained contact with him in hospital and saw him after discharge. At first Bob maintained his distant and disdainful attitude towards the psychologist as he had done to all other health professionals he had seen over the course of his illness. However, during the course of seeing him at home, it became clear that one of his major interests was chess. As the psychologist also played chess to a fairly advanced level he suggested on one occasion that they had a game. This became a habit and on succeeding visits they continued to play chess. As they were evenly matched the games proved a challenge to both players. When for the first time the psychologist emphasized the importance of taking lithium regularly to prevent further episodes of illness, Bob took some notice and arrangements were made so that he not only continued medication but also obtained further supplies when he ran out of drugs. However, Bob refused to have regular blood tests to assess serum lithium levels and on one occasion developed diarrhoea and some dehydration, which only improved after the lithium was stopped. After this occasion it was pointed out that it was likely that the episode was precipitated by excessive lithium and the only way to make sure that it would not happen again was by having regular checks of serum lithium to ensure that the level was kept within the normal range.

Again, and somewhat surprisingly in view of his former reactions to advice of this nature, Bob accepted this advice because it came from the psychologist, a man whom he had come to respect because of his chess-playing ability. Four years later he remains well on lithium carbonate alone and has recently obtained a job designing posters for an advertising agency.

This account illustrates that although Bob's withdrawn personality was not directly treated by the psychologist or by any form of drug treatment, the working relationship that developed between the psychologist and Bob enabled other treatment for his mental illness to be given successfully for the first time in Bob's life.

Other drugs

Sometimes it has been suggested that stimulant drugs such as the amphetamines may be helpful in those with this group of personality disorders. Although this may seem a good idea, actually it is not. Dependence on these drugs, of which dexamphetamine and methylphenidate are most often considered, is just as (or more) likely in these people, and will develop if treatment is prolonged (which it almost certainly will be if it is effective initially).

Anxious or fearful personality disorders

One of the difficult areas of drug treatment is that of long-term therapy for people with dependent, anankastic, depressive and anxious personality disorders. As was noted in Chapter 8, almost all drug therapies for neurotic disorders are designed for short-term treatment. People who need short-term treatment do well on both psychological and drug therapies and everyone feels a warm glow of satisfaction when the patients make their predicted dramatic responses.

We must not, however, forget the other patients who constitute a large part of those seen in community mental health teams. Such patients, with allegedly minor disorders, suffer for years from recurring phobias, anxiety, mild but persistent depression and hypochondriacal fears with somatic symptoms. Many of them have personality disorders as well, and we should not try to pretend that they are only suffering from a 'chronic' or 'resistant' anxiety, depressive or phobic disorder. In deciding on drug treatment for this group the following principles need to be observed:

- Patients with this group of disorders tend to become dependent on treatment to a greater extent than those without these personality disorders.
- Any treatment that is effective is liable to be needed for a long time (at least 1–2 years).

Table 10.4 *Summary of drug treatment in anxious or fearful personality disorders*

Drug group	Typical example	Clinical indications (if any)
Antipsychotic drugs (low doses)	Flupenthixol 0.5–2 mg daily	May sometimes be valuable in those of anxious personality who have long-term anxiety which cannot be treated by other drugs (e.g. benzodiazepines) because of the fear of dependence
Tricyclic antidepressants	Clomipramine 50–150 mg daily	May be useful in the long-term management of anankastic and anxious personalities because of persistent obsessional and phobic (avoidant) behaviour
Other antidepresants (including SSRIs)	Paroxetine 20–40 mg daily	Probably as for tricyclic antidepressants but limited information available
Lithium salts	Lithium carbonate 600–1200 mg at night	No specific clinical indications
Monoamine oxidase inhibitors	Phenelzine 45–60 mg daily	May sometimes be helpful in chronically anxious and avoidant personalities
Benzodiazepines	Diazepam 5 mg twice daily	Are generally avoided because of the risk of dependence but in some cases a conscious decision may be made to continue long-term treatment even though dependence is likely to follow
Other sedatives and hypnotics	Buspirone 10–30 mg daily	Buspirone has no risk of dependence and may be given long-term for those with anxious personality
Other drugs (beta-blocking drugs)	Propranolol 20–80 mg daily	For those of anxious and hypochondriacal personality who have excessive concern over their health and bodily symptoms such as palpitations and flushing, such treatment can be given long-term without any risks (provided that there is no respiratory disease such as asthma)

- Dependence on the therapist may be at least as common as dependence on any drugs.
- It is unwise to change therapy too often as such individuals often find it difficult to adapt to change generally.

Because so many of the symptoms experienced in this group of personality disorders are similar to those of mental illness that are treated by drugs (and the behaviours consequent on those symptoms), it is not surprising that drugs may also have a place in the treatment of these personality disorders. However, it is important to realize that this is only a limited place, and it is in this group of people that the benefits of combined psychological and drug treatment are most prominent.

Antipsychotic drugs

Antipsychotic drugs in low dosage are effective in treating anxiety. They are also safe from the risk of dependence and therefore could be used in principle for the long-term treatment of anxious personalities. Anxious (or avoidant) personality disorder describes people with persistent anxious behaviour, including avoidance of all anxiety-provoking situations, the need to live a restricted lifestyle in order to avoid anxiety being generated, and frequently persistent unremitting tension and anxious fears. This is a highly unpleasant state in acute form; it only becomes tolerable in this persistent form by a measure of adaptation to the condition.

For some people low doses of antipsychotic drugs (e.g. flupenthixol up to 2 mg daily, trifluoperazine up to 4 mg daily) may be effective and can be given long-term. However, there is a major worry about such prescribing, which is similar to that described in the previous section on flamboyant personality disorder but is more of a concern in this group because compliance with treatment is better. The syndrome of tardive dyskinesia, although almost always found when high dosages of these drugs are used, can also be created in a few cases by low-dose treatment. Although this is probably rare, the fact that a significant minority of patients with tardive dyskinesia do not improve even when their drugs are stopped makes all practitioners chary of prescribing low doses of antipsychotic drugs on a long-term basis.

Be that as it may, none of the authors have seen any cases of tardive dyskinesia, even in its mildest form, after such low-dose therapy. We see many patients who have been treated by general practitioners with low doses of antipsychotic drugs for many years and have never had any problems with movement disorders of any sort, and the risk of a dyskinesia syndrome developing in these people is probably less than 300 to 1. Bearing in mind that a small number of cases of tardive dyskinesia arise spontaneously, the incidence increasing with age, it is often difficult to decide whether the condition is a consequence of drug therapy or not. The following vignette indicates the value of such low-dose antipsychotic drug treatment in a person with an anxious personality disorder.

Case vignette 10.3
Belinda had always been anxious. She came from an anxious family and was convinced that her fears were more severe than those of her parents. She was afraid of the dark, of being on her own, and particularly of meeting people. She worked hard at school and was able to get into teachers training college, and worked afterwards as a teacher in a primary school. She led a restricted life, with little activity outside her teaching apart from necessary duties associated with the school. After a new headmaster was appointed to the school there was a reorganization of the teaching staff; she felt extremely worried about this and so anxious at times that she could not teach. She imagined that she might have a serious nervous breakdown and have to be admitted to hospital because of her inability to cope with her responsibilities. After she saw her general practitioner he became concerned that she might be developing a psychotic illness because she was so alarmed and imagined so many possible dangers that he feared she might be developing delusions. However, he only prescribed the antipsychotic drug, trifluoperazine, in a dose of 2 mg daily as he was not convinced that she had a psychotic illness and thought he would build up the dose gradually. She improved after only 48 hours and asked the doctor to continue prescribing as she felt more confident and was sleeping much better. The reorganization of her teaching was not as severe as she had expected and she adjusted quite well to her new duties. However, she continued to see the doctor for repeat prescriptions as she felt the pills were 'confidence boosters' and helped her in many different ways. When reassured that they were not habit-forming she asked why they should not be continued for many years. At this stage the doctor became alarmed and felt a second opinion was indicated. He referred the patient to a psychiatrist and asked for advice as to whether the trifluoperazine should be continued or stopped. After assessment it was felt that there were no dangers of any significance in continuing the trifluoperazine in this low dose and, even though it was possible that the drug was acting mainly in a non-specific placebo way, that it could be continued in view of Belinda's faith in its efficacy. Two years later she continued to take the drug in the same dosage and had developed a new hobby, rambling, where she had met several new friends.

In practice it is usually better to use these drugs for short periods only and combine them with other therapy wherever possible. It is also important to try to reduce the dose to the minimum effective one as tardive dyskinesia is linked to the total consumption of drugs and reductions make the risk of this syndrome that much less likely.

Antidepressant drugs

Antidepressants, as has been pointed out on many occasions throughout this book, are also effective in reducing anxiety and improving self-esteem. It is therefore reasonable to think that they may be effective in anxious and dependent individuals who suffer persistent distress because these features are part of their innate personality structure. Again, there is no good evidence to suggest that antidepressants may be effective in this population, but there are numerous examples of patients who take low doses of antidepressants, often below those required to produce antidepressant effects in people with classical clinical depression; thus antidepressants appear to be effective in enabling long-term coping to be maintained in people with anxious personalities.

Case vignette 10.4

Caroline was a 50-year-old woman who had been nervous and a frequent attendee at her doctor's surgery for many years. After her first child was born she became afraid of going out and her self-confidence deteriorated further. It was felt that she was depressed and she was prescribed amitriptyline in a dose of 50 mg at night. She improved on this regimen, and her doctor decided after 3 months that the drug was no longer needed and it was withdrawn. She became more anxious again and said she was 'returning to my usual self' and preferred to take the tablets as they 'made me a stronger person'. She continued to be prescribed this medication and the doctor was happy to continue it, as her consultations at the surgery over a variety of worries, including concern about her health, became much less frequent. However, after 15 years it was felt that a psychiatric opinion was probably necessary in view of her persistence in taking this small dose of amitriptyline. After assessment it was explained to Caroline that she had not really been taking an antidepressant for all these years, that the drug was really acting only as a sedative in the dosage that was being taken and that the only problem that she would experience if she stopped the drug was some difficulty in sleeping. It was therefore decided to reduce the amitriptyline gradually over a period of 3 weeks. Although Caroline started this programme satisfactorily, she became much more anxious and distressed after 1 week and these problems persisted after she had stopped the drugs entirely. Three weeks after stopping she attended a clinic with her husband who demanded that she be put back on the tablet as 'she had gone back to how she was 15 years ago'. Interviews with him and with other members of the family confirmed that she had been a different person since she had been on the antidepressants and that it was wrong to stop the tablets unless they became an addiction. After careful deliberation it was decided that she could return to taking her 50 mg of amitriptyline again and, after a period of 1 month she returned to the level of competence and functioning that had characterized her previous time on antidepressants. Five years later she continues to take this small dose of amitriptyline.

Textbooks on antidepressant therapy continue to tell us that low doses of antidepressants are of no value in treating depression and of limited value in anxiety. This type of response would therefore be considered to be a placebo response (i.e. to have nothing to do with the action of the drug). We personally do not accept that such a prolonged period of health could be explained entirely by a placebo response (which tends to be short-lived) and conclude that, even in this low dosage, anti-depressants can be effective and are probably acting on the underlying personality as much as on the symptoms presented by the patient.

There is some evidence that antidepressants, particularly the newer SSRIs, are effective in obsessional (obsessive-compulsive) personality disorder as well as in people with obsessive-compulsive disorders without personality problems. In fact, there is one study which demon-strates a better antidepressant response to SSRIs in patients with depression and obsessive-compulsive personality disorder than in depression alone (Ansseau *et al.*, 1991). There is also some evidence that those with obsessive personality are more likely to become depressed, and so it is far from certain whether the improvement that one sees in this group is a consequence of successfully treated depression or is related to the effects on the personality disorder itself. However, if patients with obsessional disorder are distressed enough to come for treatment for this condition (which in many cases indicates that they already have obsessional symptoms), antidepressant therapy is often an ideal method of treatment.

Monoamine oxidase inhibitors sometimes have a place in the treatment of these disorders also, particularly when other anxiety problems are present such as agoraphobia. They do not lose their efficacy in long-term use but care has to be taken over diet (avoiding cheese and fortified wines in particular) when they are taken.

Other drugs

Benzodiazepines were discussed in depth in Chapter 8 and their depen-dence problems emphasized. In this group of personalities these drugs are more prone to create dependence and should in general be avoided except for short-term intermittent use. Buspirone does not produce dependence and can be given long-term. Unfortunately, it is not a popular drug to take because of its mildly dysphoric effects, which are most marked initially. In some anxious and dependent people, however, particularly those who tend to alleviate their anxiety by taking alcohol, it may be appropriate to give buspirone on a long-term basis. The same also applies to those who show excessive anxiety accompanied by bodily symptoms, particularly palpitations, flushing and tremors. Beta-blocking drugs are effective in low dosage for such patients and these drugs may therefore be taken long-term at relatively little expense and with continued alleviation of symptoms.

Drug treatment of mental illness in the presence of personality disorder

Personality disorder and mental illness often go hand in hand. This can have a major influence on all forms of treatment. In general the presence of both the personality disorder and mental illness (often termed *co-morbidity*) makes the conditions much more difficult to treat than when a mental state disorder alone is present.

The major associations between personality disorder and mental illness are shown in Table 10.5 together with an indication of the frequency of association. Some of the figures may surprise. Schizoid withdrawn personalities have some association with schizophrenia but no more than that for flamboyant personalities, and substance use problems (alcohol and other drugs) have much higher associations with flamboyant personalities than with the anxious or fearful (and more classically dependent) personalities. Unfortunately, far too frequently in clinical practice the evidence for personality disorder creeps up on the therapist unwittingly, mainly through the problems experienced in administering treatment, and when these are identified later it is more difficult to take corrective action. This is one of the arguments for making a positive assessment of personality early on in the course of treatment (Fahy *et al.*, 1993).

The importance of knowing about both the mental state and personality dimensions of a problem cannot be overstated. The problems that can arise when both are abnormal will be illustrated mainly through examples from clinical practice, as they are often more instructive than grouping the problems together in a less personal way.

Case vignette 10.5

Eric was a 24-year-old man who was referred to a psychiatric clinic by his general practitioner because of 'severe depression'. The psychiatrist assessed him quickly and decided that he did have a degree of depression suitable for drug treatment. The main reason for his depression was the breakup of the relationship with his girlfriend. She had been living with him for 2 years but suddenly left saying that she no longer wished to have anything to do with him. This had happened 2 months earlier and he gradually became more depressed. He could not get thoughts of his girlfriend out of his mind and had been unable to concentrate because of frequent images of her. He was prescribed the antidepressant, dothiepin, in a dose of 100 mg at night and the psychiatrist made an appointment to see him in 3 weeks. When it came to his second appointment he was very much better and the psychiatrist thought when Eric walked into the room that he had done a good job of treating his depression. However, Eric was followed by his formidable mother who gave a lecture to the psychiatrist on his sloppy care. She said that he had failed to identify that her son had always been an impulsive young man with doubts about his relationships and a tendency to have frequent intense love affairs that always seemed to end in disaster. One of the reasons for the difficulties was that her son was a gambler who took drugs repeatedly, paying for them on the black market. She accused the psychiatrist of failing to find out that her son's girlfriend had left because of his gambling and drug abuse and that, under the circumstances, it was quite wrong that her son should have been prescribed 3 weeks of

Table 10.5 *Association (co-morbidity) between personality disorder and mental state disorders**[*]

Mental state diagnosis	Personality disorder	Frequency of association (%)[†]
Substance misuse	Impulsive and borderline Dependent All personality disorders	43 (in clinical practice, but only 15% in population) 30 69
Schizophrenia	Withdrawn group Flamboyant group All personality disorders	18 18 55
Bipolar affective psychosis	Anxious and fearful group All personality disorders	18 39
Neurotic, stress and adjustment disorders	Impulsive and borderline Anxious and fearful group All personality disorders	6 27 42

[*]From Tyrer (1988).

[†]Some of this association may be by chance, since around 15% of the population have a mental state diagnosis and 11% have a personality disorder (de Girolamo and Reich, 1993).

antidepressants without proper monitoring. In fact, he had taken an overdose of all his tablets 1 week after they had been prescribed and fortunately had fallen asleep with no untoward effects. His depression had dramatically improved since and already he had formed a new relationship.

This account illustrates the importance of getting additional information before rushing into treatment. Full assessment of Eric would have concluded that he had an impulsive or borderline personality disorder in which brief periods of depression are often found because such individuals tend to create negative life events for themselves, and that he also took illicit drugs. This type of depression does not normally respond to antidepressant drugs and the psychiatrist almost had a successful suicide on his hands because of his mismanagement.

Case vignette 10.6

Kendrick, a 25-year-old man, was admitted as an emergency to hospital with an acute episode of schizophrenia. This was his first episode and had apparently been precipitated by taking drugs at a party which could have included LSD. He did not know that any drugs were being administered and at interview appeared to be perplexed by everything that had gone on. He improved within 3 days of admission and it was felt that this was an isolated episode. He was discharged but did not keep outpatient appointments. Two months later he was again admitted under very similar circumstances except that on this occasion he had assaulted a policeman after a party and it was only when previous evidence of his psychiatric history was provided that he was taken to hospital and then admitted.

On this occasion a much fuller history was taken of the problem and his mother and sister were interviewed also. They gave an account of a young man who had always been headstrong and had frequently been in trouble with authority in its many forms. He had been expelled from one school for repeated fighting and had also truanted repeatedly in his last 2 years and had been seen by the Education Welfare Officer. He had become more detached from his family and preoccupied by grandiose ideas in which he saw himself as a second Superman. He believed he had the ability to see through solid objects and claimed that he had messages from a distant planet, Krypton, telling him of his mission in life. Although he had had these symptoms for 4 years they had not interfered too much in his life and he had been able to hold down a job as a postman until 2 years ago when he was dismissed for the theft of £2000 from the postal sorting office where he was based. A diagnosis of dissocial (antisocial) personality disorder was made on the basis of this information and a separate interview with the patient at which these new facts were presented. At a review with all members of both hospital and community teams it was explained to Kendrick, his mother and his sister that although he had a schizophrenic illness this was not the sole cause of his problems and he also had a personality disorder. Evidence from several sources suggested that he had deliberately exaggerated the mental illness component of his condition in order to avoid responsibility for his actions (e.g. hitting a policeman) and that the team would not excuse such actions in the future as part of his schizophrenic condition. This message was used to good effect in maintaining him on a relatively low dose of antipsychotic drugs (trifluoperazine 5 mg at night) after discharge from hospital, and to date he has remained well.

The case of Kendrick illustrates the futility of arguing at great length whether a particular individual has either a mental illness or a personality disorder. Kendrick had both a form of schizophrenia and an antisocial personality disorder, and the two were closely intertwined. Frequently in the past psychiatric services have rejected patients for treatment on the grounds that they have a personality disorder and such a condition is inherently untreatable. In Kendrick's case it was first important to establish that both conditions were present and to establish a set of 'ground rules' for treating them. Once both conditions were out in the open it was possible to achieve much more than if a sterile debate had gone on away from the patient's ears about whether or not he was genuinely schizophrenic or had only a personality disorder.

Case vignette 10.7

Wendy was 54 years old and had suffered from agoraphobia for many years. She had always been an anxious, fearful person and in retrospect she was seen to have developed her agoraphobia when moved to grammar school at the age of 11. At that time she became fearful of going to her new school and had to be treated for school refusal at a child guidance clinic. She remained anxious and fearful throughout her schooling but forced herself to attend on almost every occasion. She married at 19 and for about a year felt more secure as for most of this time she was with her husband. After the birth of the first of their two children and the need to pick the child up from the nursery she became more anxious and phobic again and dreaded her daily journeys to the nursery and back.

She was reluctant to take psychotropic drugs and went to a special hospital which had just introduced a new form of treatment called behaviour therapy (1955). She was treated by a keen young psychiatrist who was researching on 'exposure in vivo' and rapidly improved her state by accompanying her on a graded series of journeys. After she had travelled to central London in a bus while the psychiatrist followed behind in another bus she felt she was cured. She was convinced of this because the two buses became separated in traffic and for a large part of the journey she was on her own but did not feel anxious. The psychiatrist pronounced her cured and she was discharged from the clinic. Afterwards she became more anxious again and could not understand why. Rather than upset the psychiatrist she decided not to be re-referred and asked her general practitioner if she could have additional therapy. She was prescribed benzodiazepines in the form of lorazepam, 1 mg initially, rising to 1 mg 3 times a day later.

Although this alleviated some of her symptoms it did not remove the agoraphobia. Increasingly she had to take tablets of lorazepam whenever she went out of the house and over the course of several years realized that it was becoming less and less effective. The general practitioner prescribed imipramine as he thought this might also help, not least because Wendy was becoming depressed, but unfortunately she found this of little benefit and she was bothered by sedation.

Eventually she was referred to another psychiatrist in a different area with the special request that her lorazepam dependence be treated. It was recommended that she had additional pharmacological help to aid her withdrawal from lorazepam. She was prescribed phenelzine 30 mg a.m., increasing to 30 mg a.m. and 15 mg noon, and after 5 weeks was dramatically better. She insisted that she had not been so well in her life before and her husband confirmed that he had never seen his wife so optimistic and with so much self-confidence. Close examination of the apparent change in personality showed that she had been fearful and anxious ever since the age of 11 and that her new state probably was genuinely new rather than her premorbid personality. In other words her personality had always been morbid and her new well personality was a unique experience. Over the course of the next 18 months she gradually reduced her lorazepam, not without some difficulty, but 2 years after starting the drug she had been free of all benzodiazepines for 3 months and had a part-time job in the administrative division of a regional phobic society.

Wendy's case illustrates that there is such a thing as chronic agoraphobia but it is indistinguishable from (and probably the same as) anxious personality disorder in the ICD-10 classification. The main feature of anxious personality disorder is fear in, and avoidance of, a wide range of situations and the same is true of agoraphobia. The problem with short-term therapy in patients such as Wendy is that improvement is too often mistaken for cure. Cure is a dangerous word in psychiatry because few of us are foolish enough to predict that there will be no return of symptoms at any time. In Wendy's case it was clear from knowledge of her premorbid personality (i.e. the personality she had had ever since adolescence and which had accompanied her agoraphobia) that her problems would not be altered permanently by a single course of behaviour therapy, however expertly administered.

Although it may be controversial to say so, the advantage of drug treatment is that it can be given continuously and remain effective over many years. This does not mean it is more powerful than psychological treatment such as behaviour therapy; it is probably less so, since the benefits of a single course of effective psychological treatment are likely to last for a longer time than a single course of drug therapy, mainly because relapse is usually rapid after drug treatment is stopped, whereas the effects of psychological treatment may long outlast the treatment itself (see Figure 4.2). Nevertheless, for those patients who need long-term treatment, drug therapy may sometimes be the best option and when there is coincidental personality disorder, drug treatment (apart from diazepam) may be equivalent to psychological treatment in its effectiveness in the short term but better in the longer term (Tyrer *et al.*, 1988, 1993). Even though Wendy is on a drug with potential dangers she is convinced that she would much prefer to face these dangers than go back to her earlier state when she was not only dependent on lorazepam but still had her phobic fears crowding around her like wolves waiting to pounce whenever her guard was relaxed. She regards her phenelzine as a miracle drug and can't understand why it was never given before.

Compliance

Compliance is one of the major problems facing all prescribers of psychotropic drugs. In addition to the problems created by lack of insight and hostility towards drug treatment in general, personality disorder confers its own set of problems, and therefore deserves separate mention and suggestions about overcoming these difficulties.

The problem of maintaining compliance with drug treatment is most marked for the paranoid, schizoid and antisocial personality disorders. The patient with a paranoid personality disorder is naturally suspicious, and detects conspiracy and double-dealing in all social interactions. Such patients suspect they are not being given full information about treatments they have received and, in addition to asking a barrage of questions about unwanted effects, they persistently remain suspicious that they have not been given full information. This is independent of the paranoid symptoms of conditions like schizophrenia and depression; many people with paranoid personality exist in a permanent state of mild hostility with their neighbours without ever coming to the attention of psychiatric services. Drugs are not taken because of this suspiciousness but, in most cases, the person concerned will admit this to the therapist when challenged.

Patients with schizoid personality disorder are also poor at complying with medication but this is more because they are indifferent and uninterested rather than suspicious. If drugs are made available at the appropriate times (e.g. in a hostel) they will be taken passively without complaint, but if the patient has to make any effort to get tablets for themselves (e.g. by going to the doctor and obtaining a prescription) compliance is likely to be poor.

The antisocial personality is unreliable about taking all forms of treatment, both psychological and medical. Such people often forget to take their drugs or may even think they have taken them when they have not. At other times they may lie that they have taken them for the sake of convenience when challenged. In general, these individuals want an immediate and beneficial effect from taking medication, and whilst to some extent this is true about all individual suffering from any symptoms, it is present to an extreme degree in such personalities. Very few drugs in psychiatry are prescribed for their immediate effects; it is therefore not surprising that compliance is poor.

One of the reasons for making an assessment of personality status early in the course of treatment is that poor compliance can be anticipated and often avoided. The community mental health worker is usually in a key position to point out these difficulties when patients are being reviewed and plans for care are being formulated. The question 'are there any personality issues here?' is a way of introducing this topic, not only to evaluate compliance but also as an aid to choosing the best time and place to give treatment.

Conclusion

Personality disorder is a relative newcomer to drug treatment. We hope that this chapter has illustrated its importance so that whenever the community mental health worker assesses a patient both personality and mental state factors are taken into account. In case you need convincing, just think of the many occasions you have seen a close relative of a psychiatric patient and suggested a certain course of treatment. 'He couldn't possibly do that', is a common reply, 'He'd never even get started, never mind complete the treatment. Haven't you got something else you can do?' The relative or friend (or even an acquaintance) who makes these comments is telling you something about the personality of the individual concerned because he or she knows that person's habitual level of functioning much better than you do on your first visit. It is our job as community workers to try to obtain this information as quickly as possible and incorporate it into our therapeutic plans. Otherwise we, and everyone else concerned with care, will be frustrated time and time again in our subsequent care. Understanding personalities is not just an esoteric task for the specialist, it is an essential part of good community practice.

Further reading

Dolan, B. and Coid, J. (1993). *Psychopathic and Antisocial Personality Disorders.* London: Gaskell Books, Royal College of Psychiatrists.

Dowson, J. H. and Grouds, A. T. (1995). *Personality Disorders: Recognition and Clinical Management.* Cambridge University Press.

Tyrer, P. and Stein, G. (eds) (1993). *Personality Disorder Reviewed.* London: Gaskell Books, Royal College of Psychiatrists.

11

Strategies for drug treatment in the community

One of the more obvious differences between community and hospital work is that treatment can be supervised and monitored much more reliably in the hospital setting. Although this is self-evident to anyone working in the mental health services, it is often forgotten by those who promote community care from the position of the armchair. Of course people like to be treated at home or in other settings which are as near as possible to their home environment, but whilst this is all very well when the treatment is desired, it is quite another matter for those treatments which are taken reluctantly. There can also be a problem with treatments that are not only accepted but actively sought, particularly those involving substances that can create addiction. In the community mental health team we therefore need a general strategy of ensuring that, as much as possible, when one or more drug treatments are prescribed for a patient they are taken correctly.

In community work, drug treatment will always only be an approximation to the correct prescription. The authors have been involved in monitoring the consumption of drug treatment in clinical trials and have been surprised how often patients think they have taken tablets exactly as prescribed but when the actual dose taken has been calculated (by counting up the unused tablets) the consumption turns out to be only about 60–70% of the prescribed dosage. Although at first sight one is tempted to accuse (usually silently) the patient of deliberate deception, in most cases this would probably be unfair. If each of us was asked to perform an activity four times a day that was not particularly pleasant then I am sure that most of us would forget to do it occasionally. If we add to this the elements of stress, confusion and disorganization that are common in many people with mental health problems, it is easy to see how the default rate could creep up to 30–40%.

Three groups of people are involved with monitoring drug treatment to ensure it is taken more or less correctly. All begin with the same letter; they are patients, prescribers and paternalists. Although their roles are described separately, they will usually have to work together to ensure optimal drug therapy.

Patients

Patients vary tremendously in their attitude towards drugs, and this variation is far greater than is found in the other agencies that are responsible for administering them. It is therefore rather difficult to summarize strategies of helping patients to take drug treatment more effectively in a way that allows them to be generalized satisfactorily. Nevertheless, there are some general guidelines that can be helpful for the community mental health worker.

Consider, first of all, the dream patient: a person who is always in the right place at the right time to receive a prescription, observes prescribing instructions to the letter (even sometimes taking the medication on the hour exactly as the doctor has prescribed) and who also is aware of potential adverse effects and how to cope with them. This patient is a stickler for detail, is absolutely reliable – and is usually a pain to live with. Many of this type have anankastic (obsessional) personalities and some have these characteristics to the extent of having a personality disorder as described in the previous chapter.

At the opposite extreme we have the feckless individual who never keeps appointments, is either not at home or fast asleep when the community worker calls, manages to lose every appointment card and document he or she is given and who is totally disorganized in every part of living. When drugs are prescribed and, by a fortunate but rare combination of circumstances, achieve the physical form of a container containing drugs with instructions on how they are to be taken, you can be sure they will be taken only on whim and at the wrong times.

How do we change Mr Feckless into Mr Reliable? Of course we don't; personality is not so easily changed. Nevertheless, there are several ways of manipulating Mr Feckless and his drug consumption so that it is taken more effectively. These are:

- goal setting
- association
- medication management
- encouragement.

Goal setting

We are always more likely to complete a task that we do not like if there is a reward at the end of it. One of the most frustrating aspects of drug treatment in psychiatry is that it is usually open-ended. Few promises can be made about the length of treatment, and encouragement to take medication because 'it will do you good' creates the same feelings towards medication as children had towards cod-liver oil when it was given to them regularly during the war years. If it is possible to create some clear-cut goals that are linked to therapy, then even the most reluctant of drug consumers may comply with treatment.

> *Case vignette 11.1*
> *Arnold, a man of 45 years old was being treated for manic-depressive illness with lithium carbonate. Although this drug had proved very effective in preventing relapse he rarely complied with treatment for more than a few months and consequently had repeated relapses and admissions, mainly with manic episodes. He frequently moved around the country and this also made continuing care difficult. He*

had never been able to settle in any satisfactory employment since his first episode of illness when he was working as a coach driver. He had lost his heavy goods vehicle licence at that time.

As part of a collaborative strategy to try to work out a long-term plan that would be in his interests, Arnold concluded that what he would most like to do was return to work as a coach driver. It was established with the Driving and Vehicle Licensing Centre that if he was stabilized on treatment and maintaining regular contact his licence could be returned, provided there was good evidence that he would maintain treatment subsequently. It was explained to the patient that responsibility for this could only be left with him and that when he moved around the country he should ensure that he continued to received his lithium and have regular monitoring of blood levels. He agreed to this and in the next 4 years took lithium regularly and his licence was duly returned. At the time of writing Arnold is still taking lithium and has returned to work as a long-distance coach driver. He has had no relapses in the last 6 years.

This case gives a clear example of a long-term goal that was achieved with one of the most difficult drugs, lithium, to achieve good compliance because of its long-term rather than immediate benefits. However, there are many other goals that can be linked to compliance with medication. Some of these can be very short-term indeed. For example, we have often found that with drugs such as benzodiazepines, which are desired by patients because of their immediate effects and are therefore sometimes taken in dosages beyond those that are prescribed, that the next prescription can be contingent on the patient bringing back at least some tablets from the last prescription. This can be done by always giving a few extra tablets beyond those required and testing the resolve of the patients to avoid taking those extra tablets even though they are available. (In practice it is surprising how many patients are unable to resist the temptation of taking extra tablets, and so this is a good opportunity for ending therapy without being blamed by the patient.)

More commonly a goal has to be set with a rather longer time-scale. This can include a referral to a facility that the patient particularly wants (e.g. a drop-in centre or luncheon club) which can be made conditional on completing drug therapy satisfactorily, or the removal of something which is perceived as unpleasant (e.g. discharge from Section 3 of the Mental Health Act). All these approaches are really following simple learning theory in using one type of behaviour to reinforce another.

Association

Association of one activity with another is a standard way of making sure that both get carried out. Even for disorganized people, habit (as William James wrote) is the flywheel of society, and much of what we do is automatic and repetitive. For those who keep forgetting to take drug treatment, the linking of drug consumption with a regular and predictable habit is one way of ensuring that it is not forgotten. Many of our most enduring habits are in the mornings and at night just after getting out of or going to bed. Associating switching off the alarm clock, the early morning cup of tea, or brushing one's teeth with taking medication is a way of ensuring that this is not forgotten, and when the bottle of tablets is placed in a suitable position to remind the patient it also reinforces this association.

By stimulating association we are only building on a standard procedure in drug therapy, the taking of tablets as required. *Pro re nata* (p.r.n.) means 'as the need arises' and is the simplest form of association. When certain symptoms are noted the drug is taken, and this is particularly valuable for drugs in which unnecessary prescription can lead to problems, such as the benzodiazepines. In several research studies it has been shown that when drugs such as the benzodiazepines are taken only as required, the total amount of drug consumed is considerably less than when they are prescribed on a regular basis (e.g. Winstead *et al.*, 1974).

Medication management

Management of medication can be aided by a number of methods that have been stimulated by the growth of community pharmacy and which are likely to be critical in the success of community care of the severely mentally ill, even though they are rarely evaluated in assessments of community intervention (Tyrer and Creed, 1995). There are now a number of ways of administering drugs that aid proper consumption. The 'dosette box' is one of the best known. The box consists of many spaces demarcated by date and time and the tablets are placed in the appropriate spaces for each prescription. The patient is reminded when to take the tablets on each day of the week and, once a tablet has been removed and taken the possibility of 'double consumption' can be minimized. This is particularly relevant in the elderly when memory disturbance can sometimes lead people to believe they have not taken medication when they have in fact just done so. This has been recognized to be a source of accidental overdose, and the dosette box minimizes this risk considerably.

There are other, much more established ways of managing medication. The traditional pill box, often decorated elegantly so that it becomes a treasured accoutrement, is perhaps the best known. The tablets for the day are put into the pill box and, whilst the times of consumption cannot always be ensured, the daily quantity is consumed correctly.

Encouragement

Encouragement of treatment is the opposite to the setting of goals. Encouragement of drug treatment is common in hospital but is not carried out by the patient. The notion of patients 'encouraging' their own treatment may sound an odd one but can be extremely useful in maintaining therapy.

Case vignette 11.2
Bert was aged 48 and had suffered problems with alcohol dependence over a 20-year span. Despite many inpatient episodes for detoxifica-

tion, group therapy, attendance at Alcoholics Anonymous and other similar agencies, he had not been able to remain abstinent for more than 6 months. During one of his admissions to hospital he had been considered for treatment with disulfiram (Antabuse) and had received a test dose while in hospital. He had suffered a major reaction after going through the test procedure with a small dose of alcohol. His blood pressure had fallen dramatically and he had become very distressed. Because of this he had decided not to continue Antabuse afterwards because he was frightened of its effects even taken without alcohol.

Bert was seen at home following yet another relapse and insisted he was prepared to try anything in the form of treatment which had not been tried before. When his past treatment had been reviewed it was clear that Antabuse had not been given a proper trial and this was discussed with him. He was admitted to hospital for 5 days for detoxification and afterwards agreed to take Antabuse while in hospital where he was unlikely to start drinking again. He was surprised to note that Antabuse really had no effect on him while he was abstinent and so he was prepared to continue this afterwards. However, he was still extremely nervous about administering the drug himself and thought that he would be very tempted to avoid taking it after discharge. Eventually he decided himself that he would take his Antabuse (200 mg) immediately after getting up in the morning and certainly before having any breakfast or tea. He decided that he would not have anything to eat or drink until he had taken his Antabuse and set this as a fixed requirement. After discharge from hospital he continued successfully on Antabuse and at the time of writing, 9 months later, he remains abstinent.

Although there are many limits to people encouraging consumption of their own medication, imposed mainly by a lack of interest in the whole process of drug therapy, for those who are generally disposed towards the notion of drug treatment and wish to assure that it is taken appropriately the technique has attractions. It involves collaboration between patient, therapist and others in that the motivation to take the responsibility of enforcing one's own medication needs to be generated as much from other people as from patients themselves. The main advantage of the approach is that patients become responsible for their medication in a way that is not otherwise achieved. The common criticism that patients who take drug treatment are merely passive recipients of it can then be challenged.

Prescribers

Prescribers can aid compliance by:

- simplifying drug regimens
- explaining why drug therapy is being given
- testing to confirm drug consumption.

Simplifying drug regimens

The prescribing of drugs has always been invested with an air of mystery and complexity, but this is no longer necessary. In the past most drugs were ineffective and therefore much of their benefit arose from the placebo effect. If drugs of no value were prescribed with an air of authority and detailed instructions, invariably in Latin, this aided response. The medical and pharmaceutical professionals have kept hold of much of the paraphernalia of the ancient apothecaries, even though it is difficult to justify. We still prescribe drugs with Latin abbreviations which, although having some advantages in an international setting, are not normally appropriate in one country.

The common prescribing abbreviations and their meaning are shown in Table 11.1. Many of these regimens are unnecessarily complex. It may be desirable to take a certain drug before eating, but if the reasons for this are not explained to the patient they may well not take the drug merely because they do not feel hungry at the appropriate time in the day. The frequency of drug-taking is also often excessive. Psychotropic drugs such as lithium, antidepressants and antipsychotic drugs do not exert their main therapeutic effect immediately and so it is really unimportant whether they are taken once or several times a day. Far too often, complicated regimens are established in hospital, where there is much less difficulty about giving drugs on many occasions during the 24 hours, and then maintained after discharge even though they become much less easy to maintain. There sometimes can be good reasons for taking a drug on several occasions each day, and the most common is the need for intermittent sedation in a highly disturbed patient. In community mental health these occasions occur much less often and simplified drug regimens, of which *once a day* is the simplest, are more often appropriate.

Some of the more common complicated drug regimens and their simplifications for community practice are shown in Table 11.2. As compliance is likely to be so much better with such simplified regimens, we suggest that these should be adopted as the norm and more complex ones only introduced after they have been justified formally with the team workers or carers.

Explanation

Explanation of the effects of drugs, both desired and undesired, is an excellent way of ensuring compliance. Again this may be self-evident, but a great deal depends on how one goes about the explanation. Listing the positive effects of a drug as 'it successfully treats your condition', followed by a list of all the theoretical adverse effects of the drug, is likely to have the same negative effect as eulogizing the positive effects of the drug and mentioning none of its handicaps. Within days of starting the drug the patient will find that its effects are not those expected, and an important part of the trust which must exist between prescriber and patient has been lost.

Table 11.1 *Some common Latin abbreviations used in prescriptions*

Instruction	Meaning
mane	in the morning
o.m. (omni mane)	every morning
nocte	at night
o.n. (omni nocte)	every night
o.d. (omni die)	every day
b.d. (bis die)	twice a day
t.d.s. (ter die sumendus)	three times a day
q.d.s. (quater die sumendus)	four times a day
p.r. (per rectum)	through the anus (e.g. suppository)
p.o. (per os)	through the mouth (i.e. swallow)
a.c. (ante cibum)	before meals
p.c. (post cibum)	after meals
s.l. (sublingual)	below the tongue

One of the main advantages of all community mental health workers knowing about the rational use and handicaps of drug therapy is that these can be explained to the patient in an open and honest manner, emphasizing the importance of the benefit/risk ratio in all prescribing. This is a dynamic equilibrium and it always needs to be kept under review; it is not sufficient for the community mental health worker merely to reinforce the doctor's prescription. If patients feel their main worker knows about the merits and handicaps of the drugs prescribed, the treatment programme has a better chance of being completed satisfactorily.

We are well aware that a full explanation of the way in which a drug acts in the body to produce benefit is often lacking, and that even partial explanations may be so full of jargon that they are completely misunderstood by patients. For this reason we have evolved a set of explanations as to how different drugs work and their perceived effects (Table 11.3). These are not always entirely accurate because they suffer through oversimplification, but their general message is the same as if the explanation was given to a fully informed listener who had been trained in pharmacology and biochemistry.

Table 11.2   *Ways of simplifying prescriptions of psychotropic drugs*

Complex prescription	*Simple prescription*
Three or more different drugs within same class (e.g. thioridazine, chlorpromazine and haloperidol decanoate; diazepam, temazepam and chlordiazepoxide)	Reduce to one drug if at all possible in the equivalent dosage to all three combined. If one drug is given by injection try to adjust the dose so that the one given by mouth can be left out or only used in emergency
Drug prescribed to be taken three or more times each day	Most drugs can be given once a day, at night for drugs which have sedative effects, and in the morning for those that have alerting ones. For some drugs (e.g. phenelzine, paroxetine) some people can be sedated and others alerted, so it is valuable to find out by asking which are most noticeable. Some drugs (e.g. procyclidine) may need to be given twice a day but there is rarely an absolute indication for a drug being given three or more times a day regularly in community practice (in hospital frequent drug administration is more common and often necessary, e.g. in detoxification programmes)
Drug regimen in which several drugs are taken at different times in the day	This is rarely, if ever, necessary. Most drugs can be taken together and this will improve compliance.
Drug to be taken at exactly the same time each day	This too is rarely necessary. The only exception is the drug, lithium, immediately before a serum level check. The drug should be taken 12 hours before the blood test is planned. For other drugs the time taken depends on when the minimal effect of the drug is needed (e.g. 1 hour before bedtime for most hypnotic drugs). This can be left to the patient's discretion and 'taken as required'

Table 11.3 *Simple explanations of psychotic drug effects*

Drug effect	Explanation to patient
Amine retaining effect of antidepressants leading to delayed improvement in depressed mood	'These tablets help to build up natural cheerful (antidepressant) substances in the brain, and when these reach a certain level you feel less depressed'
Antipsychotic effect of major tranquillizers	'This medication helps your mind to be more efficient at sorting things out'
Antihallucinatory effects of major tranquillizers	'They help you to stand up for yourself when the voices are trying to take you over'
Antiparanoid effects of major tranquillizers	'They make you less sensitive to other people's criticisms so you can handle them better'
Mood-stabilizing effects of lithium	'They stabilize the nerves so you are neither too fast nor too slow'
Addicting properties of benzodiazepines	'Your body gets used to the tablets and stops making its natural tranquillizers to keep you calm. When you stop the tablets you have no natural tranquillizers left so you are very nervous'
Sedative effects of major tranquillizers	'Because these tablets calm your nervous system you feel more relaxed and sleepy'
Parkinsonian effects of major tranquillizers	'The tablets can interfere with your co-ordination so you become stiff or shaky'
Effects of antiparkinsonian drugs	'These reinforce the nervous system against the other tablets so your movements return to normal'

Testing

Testing for drug consumption is an obvious way of ensuring compliance. It is a regular part of treatment with one drug, lithium carbonate and its other salts, and although the main reason for testing lithium levels in the blood is to ensure that they are within the therapeutic range, it also checks whether the drug has actually been taken.

Case vignette 11.3
Catriona, aged 40, had three admissions in the manic phase of manic-depressive illness in the past 12 years. After discharge she agreed to take lithium which she had taken in the past, and to be followed up at home. She was quite well on each occasion when seen at home, but when attempts were made to see her at hospital to check her serum lithium levels she repeatedly failed appointments. Catriona insisted she was getting her lithium from her general practitioner, who happened to be based in two separate surgeries. After checking with both surgeries it was confirmed that she had not collected her prescription from either of them following her discharge from hospital. When challenged with this she admitted that she had not been taking her lithium, and would prefer to be monitored and take it at the first sign of relapse.

In the case of lithium we can check whether the drug has been taken. We are also able to check the blood levels of many other drugs without too much difficulty but this is not used in normal practice. Urine screens are more common, particularly for illicit drugs, and many laboratories combine such screens with testing for many of the psychotropic drugs that are commonly prescribed (e.g. phenothiazines, benzodiazepines). If there is doubt at any time about whether patients are taking illegal drugs or have avoided taking therapeutic ones, a random urine screen may prove extremely valuable.

There are other tests that can also check whether patients have been taking drugs regularly. One of the disadvantages of testing most drugs in the body is that patients may avoid taking medication until just before a test is due (if it is predicted) and thereby appear to be taking medication regularly when in fact they are not. Some other tests can check whether compliance is being maintained over a longer period. Antipsychotic drugs, as has been noted in Chapter 7, can create some adverse effects owing to increased prolactin levels in the body (hyperprolactinaemia). This can cause menstrual irregularities, galactorrhoea (milk production) and breast enlargement, and impotence in men. Prolactin levels can be measured fairly easily in the blood, and if the patient is having an adequate dose of an antipsychotic drug then prolactin levels will almost invariably be raised.

Despite the obvious advantages of testing drug levels in the body, which for many drugs can be done extremely accurately, there is always something a little underhand about testing patients in this way. It implies a lack of trust and, although it can be used to clarify some puzzling aspects of clinical progress or deterioration, it is not usual to keep on repeating such tests in community mental health practice. However, the threat of a random test can be used judiciously, even if never implemented, to help to maintain compliance without creating resentment.

Paternalists

'Paternalists' is a term covering a range of people who are looking after the patient's drug consumption in a benign and constructive way (i.e. they are paternalistic). This includes the patient's friends and relatives, wardens and other staff at places such as hostels and other sheltered accommodation for the mentally ill, befrienders from mental health charities, and other mental health professionals, including all those in the community mental health team. This group can help in maintaining drug treatment strategies by:

- monitoring medication
- administration of drugs
- training patients in the treatment strategy
- collecting drugs on behalf of the patient
- health promotion.

Monitoring medication

Monitoring of medication is one of the important roles of any community mental health worker, but it can be shared between several different bodies. Monitoring includes checking whether the drug has been consumed, whether supplies are available, and whether it is being taken in appropriate dosage. In general the role of the community health worker is to ensure that supplies are available and to liaise with other agencies where necessary to have confirmation that the drug is being taken. Although there used to be a philosophical abhorrence of supervising medication in many hostels and halfway houses serving as therapeutic communities, this has now been replaced by a more pragmatic approach. The extent of monitoring drug use can extend from hostels and halfway houses administering drugs from a central area within the hostel, to merely reminding patients when their next prescriptions are due.

There is considerable flexibility in supervision, and if hostel workers are backed up by a mental health professional and understand the specific reasons for closely supervising drug treatment it is possible to get a great deal of co-operation and almost as much monitoring as could be achieved in a hospital setting. Again, however, this has to be done in a sensitive way, allowing the therapeutic community to maintain its internal philosophy, which in most such communities is devoted towards empowering people to become more independent and to take greater responsibility for their actions. Such monitoring can include a relaxation as well as a tightening of supervision of medication at appropriate times.

Case vignette 11.4
Dorothy, a 37-year-old woman had a history of schizophrenia associated with rapid changes in mood as well as delusional behaviour and a history of repeated overdoses. She was placed in a Richmond

Fellowship hostel and because of her overdose history careful super-vision was made of all her medication. She made good progress but became increasingly angry at the degree of supervision she was receiving. She managed to accumulate sufficient tablets from her daily doses to take another overdose and had to be readmitted to hospital. After she returned to the hostel it was agreed that a plan to allow her more independence was worthwhile and this would include taking more responsibility for her own drug treatment. By arrange-ment with the community mental health team the hostel staff gave her increasingly long periods of leave away from the hostel during which she controlled her own medication. When Dorothy had done this successfully without taking any more overdoses other levels of supervision were relaxed and she was discharged to another hostel which allowed more independence and which was a natural progres-sion in her rehabilitation.

Monitoring can be carried out by a large range of people, extending from members of the family, friends living in the same premises, mental health professionals of all types, and neighbours and, in particular, general practitioners (Kendrick *et al.*, 1991). When untrained staff are involved in monitoring it is important to emphasize to them that they have no legal responsibility for their actions, and if something goes wrong, such as an overdose of secretly retained tablets, in no way can they be held responsible. A telephone can also be useful as a way of monitoring medication at a distance. With medication that is taken once a day it is relatively easy just to make a telephone call to remind someone of the need to take a tablet at the appropriate time. No doubt in future years the fax machine will be even more commonly used for this purpose, particularly if it can be programmed to give the same message each day.

We must also acknowledge the important role of the primary care team in helping to ensure continued compliance with medication. The general practitioner's surgery is usually the first point of contact for patients with any form of illness, and if good systems are established within primary care to ensure that prescriptions are collected regularly, a large part of care can be taken over by the primary care team with reinforcement from the community mental health team at problem times (Tyrer *et al.*, 1993).

Administration

Administration of a drug is really an extension of monitoring consump-tion of medication. Apart from occasions where administration has to be by a mental health professional (e.g. intramuscular injection), patients control their own consumption of medication. There are clearly many ways of avoiding taking medication (as every psychiatric nurse who has worked in a hospital will know), but in general once the tablet has entered the mouth most of the task of drug administration has been completed. It is surprising how often patients are prescribed medication in the community and take absolutely none of it. Rather than admit this they continue receiving tablets and disposing of them in various ways and the same may even extend to cashing of prescriptions.

A great deal of concern is often expressed over the prescription of a new drug, particularly if there are pre-existing prejudices about adverse effects. In cases of doubt it is often helpful for the mental health worker to be present while the patient takes the first dose of the new drug. In cases of real concern the worker can return within a matter of hours to check that the patient remains well and to deal with any alleged side-effects.

The role of others in administering medication is sometimes under-used. Many are happy to administer medication when asked (again with the proviso that they are not responsible if things go wrong).

Case vignette 11.5

Eddie, a 25-year-old man had the belief that he was a member of a special master race and that once this had been recognized by the rest of humanity he would be revered. He also believed that others were conspiring to kill him because of his elevated position. He improved whenever he took antipsychotic drugs in hospital but refused to take depot injections of antipsychotic drugs after discharge. He was prescribed trifluoperazine in a dose of 10 mg twice daily on discharge but rapidly deteriorated. He refused to get out of bed in the morning, said that he was waiting for the message to join his 'family' and his personal hygiene deteriorated. He insisted that he was taking his drugs but his mother, with whom he lived, thought that this was highly unlikely, as he had never taken them in her presence.

It was decided to change his trifluoperazine to 15 mg at night in the form of a slow-release capsule, and he agreed with some reluctance for this to be given by his mother. She had some difficulty at first, but under the threat of having to cook his own meals if he did not take his medication he complied and improved after 3 weeks. Two years later Eddie is still taking the same medication supervised by his mother, and is about to leave and live in more independent accommodation. There is concern expressed that he may relapse because his mother will no longer be administering his medication.

Sometimes reluctance to take medication may be unrelated to the main pharmacological contents; some patients may be unable to swallow tablets but are happy with capsules, others will not have capsules if they are vegetarians as the capsules usually contain gelatine, and others prefer their medicine in liquid form.

Training

There are some simple rules for training paternalists in exercising their role of gentle facilitators of drug treatment. Many of these are simple common sense, but are still worth listing:

- ensuring supplies are maintained
- confirming drugs are swallowed or otherwise administered
- checking that drugs can be validly administered
- recording drug administration
- recording unwanted effects.

The simplest form of non-compliance is forgetting to obtain further supplies of a drug that has not been discontinued on medical advice. Almost invariably when one sees patients after the relapse of a continuing psychiatric disorder, the relapse has followed the patient not renewing a prescription. This may be for many reasons, including a move to a new area, a change of key workers, or mere laziness. A mental health professional, a relative or even a neighbour can monitor supplies in such a way that failure to obtain the drugs should never be a reason for non-compliance. The individual concerned can obtain further supplies in several ways, including contacting a mental health professional, going directly to the general practitioner or having an arrangement that drugs can be obtained from a local pharmacy when the prescription is due. In theory with the NHS reforms it is possible for health trusts to pay individuals a small retainer to obtain and supervise medication for patients if this form of failure to take drugs is prominent and frequently leads to readmission. However, it is better for medication to be supervised by someone who has a particular concern over the patient's welfare rather than a commercial interest.

Although it is difficult to confirm that a tablet or capsule taken by mouth has actually entered the body, it is helpful for any individual supervising the consumption of medication to be present when the tablet or capsule is being taken, preferably with a drink of some sort, so that when swallowing takes place it is highly probable that the drug is swallowed as well. All nurses who have worked in hospital will know about the techniques that patients have of hiding tablets in various parts of their oral cavities and spitting them out later. However, such determined non-compliance is not so frequent outside hospital, and should be noticed by someone if the consumption of the drug is adequately supervised. It is preferable for this to be done covertly rather than the observer watching like a hawk as the drug enters the mouth.

Drugs have different 'shelf lives', the period during which they can be stored before being given. All drug supplies have an expiry date printed on them and it is important for this to be checked before the drug is given, particularly if it is an injection. Increasingly patients are given supplies of drugs such as depot injections if they move around the country, and it is important for new professionals encountering such patients to check the expiry dates of the drugs the patient have in their possession. If patients indicate the dose they are given verbally it is always wise to check this with the previous agency because often there is an error in the transfer of information.

It is always desirable to record the times of administration and obtaining of prescriptions of drugs by all those involved in monitoring their consumption. This ensures that gaps in providing medication are anticipated in advance and any overprescription is also noted. For mental health professionals it is also helpful to have one of the software packages that is linked to care management so that the administration of drugs is co-ordinated and, when medication becomes overdue, a flashing screen suitably informs the user of the importance of renewing the prescription. It is also helpful to note side-effects with medication so that they can subsequently be related to dosage. It is also important to look out for any unusual side-effects which have to be reported in the UK on the yellow forms to the Committee on Safety of Medicines.

Collection

Although the collection of drugs is also a part of training people, particularly non-professionals, to help in recording consumption of medication, it is so important an issue that it ought to be discussed separately as well. Whenever a drug that requires long-term administration is prescribed it is important for the prescriber and the mental health team to be reasonably certain as to how the patient is going to obtain further supplies of the drug. Again this is self-evident, but it is extremely common for errors to be made in the many different elements concerned with community care.

The first problem is commonly encountered after discharge from hospital. It is now commonplace for only enough medication for 7–14 days to be given to patients when they leave hospital because of the need to confine hospital drug budgets to those receiving hospital treatments. Unless there is an efficient and speedy way of informing the next supplier of the drug so that after 7–14 days further supplies are immediately available, there will be a gap, which may become a permanent cessation of treatment by prescription, which could sabotage the whole treatment plan. The community mental health team therefore needs to be informed immediately when a patient is discharged from hospital so that the need for continued medication is known. Ideally this is before the patient is discharged, when the appropriate key workers attend the meeting at which the decision about discharge is made.

If the team is reasonably confident that the patient will be able to go to a general practitioner's surgery (even though this may involve waiting some time for supplies of drugs) then this is another source of supplying continued medication. However, for many psychiatric patients it will be necessary, at least initially after discharge or after first assessment, for medication to be provided from the community mental health team, either by prescription, or in some cases, in the form of drugs actually delivered.

In many community mental health teams there is a small supply of essential drugs kept for the purposes of short-term supply until other treatment can be given. It is particularly valuable out of hours or at times of emergencies. Although these drugs will vary from team to team, depending on the individual preferences of prescribers, it is reasonable to have at least some stocks of drugs in the following groups:

- sedative antipsychotic drugs in low dosage (e.g. thioridazine 25 mg, chlorpromazine 25–50 mg)
- antipsychotic drugs (by mouth) in higher dosage (e.g. haloperidol 5–10 mg, trifluoperazine 5–15 mg)
- antipsychotic drugs by injection (e.g. haloperidol decanoate, fluphenazine decanoate, flupenthixol decanoate)
- a sedative antidepressant (e.g. amitriptyline 50 mg)

- a selective serotonin reuptake inhibitor (SSRI) (e.g. fluoxetine 20 mg, paroxetine 20 mg)
- diazepam (2 mg and 5 mg tablets), possibly with temazepam or another benzodiazepine given as a hypnotic
- antiparkinsonian drugs by injection and by mouth (e.g. procyclidine 5 mg).

Most of the other drugs given for mental disorders do not need to be given in an emergency and therefore are not included here.

Helping hands

Many people know the famous Parkinson's law (put forward by C. Northcote Parkinson in his book published in 1957) which states that the 'amount of work done is in inverse proportion to the number of people employed' and that 'work expands to fill the time available'. These are major criticisms of how organizations operate, but we think there should be another, more positive law that states 'a good organization's productivity is directly proportional to the number of additional helpers involved in carrying out its tasks'. If the community mental health worker has a caseload of 50 patients who each require supervision of medication each week then these tasks could occupy the whole of the worker's time without any other responsibilities. The more the task of monitoring this medication can be devolved to others (with confidence that the task will be carried out), the more time will be available for other tasks requiring greater skills.

The decision made by a senior psychiatrist in the course of a multidisciplinary review that a patient needs drug treatment for at least a year after discharge has many ramifications, involving many different personnel (Figure 11.1). The number of people who need to know about this decision can easily run into double figures and all could have a role in ensuring that medication is taken as prescribed. The importance of this system is that each worker should feel that the others are available for support where necessary. Whether it is the general practitioner who is unsure if a certain effect noticed by the patient is a consequence of medication, or a sleepy patient who is never awake to open the door to a visitor from a home support team who visits before midday (because of the sedative effects of medication), all need to have someone they can turn to both for advice (for those with more experience) and assistance (for those who often have less experience but more time) in maintaining an adequate level of supervision of the patient. With this help available each worker can achieve much more than if each is working alone and under pressure. Of course Figure 11.1 is not relevant only to drug treatment; good community work involves liaison with a large number of different individuals who can both reinforce good treatment and provide a rapid response when things begin to go wrong (Tyrer *et al.*, 1990a, b).

Figure 11.1 serves as a good summary of the purpose of this book. Much of good community mental health work involves liaison with a wide range of other individuals, both professionals and non-

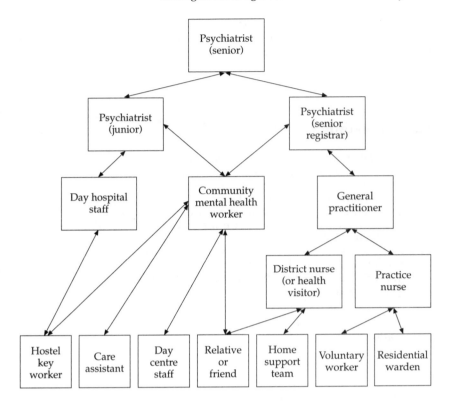

Figure 11.1 *The helping network for maintaining drug treatment in the community*

professionals with varying degrees of knowledge. In the case of drug treatment it is the job of the psychiatrist and other mental health professionals to spread appropriate knowledge throughout this network of individuals so that optimal care can be given. This is rarely a question of training an individual to carry out a task which is then performed in isolation; it is concerned with harnessing support by informing others to identify both problems and advantages in prescribing drugs. This is not an exercise in 'passing the buck', it helps us all to understand what we are doing and why. In the syndrome commonly called 'burn-out' these skills are lost and practitioners become depersonalized and uninvolved. Grasping the essentials of this book is a protection against burn-out because it helps to give greater control of the many unpredictable and sometimes harrowing events that buffet the life of the community worker in the front line (Editorial, 1994).

One of the major problems with drug treatment in psychiatry is that it has been the sole province of the psychiatrist. This view has now changed, and whilst not all community mental health workers are drug prescribers, all have a role to play in ensuring drugs are used to maximum effect for the most appropriate length of time. The message to the community mental health workers is 'you are skilled practitioners, psychotherapists, behaviour and cognitive therapists, occupational therapists and housing workers, but do not forget you are also psychopharmacologists'.

Further reading

Burns, T., Raftery, J., Beadsmoore, A., McGuigan, S. and Dickson, M. (1993). A controlled trial of home-based acute psychiatric services. II: Treatment patterns and costs. *British Journal of Psychiatry*, **163**, 55–61.

Jackson, G., Gater, R., Goldberg, D., Tantam, D., Loftus, L. and Taylor, H. (1993). A new community mental health team based in primary care: a description of the service and the effect on service use in the first year. *British Journal of Psychiatry*, **162**, 375–384.

Tyrer, P., Hawksworth, J., Hobbs, R. and Jackson, D. (1990). The role of the community psychiatric nurse. *British Journal of Hospital Medicine*, **43**, 439–442.

Tyrer, P. and Creed, F. (eds) (1995). *Community Psychiatry in Action*. Cambridge University Press.

References

Ackner, B. *et al.* (1962). Insulin treatment of schizophrenia: a three years follow-up of a controlled study. *Lancet*, i, 504–506.

Ansseau, M., Troisfontaines, B., Papart, P. *et al.* (1991). Compulsive personality as predictor of response to serotonergic antidepressants. *British Medical Journal*, **303**, 760–761.

Ashton, C. H., Rawlings, M. D. and Tyrer, S. P. (1990). A double-blind placebo-controlled study of buspirone in diazepam withdrawal in chronic benzodiazepine users. *British Journal of Psychiatry*, **157**, 232–238.

Avery, D. and Winokur, G. (1977). The efficacy of electroconvulsive therapy and antidepressants in depression. *Biological Psychiatry*, **12**, 507–524.

Balter, M. B., Manheimer, D. I., Mellinger, G. D. and Uhlenhuth, E. H. (1984). A cross-national comparison of anti-anxiety/sedative drug use. *Current Medical Research and Opinion*, **8**, suppl. 4,5-suppl. 418.

Barnes, T. R. E. and Braude, W. M. (1985). Akathisia variants and tardive dyskinesia. *Archives of General Psychiatry*, **42**, 874–878.

Barton, R. (1959) Institutional Neurosis. Bristol: John Wright.

Basoglu, M., Marks, I. M., Kilic, C., Brewin, C. R. and Swinson, R. P. (1994). Alprazolam and exposure for panic disorder with agoraphobia: attribution of improvement predicts subsequent relapse. *British Journal of Psychiatry*, **164**, 652–659.

Bebbington, P. and McGuffin, P. (1988). *Schizophrenia: The Major Issues*. London: Heinemann.

Beckman, H. and Laux, G. (1990). Guidelines for the dosage of antipsychotic drugs. *Acta Psychiatrica Scandinavica*, **82** (suppl. 358), 63–66.

Birchwood, M. J. and Tarrier, N. (1994). *Psychological Management of Schizophrenia*. Chichester: John Wiley.

Bond, G. R., Miller, L. D., Krumweid, R. D. and Ward, R. S. (1988). Assertive case management in three CHMC's: a controlled study. *Hospital and Community Psychiatry*, **39**, 411–418.

Breggin, P. (1993). *Toxic psychiatry, Drugs and Electroconvulsive Therapy: the Truth and the Better Alternatives*. London: Harper Collins.

Bristow, M. F. and Hirsch, S. R. (1993). Risk of relapse and its prevention in schizophrenia. *Clinician*, **11**, 55–67.

British Journal of Psychiatry (1992). Clozapine – the atypical neuroleptic. *British Journal of Psychiatry*, **160**, suppl. 17.

British National Formulary (printed twice yearly). London: British Medical Association/Royal Pharmaceutical Society of Great Britain.

Brown, G. and Harris, T. (1978). *The Social Origins of Depression*. London: Tavistock.

Burns, T., Raftery, J., Beadsmoore, A., McGuigan, S. and Dickson, M. (1993). A controlled trial of home-based acute psychiatric services. II:Treatment patterns and costs. *British Journal of Psychiatry*, **163**, 55–61.

Casey, J. F., Lasky, J. J., Klett, C. J. and Hollister, L. E. (1960). Treatment of schizophrenic reactions with phenothiazine derivatives. *American Journal of Psychiatry*, **117**, 97–105.

Clark, D.M. (1990). Cognitive therapy for depression and anxiety: is it better than drug treatment in the long term. In *Dilemmas and Difficulties in the Management of Psychiatric Patients* (K. Hawton and P. Cowen, eds), pp. 55–64. Oxford University Press.

Cookson, J., Crammer, J. and Leonard, B. E. (1993). *The Use of Drugs in Psychiatry*. London: Gaskell.

Cowdry, R. W. and Gardner, D. L. (1988). Pharmacotherapy of borderline personality disorder: alprazolam, carbamazepine, trifluoperazine and tranylcypromine. *Archives of General Psychiatry*, **45**, 111–119.

Crow, T. J. (1980). Molecular pathology of schizophrenia: more than one disease process? *British Medical Journal*, **280**, 66–68.

Crow, T. J. (1986). The continuum of psychosis and its implication for the structure of the gene. *British Journal of Psychiatry*, **149**, 419–429.

Crow, T. J. (1991). The origins of psychosis and 'The Descent of Man'. *British Journal of Psychiatry*, **159** (suppl. 14), 76–82.

Darke, S. (1994). Benzodiazepane use among injecting drug users: problems and implications. *Addiction*, **89**, 379–382.

De Girolamo, G. and Reich, J. H. (1993). *Personality Disorders*, pp. 11–12. Geneva: World Health Organization.

Delta Coordinating Committee (1996). DELTA: a randomised double-blind controlled trial comparing combinations of zidovudine plus didanosine or zalcitabine with zidovudine alone in HIV-infected individuals. *Lancet*, **348**, 283–91.

Department of Health (1991). *Drug Misuse and Dependence: Guidelines on Clinical Management*. London: HMSO.

Eagger, S. A., Morant, N., Levy, R. and Sahakian, B. J. (1992). Tacrine in Alzheimer's disease: time course of changes in cognitive function and practice effects. *British Journal of Psychiatry*, **160**, 36–40.

Editorial (1994). Burnished or burnt out: the delights and dangers of working in health. *Lancet*, **344**, 1583–1584.

Eisenberg, L. (1986). Mindlessness and brainlessness in psychiatry. *British Journal of Psychiatry*, **148**, 497–508.

Elkin, I., Shea, M. T., Watkins, J.T. *et al.* (1989). National Institute of Mental Health treatment of depression collaborative research program: general effectiveness of treatments. *Archives of General Psychiatry*, **46**, 971–982.

Fahy, T. A., Eisler, I. and Russell, G. F. M. (1993). Personality disorder and treatment response in bulimia nervosa. *British Journal of Psychiatry*, **162**, 765–770.

Falloon, I. R. H. and Fadden, G. (1993). *Integrated Mental Health Care: A Comprehensive Community-based Approach*. Cambridge University Press.

Frank, E., Kupfer, D. J., Perel, J. M. *et al.* (1990). Three-year outcomes for maintenance therapies in recurrent depression. *Archives of General Psychiatry*, **47**, 1093–1099.

Friedman, M. J. (1988). Toward rational pharmacotherapy for post-traumatic stress disorder: an interim report. *American Journal of Psychiatry*, **145**, 281–285.

Frith, C. D. (1992). Consciousness, information processing and the brain. *Journal of Psychopharmacology*, **6**, 436–440.

Frith, C. D. and Done, D. J. (1989). Experiences of alien control in schizophrenia reflect a disorder in the central monitoring of action. *Psychological Medicine*, **19**, 359–363.

Gaebel, W. and Pietzcker, A. (1985). Multidimensional study of the outcome of schizophrenic patients 1 year after clinic discharge. Predictors and influence of neuroleptic treatment. *European Archives of Psychiatry and Neurological Science*, **235**, 45–52.

Ghodse, A. H. and Maxwell, D. (1990). *Substance Use and Dependence: An Introduction for the Caring Professions*. London: Macmillan.

Gittleson, N. L. (1966). The effects of obsessions on depressive psychosis. *British Journal of Psychiatry*, **112**, 253–258.

Goffman, E. (1961). *Asylums*. New York: Doubleday.

Goldacre, M., Seagroatt, V. and Hawton, K. (1993). Suicide after discharge from psychiatric inpatient care. *Lancet*, **342**, 283–286.

Goldberg, D. and Huxley, P. (1992). *Common Mental Disorders: A Biosocial Model*, pp. 162–163. London: Tavistock/Routledge.

Gregory, S., Shawcross, C. R. and Gill, D. (1985). The Nottingham ECT study. A double-blind comparison of bilateral, unilateral and simulated ECT in depressive illness (Mapperley Hospital Nottingham). *British Journal of Psychiatry*, **146**, 520–524.

Hafner, H. (1987). Do we still need beds for psychiatric patients? An analysis of changing patterns of mental health care. *Acta Psychiatrica Scandinavica*, **75**, 113–126.

Hawton, K., Salkovskis, P. M., Kirk, J. and Clark, D. M. (1989). *Cognitive Behaviour Therapy for Psychiatric Problems: a Practical Guide*. Oxford University Press.

Hirsch, S. R. and Leff, J. P. (1975). *Abnormalities in the Parents of Schizophrenics*. Maudsley Monograph 22. Oxford University Press.

Hirsch, S. R., Gaind, R., Rohde, P. D., Stevens, B. and Wing, J. (1973). Outpatient maintenance of chronic schizophrenic patients with long-acting fluphenazine: double-blind placebo trial. *British Medical Journal*, **1**, 633–637.

Hogarty, G. E., Goldberg, S. C., Schooler, N. R., Ulrich, R. F. and Collaborative Study Group (1974). Drugs and sociotherapy in the aftercare of schizophrenic patients; II and III. *Archives of General Psychiatry*, **31**, 603–618.

Holton, A., Tyrer, P. and Riley, P. (1992). Factors predicting long-term outcome after chronic benzodiazepine therapy. *Journal of Affective Disorders*, **24**, 245–252.

Hudson, J. I. and Pope, H. G. Jr (1990). Affective spectrum disorder: does antidepressant response identify a family of disorders with a common pathophysiology? *American Journal of Psychiatry*, **147**, 552–564.

Huxley, P. (1990). *Effective Community Mental Health Services*. Aldershot: Avebury Gower.

Jablensky, A., Sartorius, N., Ernberg, G. *et al.* (1992). Schizophrenia: manifestations, incidence and course in different countries: a World Health Organisation ten-country study. *Psychological Medicine*, suppl. 20, 1–97.

Jackson, G., Gater, R., Goldberg, D., Tantam, D., Loftus, L. and Taylor, H. (1993). A new community mental health team based in primary care: a description of the service and the effect on service use in the first year. *British Journal of Psychiatry*, **162**, 375–384.

Johnson, D. A. W. (1988). Drug treatment of schizophrenia. In *Schizophrenia: The Major Issues* (P. Bebbington and P. McGuffin, eds). London: Heinemann.

Johnstone, E. C., Cunningham Owens, D. G., Frith, C. D., McPherson, K. and Dowie, C. (1980). Neurotic illness and its response to anxiolytic and antidepressant treatment. *Psychological Medicine*, **10**, 321–328.

Johnstone, E. C., Crow, T. J., Ferrier, I. N. *et al.* (1983). Adverse effects of anticholinergic medication on positive schizophrenic symptoms. *Psychological Medicine*, **13**, 513–527.

Johnstone, E. C., Crow, T. J., Frith, C. D. and Owens, D. G. C. (1988). The Northwick Park 'Functional' Psychosis Study: diagnosis and treatment response. *Lancet*, **ii**, 119–126.

Joyce, L. (1993). Occupational therapy: a cause without a rebel. *British Journal of Occupational Therapy*, **56**, 447.

Kendell, R.E. (1976). The classification of depressions: a review of contemporary confusion. *British Journal of Psychiatry*, **129**, 15–28.

Kendrick, T., Sibbald, B., Burns, T. and Freeling, P. (1991). Role of general practitioners in care of long term mentally ill patients. *British Medical Journal*, **302**, 508–510.

King, M. B. (1993). *AIDS, HIV and Mental Health*. Cambridge University Press.

Kingdon, D. (1994). Care programme approach: recent government policy and legislation. *Psychiatric Bulletin*, **18**, 68–70.

Kingdon, D., Turkington, D. and John, C. (1994). Cognitive behaviour therapy of schizophrenia; the amenability of delusions and hallucinations to reasoning. *British Journal of Psychiatry*, **164**, 581–587.

Kinon, B. J., Kane, J. M., Johns, C., Perovich, R., Ismi, M., Koreen, A. and Weiden, P. (1993). Treatment of neuroleptic-resistant schizophrenic relapse. *Psychopharmacology Bulletin*, **29**, 309–314.

Klein, D. F. (1967). Importance of psychiatric diagnosis in prediction of clinical drug effects. *Archives of General Psychiatry*, **16**, 118–125.

Kraemer, G. W. (1992). A psychobiological theory of attachment. *Behavioural and Brain Sciences*, **15**, 493–541.

Kringlen, E. (1987). Contributions of genetic studies on schizophrenia. In *Search for the Causes of Schizophrenia* (H. Hafner, W. F. Gattaz and W. Janzarik, eds). Berlin: Springer.

Kuipers, L., Leff, J. and Lam, D. (1992). *Family Work for Schizophrenia: A Practical Guide*. London: Gaskell.

Lader, M. and Herrington, R. (1990). *Biological Treatments in Psychiatry*. Oxford University Press.

Lader, M., Beaumont, G., Bond, A. *et al.* (1992). Guidelines for the management of patients with generalised anxiety. *Psychiatric Bulletin*, **16**, 560–565.

Laing, R. D. (1959). *The Divided Self*. London: Tavistock.

Laing, R. D. (1967). *The Politics of Experience*. London: Penguin.

Laing, R. D. and Esterson, A. (1970). *Sanity, Madness and the Family*. Harmondsworth: Penguin.

Lee, A. S. and Murray, R. M. (1988). The long-term outcome of Maudsley depressives. *British Journal of Psychiatry*, **153**, 741–751.

Leonard, B. E. (1992). *Fundamentals of Psychopharmacology*. Chichester: John Wiley.

Lewis, G., David, A., Andreasson, S. *et al.* (1992). Schizophrenia and city life. *Lancet*, **340**, 137–140.

Liddle, P. F. (1987). Schizophrenic syndromes, cognitive performance and neurobiological dysfunction. *Psychological Medicine*, **17**, 49–57.

Liddle, P. F. (1993). The psychomotor disorders: disorders of the supervisory mental processes. *Behavioural Neurology*, **6**, 5–14.

Liddle, P. F., Friston, K. J., Frith, C. D., Hirsch, S. R., Jones, T. and Frackowiak, R. S. J. (1992). Patterns of cerebral blood flow in schizophrenia. *British Journal of Psychiatry*, **160**, 179–186.

Lishman, W. A. (1993). *Organic Psychiatry*. Oxford: Blackwell.

Marks, I. M. (1987). *Fears, Phobias and Rituals*. Oxford University Press.

Marriott, S., Malone, S., Onyett, S. and Tyrer, P. (1993). The consequences of an open referral system to a community mental health service. *Acta Psychiatrica Scandinavica*, **88**, 93–97.

McEvoy, J. P., Hogarty, G. E. and Steingard, S. (1991). Optimal dose of neuroleptic in acute schizophrenia: a controlled study of the neuroleptic threshold and higher haloperiodal dose. *Archives of General Pschiatry*, **48**, 739–745.

Meltzer, H., Gill, B. and Petticrew, M. (1994). *OPCS Surveys of Psychiatric Morbidity in Great Britain. Bulletin No. 1: The prevalence of psychiatric morbidity among adults aged 16–64, living in private households, in Great Britain*. London: OPCS.

Merson, S., Tyrer, P., Onyett, S. *et al.* (1992). Early intervention in psychiatric emergencies: a controlled clinical trial. *Lancet*, **339**, 1311–1314.

Montgomery, D. B., Roberts, A., Green, M., Bullock, T., Baldwin, D. and Montgomery, S. A. (1994). Lack of efficacy of fluoxetine in recurrent brief depression and suicidal attempts. *European Archives of Psychiatry and Clinical Neuroscience*, **244**, 211–215.

Murray, R. M., Reveley, A. M. and Lewis, S. V. (1988). Family history, obstetric complications and cerebral abnormality in schizophrenia. In *Handbook of Schizophrenia*, vol. 3 (H.A. Nastralla, ed.). Amsterdam: Elsevier.

National Institute of Mental Health [NIMH] Psychopharmacology Service Centre Collaborative Study Group (1964). Phenothiazine treatment in acute schizophrenia. *Archives of General Psychiatry*, **10**, 246–261.

Onyett, S. (1992). *Case Management in Mental Health*. London: Chapman & Hall.

Ovreteit, J. (1993). *Coordinating Community Care: Multidisciplinary Teams and Care Management*. Milton Keynes: Open University Press.

Pare, C. M. B. (1985). The present status of monoamine oxidase inhibitors. *British Journal of Psychiatry*, **146**, 576–584.

Pilowsky, L. S., Ring, H., Shine, P. J., Battersby, M. and Lader, M. (1992). Rapid tranquillisation: a survey of emergency prescribing in a general psychiatric hospital. *British Journal of Psychiatry*, **160**, 831–835.

Post, R. M., Uhde, T. W., Ballenger, J. C. and Squillace, K. M. (1983). Prophylactic effect of carbamazepine in manic-depressive illness. *American Journal of Psychiatry*, **140**, 1602–1604.

Post, R. M., Uhde, T. W., Roy-Byrne, P. P. and Joffe, R. (1986). Antidepressant effects of carbamazepine. *American Journal of Psychiatry*, **143**, 29–34.

Puri, B. and Tyrer, P. (1992). *Sciences Basic to Psychiatry*. Edinburgh: Churchill Livingstone.

Sachs, O. (1995). *Awakenings*. London: Picador.

Sartorius, N., Jablensky, A., Gulbinat, W. and Ernberg, G. (1980). WHO collaborative study: assessment of affective disorders. *Psychological Medicine*, **10**, 743–749.

Seivewright, N. and Dougal, W. (1993). Withdrawal symptoms from high dose benzodiazepines in polydrug users. *Drug and Alcohol Dependence*, **32**, 15–23.

Seivewright, N. A. and Greenwood, J. (1996). What is important in drug misuse treatment? *Lancet*, **347**, 373–375.

Schmidt, U. H. and Treasure, J. (1993). *Getting Better Bit(e) by Bit(e)*. London: Laurence Erlbaum.

Szasz, T. (1960). The myth of mental illness. *American Psychologist*, **15**, 113–118.

Treasure, J., Schmidt, U., Troop, N. *et al.* (1996). Sequential treatment for bulimia nervosa incorporating a self-care manual. *British Journal of Psychiatry*, **168**, 94–98.

Trimble, M. R. (1988). *Biological Psychiatry*. Chichester: John Wiley.

Tyrer, P. J. (ed.) (1982). *Drugs in Psychiatric Practice*. London: Butterworth.

Tyrer, P. (1985). Neurosis divisible? *Lancet*, **i**, 685–688.

Tyrer, P. (1986). *How to Stop Taking Tranquillisers*. London: Sheldon.

Tyrer, P. (1989). Treating panic – psychological treatments are preferable to drug treatments. *British Medical Journal*, **298**, 201.

Tyrer, P. (1991). The nocebo effect – poorly known but getting stronger. In *Side Effects of Drugs Annual 15* (M. N. G. Dukes and J. K. Aronson, eds), pp. 19–25. Amsterdam: Elsevier.

Tyrer, P. and Creed, F. (1995). *Community Psychiatry in Action*. Cambridge University Press.

Tyrer, P. and Harrison-Read, P. (1990). New perspectives in treatment with monoamine oxidase inhibitors. *International Review of Psychiatry*, **2**, 331–340.

Tyrer, P. and Seivewright, N. (1988). Pharmacological treatment of personality disorders. *Clinical Neuropharmacology*, **11**, 493–499.

Tyrer, P. and Stein, G. (1993). *Personality Disorder Reviewed*. London: Gaskell/ Royal College of Psychiatrists.

Tyrer, P. and Steinberg, D. (1993). *Models for Mental Disorder: Conceptual Models in Psychiatry*. Chichester: John Wiley.

Tyrer, P., Owen, R. and Dawlings, S. (1983). Gradual withdrawal of diazepam after long-term therapy. *Lancet*, **i**, 1402–1406.

Tyrer, P., Seivewright, N., Murphy, S. *et al.* (1988). The Nottingham study of neurotic disorder: comparison of drug and psychological treatments. *Lancet*, **ii**, 235–240.

Tyrer, P., Ferguson, B. and Wadsworth, J. (1990a). Liaison psychiatry in general practice: the comprehensive collaborative model. *Acta Psychiatrica Scandinavica*, **81**, 359–363.

Tyrer, P., Hawksworth, J., Hobbs, R. and Jackson, D. (1990b). The role of the community psychiatric nurse. *British Journal of Hospital Medicine*, **43**, 439–442.

Tyrer, P., Casey, P. and Ferguson, B. (1991). Personality disorder in perspective. *British Journal of Psychiatry*, **159**, 463–471.

Tyrer, P., Higgs, R. and Strathdee, G. (1993). *Mental Health and Primary Care: A Changing Agenda*. London: Gaskell/Royal College of Psychiatrists.

Tyrer, P., Ferguson, B., Hallström, C. *et al.* (1996). A controlled trial of dothiepin and placebo in treating benzodiazepine withdrawal symptoms. *British Journal of Psychiatry*, **168**, 457–461.

Vaughn, C. and Leff, J. P. (1976). The influence of family and social factors on the course of psychiatric illness. *British Journal of Psychiatry*, **129**, 125–137.

Winstead, D. K., Anderson, A., Eilsers, M. K., Blackwell, B. and Zaremba, A. L. (1974). Diazepam on demand: drug-seeking behavior in psychiatric patients. *Archives of General Psychiatry*, **30**, 349–351.

World Health Organization (1979). *Schizophrenia: An International Follow-up Study*. Chichester: John Wiley.

World Health Organization (1992). *ICD-10: Classification of Mental and Behavioural Disorders*. Geneva: World Health Organization.

Index

Note: references in *italics* indicate tables or figures; there may also be textual references on these pages